DEEP BRAIN STIMULATION: APPLICATIONS, COMPLICATIONS AND SIDE EFFECTS

DEEP BRAIN STIMULATION: APPLICATIONS, COMPLICATIONS AND SIDE EFFECTS

MARK H. ROGERS
AND PAUL B. ANDERSON
EDITORS

Nova Biomedical Books
New York

For permission to use material from this book please contact us:
Telephone 631-231-7269; Fax 631-231-8175
Web Site: http://www.novapublishers.com

Library of Congress Cataloging-in-Publication Data

Deep brain stimulation : applications, complications, and side effects / [edited by] Mark H. Rogers and Paul B. Anderson.
p. ; cm.
Includes index.
ISBN 978-1-60692-895-0 (hardcover)
1. Brain stimulation--Therapeutic use. I. Rogers, Mark H. II. Anderson, Paul B., 1962-
[DNLM: 1. Deep Brain Stimulation--adverse effects. 2. Deep Brain Stimulation. 3. Brain Diseases--therapy. 4. Mental Disorders--therapy. WL 368 D311 2009]
RC350.B72D44 2009
616.8'046--dc22

2009007908

Published by Nova Science Publishers, Inc. ✢ New York

Contents

Preface

In neurotechnology, deep brain stimulation (DBS) refers to a surgical treatment involving the implantation of a medical device called a brain pacemaker, which sends electrical impulses to specific parts of the brain. DBS in select brain regions has provided remarkable therapeutic benefits for otherwise treatment-resistant movement and affective disorders such as chronic pain, Parkinson's disease, tremor and dystonia. Despite the long history of DBS, its underlying principles and mechanisms are still not clear. While DBS has proven helpful for some patients, there is potential for serious complications and side effects. This book presents current research on this cutting edge treatment. Success of functional stereotactic procedures is shown to depend on a variety of factors, including patient selection, methodology of choice and localization of the target, and the experience of the neurosurgery team. Complications on the use of the procedure in the treatment of Parkinson's disease are also presented. The use of aagus nerve stimulation on treatment-resistant patients with major depression is discussed as well.

Chapter I - When a new technique is introduced, a certain period of time is required for it to be improved and adjusted. The success of functional stereotactic procedures depends on a variety of factors: patient selection, methodology of choice and localization of the target, and the experience of the neurosurgery team. The learning curve resulting from the neurosurgery team's acquired knowledge is also notable.

After 12 years of working with deep brain stimulation (DBS), operating on over 200 patients and implanting more than 380 DBS electrodes for different illnesses, Parkinson's disease, dystonia, tremor and Horton's headache, the authors believe that their experience may be useful to others who are starting out in functional stereotactic procedures.

Chapter II - Over the last twenty years, deep brain stimulation (DBS) has been increasingly accepted as an effective alternative treatment to the selective lesioning methods previously used in stereotactic and functional neurosurgery. This method, based on its reversibility and adaptability, has currently been used for the alleviation of medically-refractory cases of movement disorders, epilepsy, pain, and psychiatric diseases. In the present commentary, data comparing DBS with other brain stimulation methods such as electrical cortical stimulation (CS) and transcranial magnetic stimulation (TMS) are analyzed and the perspectives of the field are outlined. Progress in the related fields of neuromodulation, functional neuroprosthetic surgery, neuroinformatics, neurocomputation, and developments in neuroengineering that are expected to refine, enhance and widen the therapeutic applications of DBS are also discussed.

Chapter III - Therapeutic brain stimulation can be applied: a) in networks that are located in cortical and subcortical layers, b) in deep nuclei groups (relay nodes) or c) in combination. CS and DBS belong to the domain of *operative neuromodulation* and particularly to the field of *neural networks surgery* (Sakas et al., 2007a), defined as the field that studies and applies advancements in neural networks research, digitized stereotactic brain imaging and implantable electrical or electronic devices in order to alter electrically the signal transmission in the nervous system, modulate neural networks and produce therapeutic effects.

Therapeutic brain stimulation methods are currently distinguished into two major categories: a) noninvasive and b) invasive. The *noninvasive* methods (rTMS, tDCS) stimulate electrically the brain cortex after applying electrical currents on the human scalp. The *invasive* methods require the surgical implantation of specially designed electrodes either in contact with the cortex of the brain, i.e., CS, or in deeply located selected targets, i.e., DBS. Instead of *invasive*, the terms *implantable* or *by implantable devices* are much more appropriate, as they do not carry the negative association of a traumatic intervention that is implied by the term *invasive CS*. In this chapter, the authors describe and compare the current state and future prospects of DBS and CS in the fields of neurology and psychiatry.

Chapter IV - Ever since the observation that motor cortex (MI) stimulation (MI ECS) could relieve some patients suffering post-stroke movement disorders (Katayama et al., 1997, 2002) and, above all, the successful introduction of MI ECS for the treatment of Parkinson's disease by Canavero in 1998 (Canavero and Paolotti, 2000), extradural MI ECS has been employed for the treatment of several movement disorders. This chapter reviews this field.

Chapter V - About 30% of epileptic patients do not respond to antiepileptic drugs (Kwan & Brodie, 2000), of whom only a minority can benefit from resective surgery. Such a therapeutic option is considered only in patients who suffer from focal seizures with an epileptogenic zone clearly identified and safely removable. Therefore, patients with seizures arising from eloquent cortices, or which are multifocal, bilateral, or generalized, represent a particular challenge to "new" or "alternative" therapies. For these patients, neurostimulation appears to have great potential (Polkey et al., 2003; Theodore and Fisher, 2004). Different approaches to neurostimulation in epileptic patients now exist and depend on (i) the brain region which is targeted and (ii) the way the stimulation is applied (Oommen et al., 2005; Morrell, 2006; Theodore and Fisher, 2004; Vonck et al., 2007). The aim of neurostimulation in epilepsy is to reduce the probability of seizure occurrence and/or propagation, either by manipulating remote control systems (vagus nerve stimulation, deep brain stimulation), or by interfering with the epileptogenic zone itself (repetitive transcranial magnetic stimulation, cortical stimulation). In most cases, stimulation is delivered continuously or intermittently according to a scheduled protocol. In particular, new progress in biotechnology and EEG signal analysis now allows stimulation in response to detection of electrographic seizures (e.g., closed-loop stimulation). Here, the authors review the various experimental and clinical attempts that have been made to control epileptic seizures by the means of deep brain electrical stimulation.

Chapter VI - Obsessive-compulsive disorder (OCD) is a relatively common psychiatric condition with an estimated lifetime prevalence of 2–3% of the general population. It is generally characterized by a chronic course leading to a profound impairment in psychosocial functioning and quality of life. Although its pathophysiology is still far from resolved, an ample body of literature suggests the role of an overactivity in the frontal-subcortical loops originating in the orbitofrontal cortex and the anterior cingulate cortex, respectively. Today, the well-established efficacy of antidepressants, acting preferentially by blocking serotonin reuptake, in addition to psychological treatments, have considerably changed the poor prognosis of the illness. However, both conventional therapeutic approaches failed to substantially alleviate obsessive-compulsive symptoms in 20–30% of cases. From these considerations, several surgical strategies have been successfully proposed for treating the resistant forms of OCD, including anterior capsulotomy, anterior cingulotomy, subcaudate tractotomy and limbic leucotomy. They have been performed in order to interrupt the orbitofrontal and anterior cingulate loops at either cortical or subcortical level, which have been found as disrupted in OCD. Despite these lesion-producing techniques have a relatively low incidence of serious complications or undesirable effects, deep brain stimulation, as a reversible procedure, has recently been introduced in the field of OCD, primarily targeting the limb part of the internal capsule or the ventral caudate nucleus. It has been shown to be of promising benefit that should be considered with caution and confirmed by further research in this area.

Chapter VII - In numerous medical conditions, abnormal movements (dystonia, dyskinesia, myoclonus and tremor) are present, isolated or associated to other neurological deficits. Deep brain stimulation has been validated as a safe and efficient neurosurgical procedure in treating Parkinson's disease and essential tremor. Following the experience with ablative surgery for dystonia and high frequency stimulation for Parkinson's disease, chronic electrical stimulation of the internal globus pallidus (GPi) has been proposed to treat dystonic syndromes. Based on etiology and spread of symptoms, 82 patients were divided in subgroups separating, for each of them, children and adults: primary DYT1 dystonia, primary dystonia without DYT1 mutation, primary segmental dystonia, post anoxic cerebral palsy, pantothenate kinase associated neurodegeneration (PKAN) and mitochondrial diseases. Assessment was performed pre- and postoperatively by the Burke-Fahn's Marsden Dystonia Rating Scale, motor and disability sections. Bilateral electrode implantation was performed under general anaesthesia. High frequency (130 Hz), 450 microseconds pulse width and monopolar stimulation were used. Clinical improvement at three years was comparable for the groups of primary dystonia (82% for the motor scores) and for secondary dystonia and degenerative diseases, improvement was less important but still interesting (40%). The originality of the method consisted in the use of stereotactic MR imaging for the target selection without microelectrode recordings. This reduced the duration of the procedure and the risk of haemorrhage. Chronic high frequency stimulation of the GPi can be considered as an efficient and lasting treatment in primary dystonia and proposed in selected cases of secondary dystonia and degenerative disease.

Chapter VIII - The basal ganglia were considered as a site for integrating diverse inputs from the entire cerebral cortex and funneling these influences via the ventrolateral thalamus to the motor cortex (Alexander, 1994). The subthalamic nucleus (STN) has generally been considered as a rely station within frontal-subcortical motor control circuitry. The function of the STN in the current model of the basal ganglia organization was developed from animal model and neurodegenerative diseases with hypo- and hyperkinetic movement disorders (Alexander et al., 1986): in this model, the STN represents a relay in the so-called "indirect" pathway of the parallel basal ganglia-thalamocortical circuits. STN excitatory efferents reinforce the inhibition of basal ganglia output nuclei, the internal globus pallidus (GPi) and the reticular substantia nigra (SNr) on thalamo-frontal neurons. A "direct" striato-pallidal pathway opposes the STN by normally inhibiting basal ganglia outflow, facilitating thalamo-frontal drive (Schroeder et al., 2002).

Clinicians maintain firm conviction on the fundamental role of the basal ganglia, and of STN, in motor syndromes such as Parkinson Disease. Lesions at the level of STN lead to hemiballism and involuntary movements of the contralateral extremities (Guridi and Obeso, 2001).

Chapter IX - Background: Subthalamic high-frequency deep brain stimulation (STN DBS) has during the last decade been widely used in the treatment of Parkinson's disease (PD) complicated by motor fluctuations and medicine-induced adverse effects. The exact mechanism of STN DBS is, however, still unelucidated. Objective: To evaluate whether STN DBS changes regional cerebral blood flow (rCBF) and oxygen consumption, by positron emission tomography (PET) in a non-primate large animal PD model of STN DBS. Methods: Three MPTP (1-methyl-4-phenyl-1,2,3,6-tetrahydropyridine) intoxicated female Göttingen minipigs (age 8–12 months, weight 16–20 kg) were stereotaxically implanted unilaterally with a DBS electrode (Medtronic, model 3387) connected to a pulse generator (Medtronic, model 7424) placed subcutaneously in the neck region. Four to six weeks later the animals were anesthetized and placed in a PET scanner. Three water ($H_2{}^{15}O$) and three oxygen ($^{15}O_2$) scans were performed, before stimulation with clinical parametres (continuous unipolar stimulation (electrode negative, case positive), amplitude 3V, frequency 160 Hz, and pulse-width 60 μs) was initiated and followed by 5 water and oxygen scans 5, 30, 60, 120 and 240 min thereafter. The obtained data (the three baseline scans versus the five poststimulation scans) were analysed by parametric DOT-analysis after semiautomatic coregistration to an average MRI pig brain. Results: rCBF was significantly increased (t-value = 5.47, p-value < 0.05) at the electrode tip after initiation of stimulation, and non-significant increases of oxygen consumption occurred in the ipsilateral- (t-value = 3.67, p-value < 0.1), and contralateral cortex (t-value = 3.34, p-value < 0.1). Conclusion: The authors' results indicate that STN DBS increases local midbrain rCBF and oxygen consumption in centrally placed cortical areas. The minipig may thus be a well-suited animal model for further studies of the mechanism of STN DBS in PD.

Chapter X - Treatment-resistant depression (TRD) is a leading cause of disability and therapeutic strategies used for this prevalent and impairing condition include pharmacological augmentation strategies and brain stimulation techniques. Vagus nerve stimulation (VNS) is a brain stimulation intervention that has shown to decrease seizure frequency in partial-onset seizure patients. Subsequent trials performed on treatment-resistant patients with major depression indicated that VNS may be an effective and safe treatment. VNS involves minor surgery in which an electrode pair is wrapped around the left vagus nerve in the neck and connected to a generator implanted in the chest wall subcutaneously.

Several methodological approaches have been employed in order to better understand the mechanism of action of VNS and its effects on neurobiological circuits involved in mood regulation. Despite its invasive nature, the tolerability profile of VNS seems to be favourable given that, differently from other brain stimulation interventions (i.e., ECT, rTMS, tDCS), VNS is a continuous and chronic stimulation. Even though previous positive results from clinical trials have led VNS to be approved by the FDA and the EMEA for the use in TRD, researchers are now focusing their efforts in the identification of possible predictors of response to VNS. Further investigation of the effects of VNS in the long-term treatment (>2 years) of TRD is also required.

In: Deep Brain Stimulation
Editors: Mark H. Rogers and Paul B. Anderson

ISBN 978-1-60692-895-0

Chapter I

Common Questions and Answers to Deep Brain Stimulation Surgery

Fernando Seijo[1*], Marco Alvarez-Vega[1], Beatriz Lozano[2], Fernando Fernández-González[2], Elena Santamarta[3] and Antonio Saíz[3]

[1]Functional Neurosurgery Unit, Neurosurgery Department
Hospital Universitario Central deAsturias, Oviedo, Spain
[2]Clinical Neurophysiology Department. Hospital Universitario
Central deAsturias, Oviedo, Spain
[3]Radiology Department. Hospital Universitario Central deAsturias, Oviedo, Spain.

Introduction

When a new technique is introduced, a certain period of time is required for it to be improved and adjusted. The success of functional stereotactic procedures depends on a variety of factors: patient selection, methodology of choice and localization of the target, and the experience of the neurosurgery team. The learning curve resulting from the neurosurgery team's acquired knowledge is also notable.

After 12 years of working with deep brain stimulation (DBS), operating on over 200 patients and implanting more than 380 DBS electrodes for different illnesses, Parkinson´s disease, dystonia, tremor and Horton's headache, we believe that our experience may be useful to others who are starting out in functional stereotactic procedures.

* Servicio de Neurocirugía,Hospital Universitario Central Hospital de Asturias,33006, Oviedo, Spain. Tfno: 00-34-98510800- Ext. 38164 Fax: 00-34-985 273657,E-mail: fseijo@uniovi.es

Question One: Patient Selection

Many patients are referred to surgical centres to be considered for DBS. It is essential to establish criteria that will effectively predict the outcome of DBS before the therapy is applied. It is then necessary to use a rigorous selection process that will successfully identify candidates who will obtain the greatest benefit from this therapy and who will maintain this benefit for long enough to justify the time and expense involved. Candidates must also be in a suitable physical, cognitive and emotional condition to tolerate surgery [24].

The following protocol is used for DBS surgery candidates: a) a clinical diagnosis of idiopathic Parkinson´s disease (PD) with Core Assessment Program for Intracerebral Transplantations (CAPIT) [25], Unified PD Rating Scale (UPDRS, part III, version 3) [9], > 30% improvement after administration of levodopa or apomorphine, OFF phase Hoehn & Yahr stage 3 or above, severe motor fluctuations and/or dyskinesias secondary to medication; absence of severe disease that could interfere with the surgery or concomitant medication that is incompatible with surgery;, stabilised antiparkinsonian treatment 6 months before surgery; dystonia [8], tremor (essential tremor, rubral tremor, PD´s tremor) [16, 34], cluster headache [29]; b) less than 70 years of age; c) absence of dementia, psychosis, severe depression and drug dependence; d) brain magnetic resonance imaging within 6 months of surgery without severe atrophy or any anomalies that could prevent surgery; e) written informed consent.

Depending on the clinical diagnosis, patients underwent the following neurological, neurophysiological and psychological battery before surgery: 1) pharmacological tests and UPDRS scale in ON and OFF states, 2) chronometric tests consisting of right and left hand tapping and gait, 3) video recording, 4) electroencephalogram, 5) mapping of somatosensory, visual and cognitive evoked potentials, (P-300), 6) cognitive evaluation with the Mattis dementia scale, Hanoi tower, Rey oral auditive learning test, Benton visual retention test (VRT form 1), words and colours test (Stroop test), letters and numbers test (Wais-III), oral fluency test, Benton line orientation test, 7) behavioural test with the ISRA anxiety test and the Montgomery Asberg depression scale, 8) functional evaluation with the PDQ-39 Quality of Life questionnaire.

A patient with a third ventricle width of more than 9 mm is not a candidate for DBS surgery in our opinion because of the shift that occurs in the brain from the loss of cerebrospinal fluid and pneumoencephalus. Cortical atrophy is also a major handicap to surgery because of the risk of subdural haematoma.

Also, although it has been suggested in the literature that patients with pacemakers are not candidates for this type of surgery because of incompatibility with magnetic resonance imaging (MRI), we had a patient with a pacemaker due to bundle branch block, and we obtained the stereotactic coordinates with computed tomography (CT) imaging alone. The patient did not have any problems peri- or post-surgery when the brain neurostimulator was implanted, because of the distance from the pacemaker. Likewise, a history of myocardial infarction or diabetes increases morbidity/mortality but are not exclusion criteria for intervention. We have operated on three patients with a history of myocardial infarction as well as patients with previous controlled diabetes, with good results.

Exclusion criteria are: serious systemic disease, carotid stenosis, cerebral atrophy, dementia or major psychological disorder, lack of collaboration on the patient's part, or unsigned informed consent.

Question Two: There Are Different Stereotactic Devices with Different Properties, Depending on the Type of Surgery in Question. Which Device Is the Most Suitable for Deep Brain Stimulation Surgery?

Stereotactic surgery is a surgical method that provides access to any part of the brain with the utmost accuracy. The safety of these devices is ± 1 mm for the X and Y coordinates, and 1.5 mm for the Z coordinate [7, 12]. To achieve their objective, stereotactic devices are based on two different systems: the arch-centre system and the polar coordinate system.

The arch-centre system means that any given point of the brain expressed in Cartesian coordinates (X, Y, Z) can be reached from anywhere in the cranial area. In other words, there may be multiple entries on the skull for a particular site in the brain.

These coordinates are bound by three planes. First, a midsagittal plane to the brain passes through the septum pellucidum and commissure anterior-commissure posterior line (Y coordinate). Second, a plane that is perpendicular to the previous basal plane and passes through the upper edge of the external auditory canal-edge lower orbits (X coordinate). And third, another plane perpendicular to the midsagittal plane and the basal plane called the coronal plane (Z coordinate).

This system is used in stereotactic devices such as the Leksell apparatus (Elekta Instruments, Stockholm, Sweden) and the Cosman-Roberts-Wells stereotactic apparatus (CRW) (Radionics, Burlington, MA, USA).

The coordinate system or spherical polar point target is defined by a distance (R) and two angles (Δ, Ω) from a reference point known as 0. This is the system that is used in astronomy. R is the distance between point 0 and the target, the Δ angle is the angle on the sagittal plane, and the Ω angle is on the horizontal plane. This system enables any point in the brain to be reached through a previously selected burr-hole. The mathematical calculations are complex because of its operability-specifying trigonometric calculations. This system is used less than the arch-centre system.

An example of stereotaxy apparatus using this system is the Riechert-Mundinger apparatus. It has an accuracy of ± 0.5 mm [39].

During the first few years we used the Riechert-Mundinger apparatus, and we then went on to use the CRW-FN frame (CRW improved) and the G model Leksell frame. Despite the safety of using the polar coordinate methodology in the Riechert Mundiger-frame, its practical complexity led us to replace it with appliances that use the simpler arch-centre system.

The first of these devices we used was the CRW frame that can only be used with CT. When a CRW frame was used in MRI, unpredictable geometric shifts were observed.

However, images obtained using a Leksell stereotactic frame was virtually free of these geometric shifts [15]. Then we used the CRW-FN frame and the Leksell G frame. These two models have the advantage that they can be used equally with CT and MRI alike. We also observed that there is greater distortion in MRI studies with the CRW FN-frame than with the Leksell frame. Using the Philips MRI scanner (Philips Medical Systems) and Siemens MRI scanner (Siemens Medical System) with the Leksell frame the mean values of the maximum errors for the X, Y, and Z axes were 0.9-1.0 mm, 0.2-0.4 mm, and 1.6-3.8 mm respectively [56]. In our experience using MRI (General Electric, 1.5 teslas) the largest distortion was found around the periphery (2-3 mm) and the least distortion was present in the middle (1-2 mm). A number of factors cause the spatial distortion, heterogeneities in the scanner's constant static magnetic field, nonlinearity of the gradient field, linear scale error, instrument imperfections, magnetic susceptibility artefacts, effects of local magnetization [42], and the magnetic properties of the stereotactic frame [5]. Magnetic susceptibility perturbations introduced by human head anatomy and by stereotactic frames can produce geometric shifts of up to several mm [5].

The head ring of the CRW-FN frame and Leksell frame have earplugs to help stabilise the frame and prevent significant tilt ("roll" in the coronal plane) or rotation ("yaw" in the axial plane) of the frame with respect to the brain [22], but they do not affect the anterior-posterior axis. To minimise the sagittal pitch angle, the axial plane is aligned with the anterior commissure-posterior commissure line (AC-PC line) by angling the base ring parallel to an imaginary line between the external auditory meatus (EAM) and the orbital floor.

We have avoided this problem by developing a frame for the CRW-FN that is fixed from the head ring on the CRW-FN and has two earplugs and a nose bar. With this mechanism, the CRW-FN's head ring is fixed to the head by three points and it can therefore define an axial plane parallel to the anterior commissure-posterior commissure plane (AC-PC plane). In the case of Leksell frame we fixed the ring head to the head with three points, on a parallel to the AC-PC plane, by adding another earplugs at the front of the head ring, so that the three earplugs on the Leksell frame could set the ring head on a parallel to AC-PC plane (figure 1).

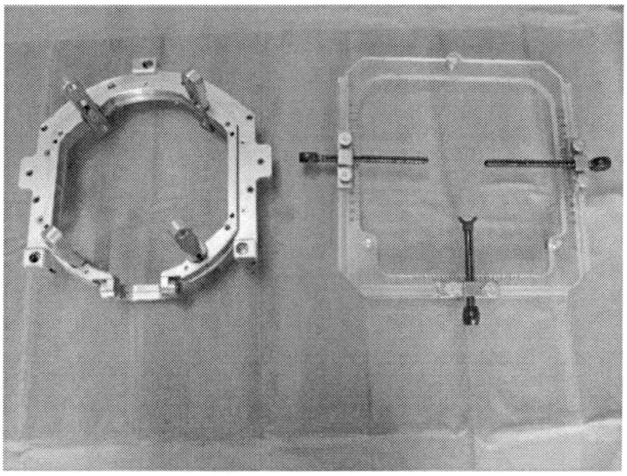

Figure 1. A) CRW head ring with adapter to earplugs and nose bars. B) Leksell head ring with earplugs.

Question Three: What Is the Best Method for Placing the Stereotactic Ring in the Correct Position?

Good identification of the AC-PC line in the CT or MRI requires correct frame placement. In theory the AC-PC line is parallel to a line connecting the EAM with the inferior orbital wall but not in all cases. Some authors believe that the AC-PC line draw an angle of -10° with the orbit-meatal line, which is the vertex angle of the line joining the EAM [57]. It is essential to place the frame with its axes orthogonally to the standard anatomic planes of the brain, to ensure that preoperative images as well as the intraoperative microelectrode-derived brain maps are interpretable in terms of familiar anatomy corresponding to standard brain atlases [48]. Then, the frame must be placed on the head on a parallel with the AC-PC plane.

The stereotactic frames have earplugs to help stabilise the frame and prevent any "roll" or "yaw" with respect to the brain, but they do not affect the anterior-posterior axis. It is also possible that the EAMs may not be symmetrical. To minimise the sagittal pitch angle, the axial plane is angled on the base ring parallel to an imaginary line between the EAM and the orbital floor. In theory, the plane of frame is parallel to the AC-PC plane.

In order to place the stereotactic ring as parallel as possible to the AC-PC plane we use a methodology that can be performed directly on the MRI console or MRI images. Days before surgery on a sagittal image MRI slide taken beforehand, we mark the EAM. Then, this point (EAM) is moved to midsagittal image MRI slide where it shows the AC-PC line. Once this point (EAM) is marked on the midsagittal image MRI slide where the AC-PC line is displayed, we draw a line that starts at the point of the EAM that is parallel to the AC-PC line and runs through the patient's nose. Then, we measure the distance between the nasion and the point where the parallel line cuts the patient's nose. The distance between the nasion-intersection of the line parallel to the AC-PC line and the patient's nose gives us the point on the nose where we put the head ring nose bar. A mark is done in this point.

Once this is done, on the morning of surgery, we fix the head ring to the patient's head so that the earplugs are fixed on the EAM, and the nose bar is fixed to the mark that has been made on the patient's nose. Thus, the head ring forms an axial parallel plane to the AC-PC of the patient's head and the frame is parallel to the axis of scanning (Figure 2).

Example (Figure 3). The first image in Figure 3 shows the EAM mark and determines its position on the sagittal MRI images display using the radiological scale. In the second image in Figure 3, having moved the point representing the EAM, we draw a parallel line to the AC-PC line. This line starts at the point where the EAM crosses the patient's nose. Then, we measure the distance from the nasion-parallel line intersection point to the AC-PC line on the patient's nose. This distance measures 18 mm. Then, we mark this point on the patient's nose and the head ring is placed on the patient's head. The earplugs are placed in the EAM and the nose bar on the mark of the nose. Thus the head ring is parallel to the AC-PC plane. In this patient the AC was lower than PC (Figure 4).

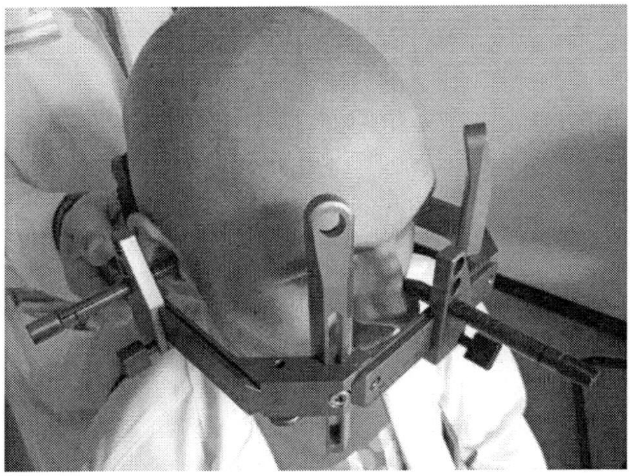

Figure 2. A) CRW head ring with adapter to earplugs and nose bar. B) Leksell head ring with earplugs. The head ring forms a parallel plane to the anterior commissure-posterior commissure plane.

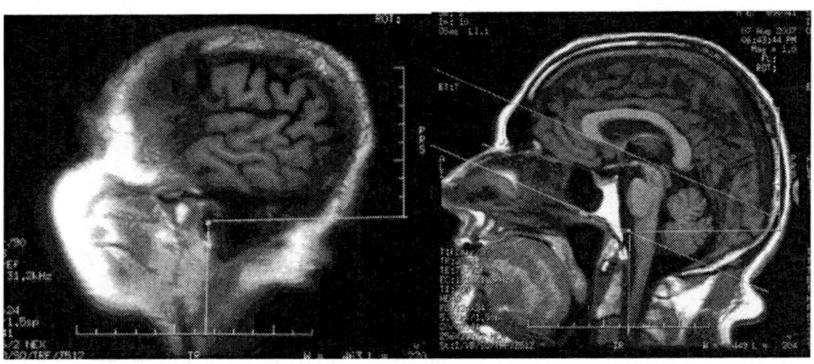

Figure 3. A) Position of the external auditory canal. B) Line parallel to anterior commisure-posterior commisure line and its intersection with the nose.

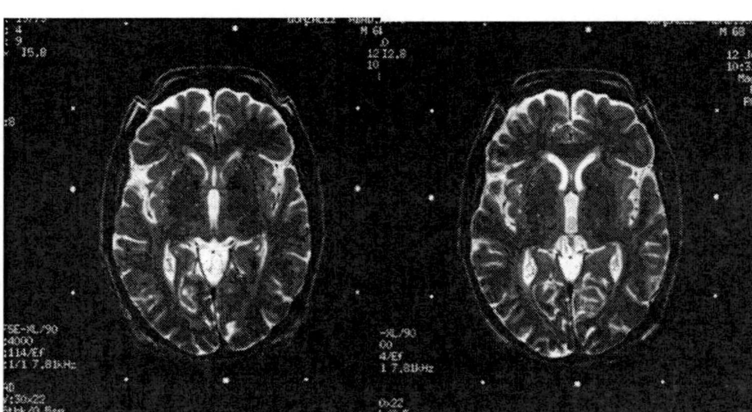

Figure 4. A) The first slide shows the anterior commissure alone. B) The second slide shows the posterior commissure. The two slides are separated by 3 mm.

Therefore, the angle formed between the head ring and AC-PC plane was 2.5°. During surgery, the subthalamus nucleus was identified in the first track. The neurophysiological identification was observed on the AC-PC plane rather than 2 mm below the level of the AC-PC line which is more commonly reported [2].

Having performed this method in over 180 patients with PD, we have obtained a half deviation angle between the AC-PC plane and the ring plane of 1° ± 3°. Others authors have reported a mean pitch angle of 7.5° [58].

Question Four: What Is the Best Radiological Procedure for Fixing the Target, CT, MRI or a Fusion of Images? How Are the Coordinates Calculated? Is There a Specific Computer Program or a Direct Method?

Accurate target localisation is of prime importance in functional stereotactic neurosurgery. Classically, localization of subcortical nuclei (targets) has been performed indirectly, based on fixed distance from an internal reference that can be visualized on a stereotactically-acquired brain imaging study. The internal reference used to obtain the stereotactic coordinates of target is the AC-PC line.

Normally the targets are obtained from different stereotactic atlases. Human brain atlases are used to measure the distance in each dimension [47]. The atlases have been written from the anatomical examination of a limited number of post-mortem brains. They are of limited statistical value and artefacts due to fixation and sections are difficult to assess and correct. Adaptations have to be made to an individual patient's dimensions.

In the Schaltenbrand and Wahren atlas the AC-PC line is 23 mm [43], in Tailarach and Tournoux atlas it is 24 mm [49], by Van Buren and Maccubbin it is 25 mm [54], by Riechert it is 20.9-27.3 mm [40] and by Taveras it is 23-28 mm [51]. Schaltenbrand et al [43] and Talairach et al [49] are the most human atlases used. However, if we use this method, we make an intrinsic error of calculation because the length of the AC-PC line differs between post-mortem brains (atlas) and brains of living persons (patients) [43, 49]. On the other hand, in the Schaltelbrand et al atlas [43], the AC-PC line is measured between the upper border of AC (length 2.5 mm) [55] and the lower border of PC. CT and MRI images of the AC-PC line are measured between the posterior edge of the AC and the anterior border of the PC. To standardise measurements, the length of the AC-PC line is established as 24 mm.

Finally, another error factor is the wide diversity of coordinates for the same target [23].

The aim of radiological studios is able to calculate coordinates of stereotactic frame from the AC-PC line. First of all, the stereotactic frame coordinates of the patient's reference AC-PC line must be determined. The X axis is defined as a perpendicular line to the AC-PC line on an axial plane, the Y axis is defined as a line crossing the midpoint of the AC-PC line in the anteroposterior direction on an axial plane, and the Z axis is defined as a perpendicular line to the AC-PC line on a midsagittal plane. Then, the target coordinates that have been determined in the patient´s AC-PC line must be transcribed into the frame stereotactic coordinate system.

To display the AC-PC line, ventriculography [5] was initially used, then CT [26] became more popular and recently MRI is used [36]. Although ventriculography is still used at several medical centres and is considered the gold standard for localisation in stereotactic coordinates calculation [3], it has since been replaced by CT and MRI. The advantages of ventriculography are that it provides accurate and rapid localization of the commissures and is free of image distortion. Its disadvantages are: there can be inaccurate imaging if the geometrical radiological set-up is not perfect, leading to potential morbidity [44]. Finally, there is a displacement of structural fiducial markers and an enlarged width of the third ventricle [14].

At present, CT and MRI are the most commonly-used methods in functional stereotactic neurosurgery, but there is no universal consensus as to which is the most advantageous.

CT provides spatially accurate imaging of the AC and PC, but does not provide the necessary resolution of anatomic detail for direct observation of the target, and final target coordinates must be derived from atlas predictions based on the AC-PC line. On the other hand, MRI can provide neuroanatomic detail and could be used to directly target desired structures, but MRI images are subject to spatial distortion [4, 7, 15]. Moreover, the average difference in level between the axial CT and MRI is about 3.29 mm, 3.52 mm in the coronal plane and 4.28 mm in the sagittal plane [12, 19]. The maximum error distance between CT and MRI is between 1.2 mm in the mediolateral dimension to 2 mm in the anteroposterior dimension [58].

On the other hand, there are significant differences in coordinates obtained by MRI performed concomitantly with ventriculography (anteroposterior coordinates, mean error: 2.6 mm, range 0.5-6.8 mm) [33]. Therefore, the use of MRI alone for the determination of stereotactic targets has been questioned.

To summarise the advantages of ventriculography are good AC-PC display, without distortion. Its disadvantages are that it is an invasive method, involves radiation exposure, does not show the surrounding structures of AC-PC and it distorts the shape and size of the third ventricle.

The advantages of CT are that it provides a good AC-PC display, does not produce distortion, does not distort the third ventricle, and it is not an invasive method. Its disadvantages are that it involves radiation exposure, and does not show the surrounding structures of AC-PC.

The advantages of MRI are that is provides a good AC-PC display, it is non-invasive, does not involve radiation, and it displays the surrounding structures of AC-PC well. Its disadvantages MRI images are subject to spatial distortion

In order to eliminate the disadvantages of these studies and only retain their advantages, software has been designed to merge the images of CT and MRI [27, 41]. These programs have two disadvantages which lie in the economic cost and that the fact that MRI images are not in real time.

The philosophy of our surgical method is to calculate stereotactic coordinates in real time. An MRI and CT are performed on the day of the operation to fix the stereotactic frame to the patient's head. Then, we calculate the stereotactic coordinates on CT and MRI. The great advantage of this method is that the stereotactic coordinates in the CT and MRI are calculated in real time and can be made on the same slide.

On the other hand, with the aim of avoiding this error several authors recommend direct localization of target [6, 18]. This method seems the most logical and correct, but, it also entails mistakes. The targets are difficult to identify in MRI and it has the problem of distortion [7, 28, 47].

In the actuality, we believe that the current method which provides a more operational, fast and safe way to calculate the stereotactic coordinates of different targets is the indirect method based on real time images obtained with CT and MRI.

Then we choose MRI scanning and CT as the routine imaging procedures to guide the implanted DBS electrode. We compare the two imaging methods used frequently in stereotactic neurosurgery for anatomical localization of the target: CT and MRI. Once the patient is selected for DBS procedure we perform a standard MRI to disclose the presence of anatomical variations or unexpected pathology. On the MRI monitor and using the middle sagittal T1 MRI as a reference, we find the AC-PC line and translate it to the EAM level. We project this line to the nasal bridge. In this way, (so) we obtain the superficial nasal reference and calculate the nasion-nasal point distance (about 2 cm). In this plane, the neurosurgeon will fit the patient with the stereotactic frame.

Under local anaesthesia, this device will be temporarily affixed to the skull by four shallow screws so that the patient's head will not move during diagnostic imaging, or the actual DBS procedure. Following placement of the stereotactic frame, we performed a CT scan (Toshiba Aquilion 16) on all our patients prior to the MRI. After fixing the frame onto the CT table serial CT scans were obtained at a 1 mm interval and a scan thickness of 2 mm, with the CT gantry parallel to the stereotactic frame. We obtained an AC-PC plane where the AC and PC were identified.

After CT scan, four MR image sets were obtained using a GE MR 1.5 T. A stereotactic T2 magnetic resonance sequence was performed on the three spatial planes (first sagittal, then coronal and finally the axial plane) with the following parameters: (TR/TE) repetition time msec/echo time msec, 4000/113.8; number of sections acquired 15; section thickness, 2.5 mm; spacing 0.5; NEX 2; matrix, 320 x 256; field of view, 30x30; and receive bandwidth, 7.8 KHz. In addition to the images above, imaging with a three-dimensional data set for the purpose of anatomic localization was performed using 3-dimensional T-1-weighted 2.6 mm thick gradient-echo images to obtain 110 contiguous axial slices (MPRAGE) 3D/FGR (magnetization-prepared rapid acquisition gradient-echo transverse acquisition). Parameters were as follows: 11.1/4.2/500 msec TR/TE/TI; flip angle 15°; number of sections acquired 112; spacing 1.3; matrix 256x192; field of view, 28x21; and receive bandwidth, 15.6 KHz. This 3D sequence optimizes the surgical approach, avoiding traversing sulci, cortical veins, dural venous lakes and lateral ventricles. Images were reconstructed in a 3-D GE-workstation (Advantage Windows, Version 4.0, software (GEMS, Milwaukee, WI. USA).

To account for a potential shift in the AC-PC coordinates and the ICP of the patient's head with respect to the stereotactic frame, we calculated the following measurements on the 2D T2-weighted images. In the axial AC-PC plane on T2-WI, we measured AC-PC distance and ICP. We also measured the width of the third ventricle. To find the geometrical centre of the stereotactic frame, we intersected lines from peripheral reference points on the stereotactic frame, thus, fixing the coordinate axis (X, Y). To calculate Z axis of ICP we used the measurement of the lateral oblique fiducial markers on the stereotactic frame as a reference. After this, we compared the patient coordinates to the real centre of the stereotactic frame *(Scanner localization guidelines with Leksell stereotactic frame. Elekta Instrument. Stockholm, Sweden)*. We then verified the AC-PC distance on the reformatted sagittal plane of the volumetric MPRAGE images. We calculate α and ß angles on the coronal and sagittal reformatted planes, respectively (Figure 5).

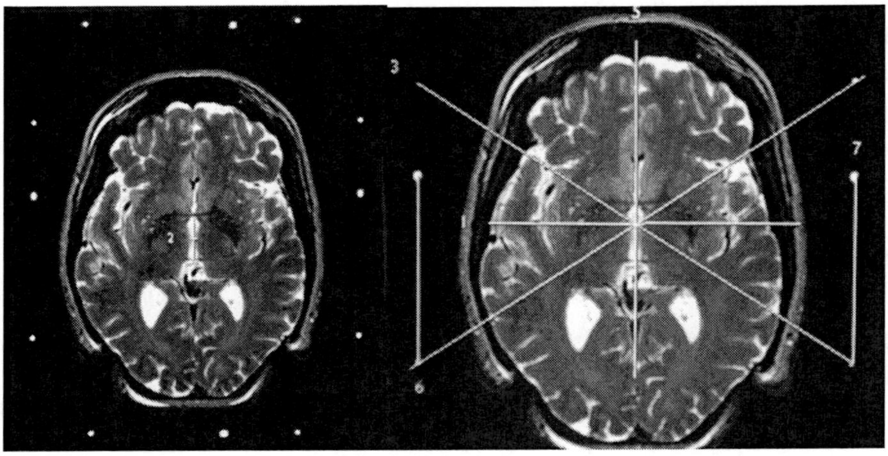

Figure 5. Axial AC-PC plane on T2 magnetic resonance sequence. A) The first image shows the width of the third ventricle. B) The second image shows target localization with Leksell stereotactic frame.

Question Five: Which Is the Best Anesthesia for Functional Neurosurgery?

DBS is a long operation that usually requires the collaboration of the patient. Moreover, the patient's personality, the uncomfortable position on the operating table and the anxiety it produces throughout the long surgical process leads to discomfort and less collaboration with the patient's medical team. Therefore, anaesthesia in functional neurosurgery must meet three strategic objectives, to keep the patient awake, cooperative and comfortable (no pain, no anxiety, etc.). Thus, the surgeon can assess the patient throughout the operation as well as his/her response to neurostimulation. In exceptional cases, such as generalized dystonia, general anaesthesia will be essential.

We have operated on more than 200 patients and only 4 patients needed general anaesthesia; three with generalized primary dystonia and one 51 year-old patient with PD who had painful dystonia that prevented CT and MRI-imaging from being performed. Generally, we use the following anaesthesia protocol: Antiparkinsonian drugs are discontinued 12 hours before surgery.The patient is placed in a semi-seated position to minimize cerebrospinal fluid loss and facilitate neurological examination. Monitoring included electrocardiography, pulse oximetry, arterial pressure (non invasive), end-tidal CO2, urinary catheter and entropy (it informs us of the degree of sedation of the patient). Control of fluids and electrolyte imbalances. Analgesics that do not interfere with coagulation (paracetamol).

Opioid analgesics (fentanyl) administered in IV bolus. We do not use remifentanyl because of the potential side effect of respiratory depression. This side effect is difficult to resolve by the patient's position and his head placement and fixation in the stereotactic frame.

Benzodiazepines (potassium clorazepate) are administered intravenously. It keeps the patient sedated but able to give verbal responses.

Hypnotic sedatives derived from benzodiazepines (midazolam) administered in IV bolus. The potent effect of anxiolytics enables us to keep the patient asleep at certain times.

The long duration of the surgery and fixing the head is difficult to endure for some patients.

We try not to use propofol because it interfered with parkinsonian symptoms even when used in low amounts. It also elicited abnormal movements in individual patients [21]; the most adverse event is its interference with neurophysiological monitoring (personal experience).

Once the surgery is finished, a CT control is done and the patient is transferred to the intensive care unit where he is hospitalized 24 hours.

Question Six: Neurophysiological Recordings in the Surgical Procedure. What Are the Advantages and Disadvantages of the Microelectrode and the Semi-Microelectrode?

In any functional neurosurgery scenario, the neurophysiological targeting is still controversial and is identified as a luxury, research or a risk. In our experience, stereotactic imaging is used only to define the general location of the target then intra operative neurophysiological monitoring (IONM), to avoid neurologic impairment, is currently used for surgical decision-making. The average distance error between the final physiological targets and the magnetic resonance imaging-derived targets is 2.6 ± 1.3 mm [46] and IONM improved the initial accuracy from 64% to 100% [53]. The identification, localization and preservation of anatomically ambiguous nervous tissue and the continuous “on-line” assessment of functional integrity of neural pathways are the IONM’s neurological primary objectives.

In this context, IONM is a cooperative process between anaesthetist, neurophysiologist and neurosurgeon in the operating theatre. The classical reference to Functional Neurosurgery as Applied Neurophysiology is representative of the neurophysiologist-neurosurgeon teamwork outside and/or inside the operating room. This cooperative expertise optimises the final decision. Moreover, today, surgical processes require candid communication, checking time-tables and quality assurance of the implemented procedures. Hence, the accurate placement of the electrode in specific brain nuclei for ablative procedures or DBS require IONM to identify, to register and to document each trajectory's incidences and to correlate the trajectories with the relevant post-operative neurophysiological assessment. Furthermore, the physical dilemma of accuracy versus sharpness is present during target neuroimaging-based planning. The reconstruction from MRI and CT needed to measure the coordinates of the direct or indirect theoretical target, would be regarded as a technical approach to the localization of the ambiguous tissue. In this context, the role of IONM is related to the improvement of the detected planning inaccuracies since they are in relationship to millimeters.

To summarize, neuroimaging techniques for stereotactic planning, neurophysiological mapping to confirm the target and the exploration of the target's adjacent structures before placement of a DBS lead are essential to improve the accuracy of the process and to reduce side effects. This is the reason we think the recording techniques are mandatory in order to accurately localize the optimal target site.

From Albe-Fessard and Pendfield, as early as 1920-1970 [1, 37], a set of neurophysiological procedures, from microelectrode recording to evoked potentials, have been used for localizing cortical and subcortical targets for stereotactic brain surgery. Years ago, to cover these technical procedures, a set of sophisticated laboratory equipment was required in the operating room, but at the present time, standard IOM equipment with any facility can be used. In our opinion, requirements such as easy application and easy interpretation, unimpaired and unimpeded surgery, uninterrupted and continuous monitoring, no risk and low rate of failure, affordable costs, high sensitivity and specificity should be kept in mind when doing IONM planning [10].

The neurophysiological methodologies used in the operating theatre require trained and skilled personnel, not only to collect but also to interpret the data and to cooperate with the neurosurgeon in decision-making. Different IONM protocols for subcortical targets are available in the medical literature.

The present opinion is based on our monitoring, assessment and research experience at the Hospital Universitario Central de Asturias, Spain, from 1996 to July 2008, with more than 400 hemispheric procedures. We implemented IONM's protocol based on standard IOM criteria plus specific software tools. Somatosensory evoked potentials (SSEP), visual evoked potentials (VEP), integrated-interference pattern and turn-amplitude analysis in electromyography (EMG), motor evoked potential (MEP), spectral filters, threshold and delay facilities, etc., available as standard hardware and software in IONM equipment, are used for monitoring and mapping an optimal and impeded target. Special software tools could be implemented to improve the standard IOM equipment performance. In general, these tools are related to neuronal single-unit and/or multi-unit microelectrode recording (MER) on-line analysis and the data displayed on a MER/atlas background.

Neuroimaging techniques for stereotactic planning, neurophysiological mapping to confirm the target and the exploration of the target's adjacent structures before placement of a DBS electrode are essential to improve the accuracy of the process and to reduce side effects. However, opinions differ not only in regards to the inaccuracies of the CT-MR imaging fusion techniques for direct or indirect planning, but also which neurophysiological methods should be considered for target mapping and DBS electrode securing after identifying an appropriate track and target.

Our procedure has four steps: Pre-surgical, intra-operative, inter-operative and post-surgical:

1. Pre-surgical: Patients considered for surgery are also selected for pre-surgical neurophysiological assessment. A standard EEG, afferent evoked potentials -PEV for the internal globus pallidus (GPi) target; SSEP for the ventralis intermedius nucleus (Vim) and subthalamic nucleus (STN)-, P30 and P300 event related potentials and motor evoked potentials (MEP magnetic stimulation) are performed. Patients should be willing and able to undergo a conscious, long and noisy surgical procedure in which the exploration of patient behavioural responses are empirically assessed and recorded.

2. Intra-operative: This concerns monitoring, mapping and securing the DBS electrode at the selected target site. Because the differences between the type of anatomic planning and the functional information needed to locate the optimal target vary from patient to patient, free and evoked deep brain macro- and micro-electrode recordings, EMG polygraph recordings, SSEP or VEP and MEP are performed. In regards to equipment, over the course of 12 years we have changed the IOM equipment from an initial low cost four-channel Premier (MEDELEC, England) to a moderately priced Keypoint plus Lead-Point facilities (DANTEC-MEDTRONIC, Denmark) and/or a 10Ch. XLTECH (Canada). The MER continuous on-line recording is analyzed and displayed on an auxiliary laptop with NDRS (CIREN, Cuba) software. We use an Ohye's electrode (Unique Medical, Japan) for multi-unit MER [30] and two types of DBS tetraelectrodes (MEDTRONIC, USA), Model 3389 for STN and hypothalamus surgery and Model 3387 for Gpi and thalamus ones for macro-electrode recording and stimulation. We also used to include mapping performed by MER of extracellular single-unit activities (neuronal activities), but only for research purposes. An ISO-80 (WPI, England) isolated differential amplifier is used as a preamplifier to secure deep brain intrusion and to optimize the high impedance noise from microelectrodes [10].

Neurophysiological measurements in a hostile operating theatre environment, with a conscious patient, face strong limitations when compared to the freedom we can find in a physiological laboratory. Thus, MER-IONM requires not only surgical time but skills, knowledge and neurophysiological expertise. In order to answer the neurosurgeon's questions and to make decisions in the operating room, the neurophysiologist needs to select, record and compare all the neurons recorded so far in a track, in order to detect the transition between the various structures crossed by the microelectrode and to identify the abnormal pattern of discharge and synchronization of the neuronal activities of different nuclei. Not all centres use MER-IONM, and not all centres that use MER, have a physiologist-surgeon team. As a result of our experience, we can confirm that the interplay between neurosurgeon and neurophysiologist optimizes safety, accuracy, constraints, knowledge and final outcomes. In our opinion, the use of the different mapping methodologies depends upon the circumstances and characteristics of the medical team involved in the neurosurgery, such as their level of expertise-training, skills-knowledge, research-clinical background and medical specialization, as well as the degree of their relationship. In our experience, if an IOM criterion is applied, in order to facilitate the neurophysiological intraoperative assessment after frame placement, image acquisition, theoretical target and initial trajectory planning, a set of electrodes is distributed with a 10-20 IS criterion over the patient's scalp and respectively, on the extensor digitorum communis and tibialis anterior muscles in the operating room. Ocular movement and facial expression video-recording are performed for monitoring purposes.

The extracellular single-unit MER is a well-designed mapping technique whose analysis includes a minimum of three steps: A subjective characterization of the neuronal discharge pattern, an empirical amplitude threshold selection and an objective quantification of the selected single-unit. This technique uses sharp 5-30 μm diameter, high impedance (> 1MΩ) micro-electrode tips. By recording on-line single-unit activity, we can identify the free and evoked activities from different nuclei and characterize the superior and inferior borders of the ambiguous nervous tissue. The sporadic or rhythmic neuronal discharge patterns are auditory discriminated and quantitatively analyzed. Usually an amplifier 500 Hz filter is used for single-unit MER. It is a time-consuming technique if properly performed (30-40 min by track), because the microelectrode must advance along the recording track by small steps (<0.5 mm) and frequently not all steps show a useful signal.

However it is very efficient when the limitations of this methodology are known by the neurosurgeon and the technique is mastered with experience and patience by a neurophysiologist.

Another IONM point of view or physiological mapping alternative is the multi-unit MER analysis, a methodology we normally use. This technique uses a concentric bipolar sharp microelectrode that has a 0.2 mm^2 active area with a 5 μm tip, referred to as a *semi-microelectrode.* This active area is separated from the reference area by 1 mm to 0.8 mm^2 (Ohye's electrode). This MER detects the activities of 10 to 40 perceptible neurons localized in a small volume (100-200 μm^3) around the sharp and facilitates the bipolar recording of local-field evoked potentials. The EMG standard software is useful for multi-unit MER analysis. Our procedure resembles that of EMG pattern analysis applied to assess recruitment and synchronization/interference of motor unit potentials. Therefore, amplitude, time and frequency domain analysis are considered for on-line identification and characterization of ambiguous nervous tissue.

Compared to single-unit MER, multi-unit MER has lower spatial resolution and cannot specify the pattern of neuronal discharge. Conversely, multi-unit MER better estimates the number of active neurons within certain areas and enables easy and reliable quantification of neuronal activity with a few sources of technical pitfalls [11]. The amplitude change or "*integrated*" multi-unit values of the recorded interference pattern significantly distinguishes between inside and outside the nucleus. The use of other standard on-line automatic EMGs such as turn-amplitude measurements of the interferential multi-unit MER pattern show specific features. Usually multi-unit MER is a timeless technique that consumes 10 to 15 min. per track.

For our mapping proposes we implement both multi-unit and local-field potential using MER, but in special research cases, a single-unit study was performed. The standard amplifier settings are carried out usually through a 100 Hz-5 KHz band pass for multi-unit

MER and 10 Hz-5 KHz for local-field potential MER or beta-band MER signal analysis. The intraoperative MER is performed with the patient awake, but occasionally low doses of fentanyl are required and, if necessary, a reduced infusion of propofol. In our experience, both sleep and propofol modify multi-unit neuronal activity pattern. Once the duramatter has been opened, the Ohye's electrode is inserted through the burr hole and is then advanced by 1 mm steps using a microdrive device. In order to identify and localize ambiguous tissue, mapping for deep brain multi-unit MER is performed from the striatum to the inferior border of the expected nuclei. After two seconds, using the new step-impact, two seconds of free of artifacts multi-unit patterns are recorded and then the two-second "*integrated*" multi-unit value is graphically displayed as a step-related histogram on the theoretical outlined atlas-plane background (Figure 6).

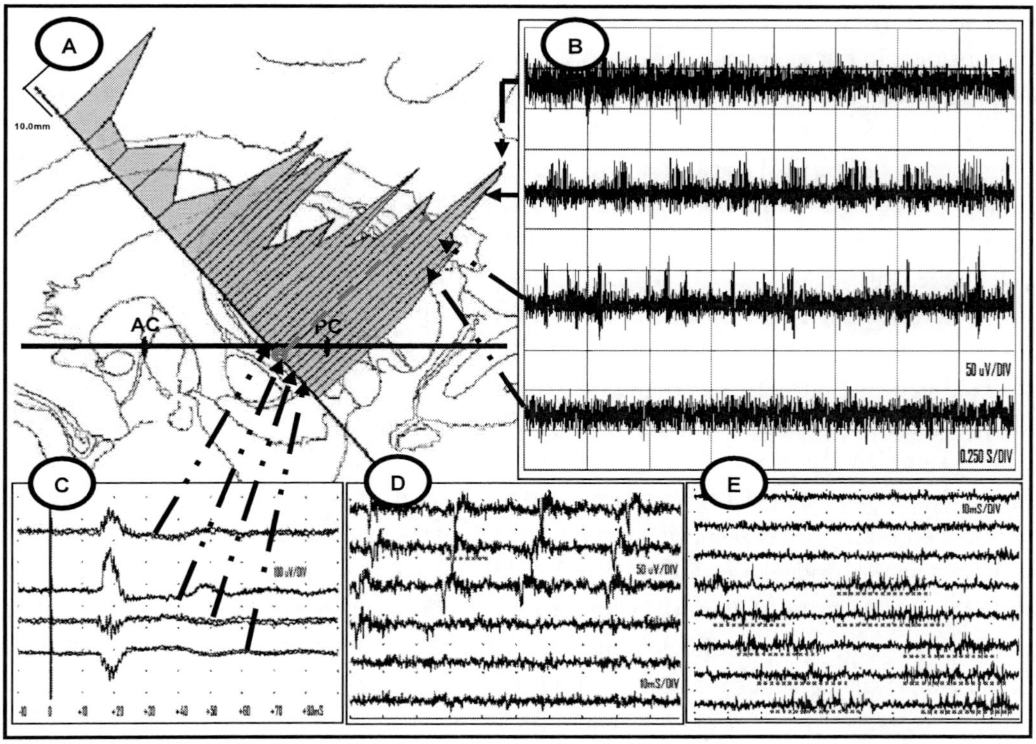

Figure 6. Mapping of the thalamic ventral intermedius nucleus (Vim). A) Display of the processed micro-electrode "*step by step*" multi-unit recording histograms and anterior commisure (AC) – posterior commisure (PC) plane over a 12 mm sagital plate of Schaltebrand and Wahren Atlas. B) Four traces of two seconds free run multi-unit recording from thalamic track showing tremor related multi-unit recruitment at a frequency of 4 Hz. C) Vim-ventroposterolateral nuclei (VPL) transition identify by median nerve somatosensory evoked potentials polarity reversal. D) Scrolling of three underlines consecutive traces of tapping event related somatosensory evoked responses. E) Scrolling of five underlined consecutive traces of rushting event related responses.

In a downward direction, the abrupt amplitude, frequency and pattern changes of multi-unit MER significantly distinguish between the inside (top) and outside (bottom) of the nucleus or nuclei transitions, and the length of the track in the nucleus measurement. This methodology makes the spatial abstraction of the three-dimensional track easier. The 3D displayed neurophysiological trajectory is a user-friendly and useful tool for decision-making by the neurosurgeon-neurophysiologist .

Usually, in 78.3% of the explored hemispheres in DBS tetraelectrode implantation, we perform no more than five MER tracks plus the final DBS tetraelectrode track (5.93 tracks ±1.82). It can be useful to perform local-field SSEP and VEP-MER when, for example, the STN nucleus can not be located or we need to know the inferior border of the GPi. In this context, if the first STN track shows a thalamic trajectory and the nuclei were not detected, then, we perform a median nerve SSEP-MER. In the case of clearly identified SSEP-MER responses, we do a rectification for the next track, 6 mm anterior and 2 mm lateral from the previous one. In our experience, the theoretical initial target result of the neuroimaging-based planning needs to be corrected. For example, in STN mapping, when the correction of inaccuracies were related to a necessary rostro-dorso-lateral displacement (75% of explored hemispheres) of the final track, the corrections were in the order of 1.91 mm±0.79 (median 2.0 mm) lateral, 3.24 mm±1.64 (median 2.5 mm) rostral and 1.04 mm±0.66 (median 1.0mm) dorsal. Conversely, when we need a caudo-ventro-medial displacement (25% of explored hemispheres) to localize the best final target, the corrections were in the order of 1.62 mm±0.60 (median 2 mm) medial, 2.96 mm±1.6 posterior (median 2.25 mm) and 1.0 mm±0.65 ventral (median 1 mm). In this context, the precise and effective functional localization of the nucleus is only possible using the mapping of the single-unit or multi-unit MER neuronal activity. However, the definitive implant of the DBS tetraelectrode can deviate significantly from the selected neurophysiological target due to the variability introduced by the manual neurosurgery method. An integrative methodology is needed to allow the correction of the inaccuracies between the target identified and the final implant of the DBS tetraelectrode. In order to optimize this objective, a bipolar macro-recording from the DBS tetraelectrode is performed to check the correct final position of the implant. To achieve this goal, the recordings from 0-1, 1-2 and 2-3 tetraelectrode contact, when the bottom contact is named as 0 and the top one as 3, were analyzed and displayed respectively on three channels. The "*integrated*" macro-recording signal from 0-1 contact derivation was correlated with the data of the final-track

Although many MER systems allow the surgical team to switch between recording and stimulation modes, we do not perform micro-stimulation to identify motor bundles or motor nuclei during IONM. In our experience, the "integrated" multi-unit value change identifies nucleus limits without requiring this assurance technique. Secondly, as Shils et al [46] points out, "*the volume of tissue that can be affected with microelectrode stimulation is so small that gross clinical changes are rarely observed with this technique*".

3. Inter-operative: This period refers to the 6 days between DBS tetralectrode implantation and the surgical act for definitive plug-in to the impulse generator stimulator (IGS). After 72 hrs with the DBS tetraelectrode and during the 3 days before the IGS implants, we perform a set of neurophysiological techniques to find the best contact and any possible inaccuracies. The relative distance between the different DBS tetraelectrode contacts and the efferent motor fibres is assessed by low rate monopolar DBS tetraelectrode contact stimulation and EMG recording. From a 0.5 mA intensity, 5 Hz frequency and 200 μS duration initial pulse, the threshold MEP from masseter, extensor digitorum communis and tibialis anterior muscles is identified and the intensity/duration characteristics of the stimuli measured. If the necessary stimulus to induce a response is low, an abnormal placement of the electrode is confirmed. The anatomo/functional relationship between DBS tetraelectrode and the lemniscus medialis and ventro-postero-lateral (VPL) thalamus is assessed by SSEP for Vim and STN targets [11]. In this way, the median nerve and/or tibialis anterior nerve stimulation evoked event-related potentials can be recorded as far-field potentials from the DBS tetraelectrode contacts. From the 0-1, 1-2, 2-3 bipolar derivations, we measure the amplitude, polarity and configuration responses. This data is correlated with the MEP. Macro-recordings from these bipolar derivations in addition to a standard polysomnography (PSG) are performed and the polarity of the beta rhythms and the sharp waves recorded during the REM sleep are measured to make a final decision. When the target is the GPi to assess the position of the DBS tetraelectrode with respect to the optic bundle, VEP are performed. If the results from SSEP or VEP, MEP and STN-PSG indicate an adequate 3D-location of the DBS tetraelectrode on the subthalamic volume, the IGS is implanted.
4. Post-operative: The initial contact for therapeutic DBS is selected based on interoperative neurophysiological data previously described. After one year, the outcome is evaluated by an adequate clinical assessment [20] and a scalp-recorded STN, Vim or GPi evoked potentials by bipolar DBS tetraelectrode stimulation. Short latency and cortical mapping can be evaluated and correlated with the clinical improvement.

Question Seven: How Do You Implant the DBS? Is an Introductory Cannula Necessary? Is a Radiological Control Necessary? How Can We Check the Correct Positioning of the DBS in the Operating Room?

Currently, there are only two DBS leads models available, Model 3387 and 3389 (Medtronic Inc, Minneapolis, MN, USA). The Model 3387 lead has four electrodes, of which each one is 1.5 mm long, separated by 1.5 mm, thus spanning a linear distance of 10.5 mm.

The Model 3389 lead has the same four electrodes separated by only 0.5 mm, spanning a total of 7.5 mm. In both cases, the leads are 1.27 mm in diameter.

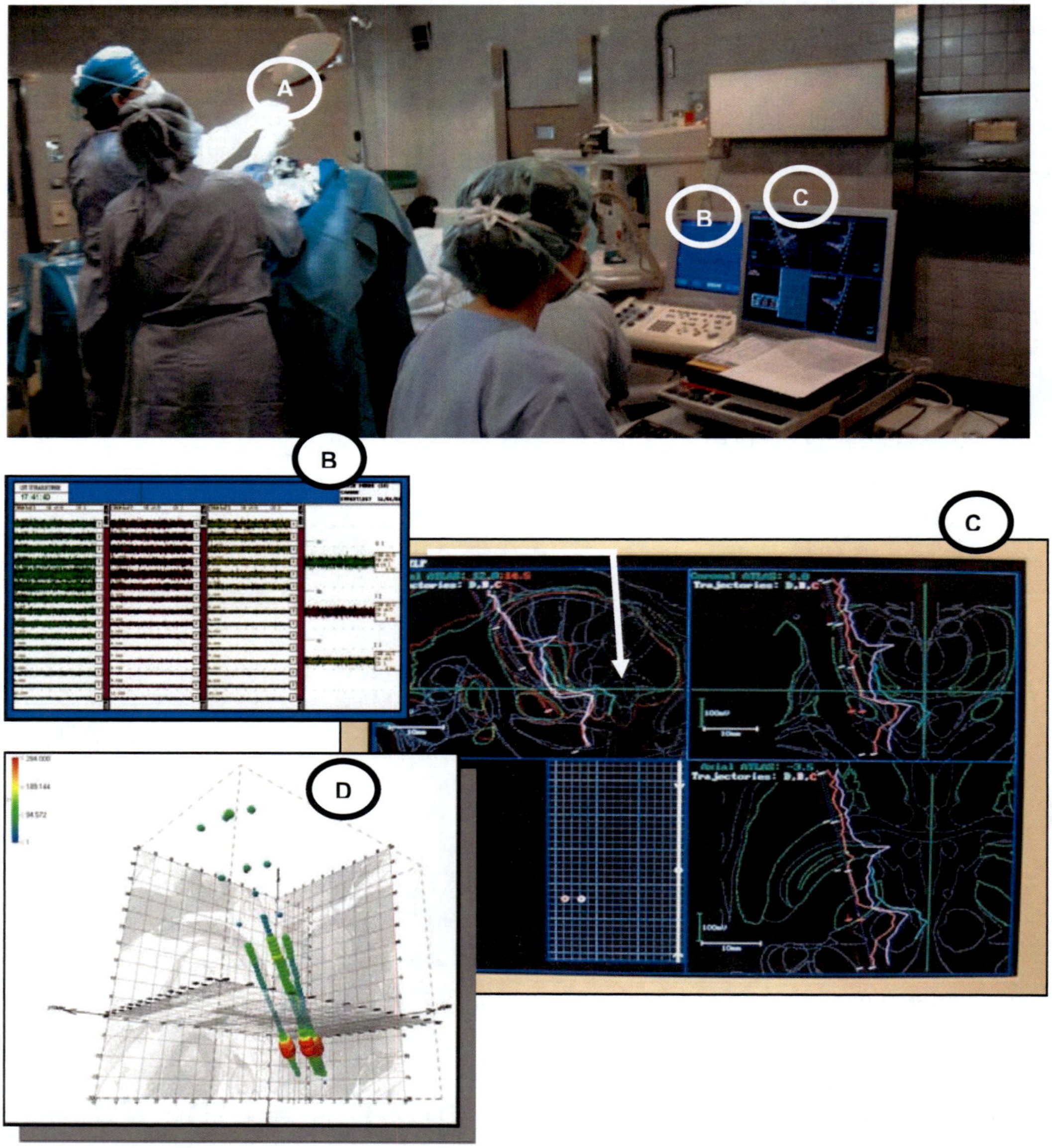

Figure 7. Operating room. A) Micro- tetra-electrode tower. B) Identification and recording of subthalamic nucleus (STN) activity and bipolar tetraelectrode activity display recording from EMG/PE equipment. C) On-line sagital. Coronal and axial display of the processed micro- and tetra-electrode *"step by step"* recording histograms superimposition from the STN multi-unit recording (red and blue traces) and the tetraelectrode 0-1 bipolar recoding (red trace) to identified final DBS tetraelectrode position. D) 3D-display mapping of three tracks. Color and size indicate *"integrated"* multi-unit MER values where red color points correspond to STN.

Even though it seems logical to think that the higher number of trajectories would increase the risk of bleeding, in our experience, no statistical significance was found between the number of sites and bleeding [45]. An increased number of tracks have a higher risk of brain edema that spreads along the longitudinal direction of the axons and generates a shift in midline structures. In our series, such edema did not produce morbidity (Figure 8).

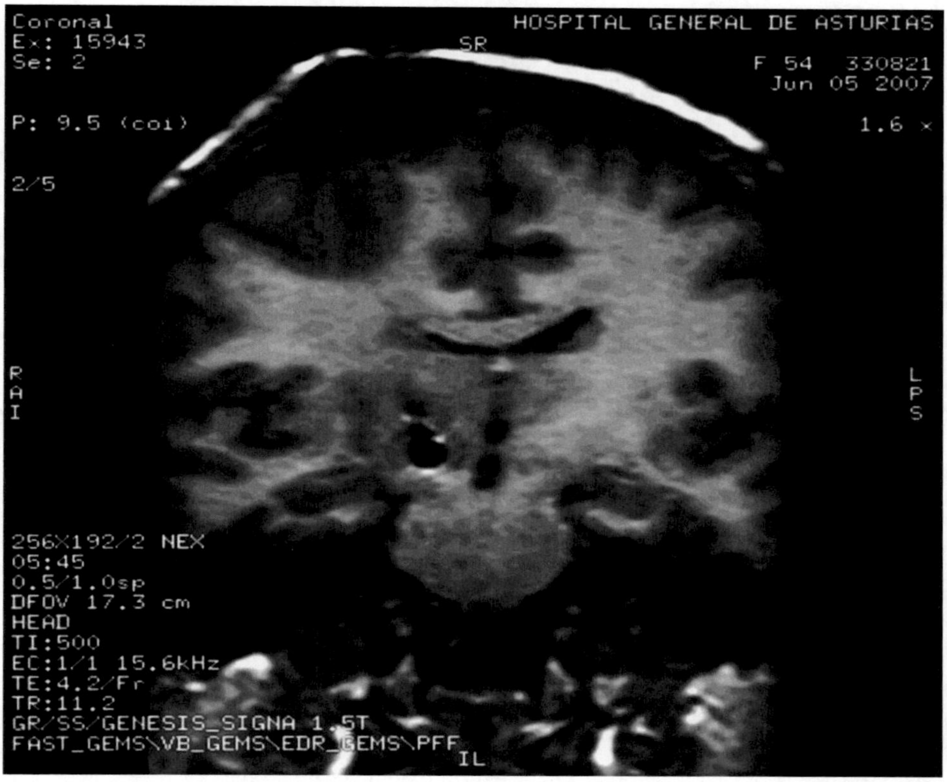

Figure 8. Shift by cerebral brain after DBS lead implanted

Once semi-microelectrode recording confirms the target, we checked its position with control X-ray films. After the semi-microelectrode and its guiding cannula are withdrawn and replaced by the guiding cannula for the DBS lead in the same place. This cannula is inserted to the brain slowly and gently until 10 mm above the target. Then, the DBS lead is deployed and DBS lead electrode recording is performed to confirm the physiology of the neural activity of the target. Its position is checked by X-ray films and compared with the position of the semi-microelectrode. If DBS lead´ electrode recording, radiological position and the macrostimulation test are correct, we implant the DBS lead.

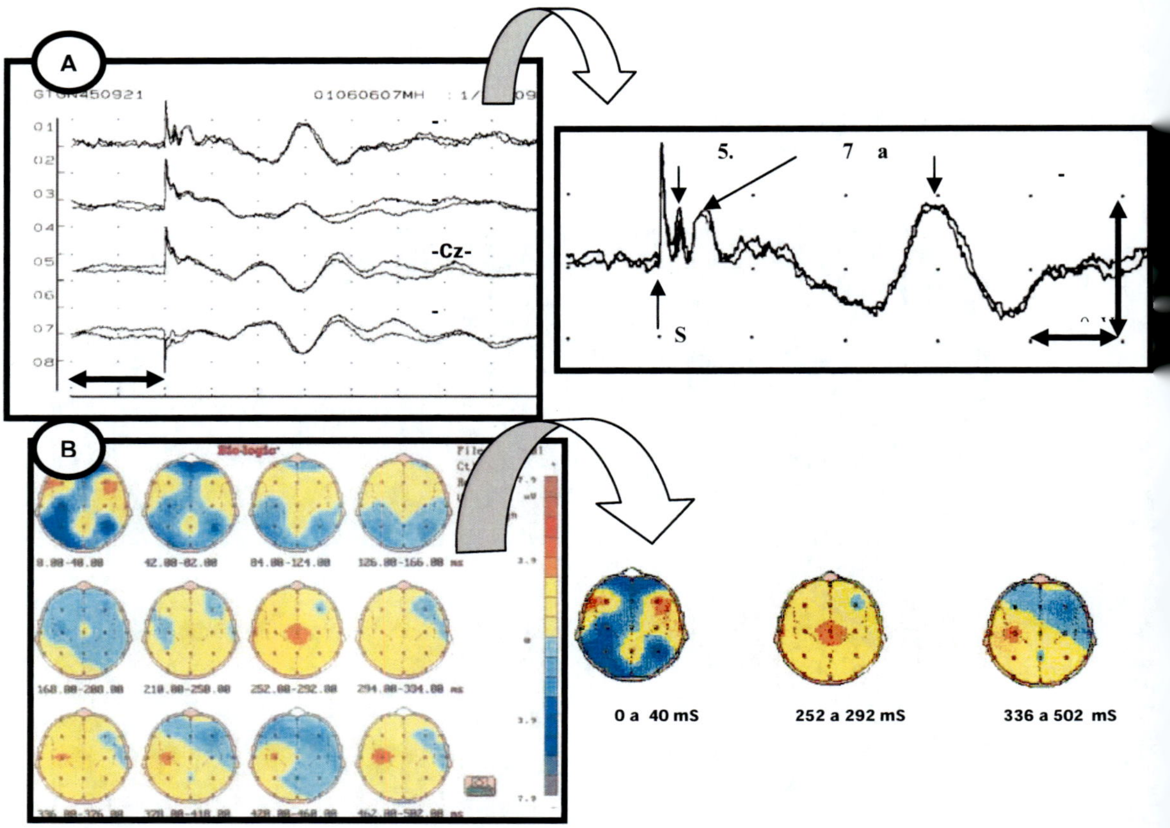

Figure 9. Scalp evoked responses after low frequency subthalamic nucleus (STN) stimulation of the therapeutically effective DBS tetraelectrode contact. A) Short and middle latency responses showing frontal predominance of the 5 to 12 ms potentials and polarity change over Cz 10-20 IS electrode. B) Display of twelve consecutive relative amplitude/fourteen second maps of the scalp recorded event related responses showing as red color higher amplitude.

We always implant the DBS lead with a guiding cannula because the DBS lead stylet that facilitates stereotaxic placement of the lead is weak, thus, there is a potential for a breach of procedure. In the beginning, after getting the final trajectory with semi-microelectrode, a lateral X-ray film was taken for attitude control of the implant. Then the semi-microelectrode is withdrawn and a lesion probe with a 1.1x3 mm exposed tip (Radionics, Burlington, Mass, USA) is introduced into the same site. We take another X-ray film to check that the lesion probe remained in the same position as the semi-microelectrode. Afterwards, the lesion probe is removed and the DBS lead, Model 3387 or Model 3389 is introduced with its stylet, tracing the path undertaken by the lesion probe. Finally, an X-ray film was taken to verify that the DBS was in the same position as the semi-microelectrode (Figure 10).

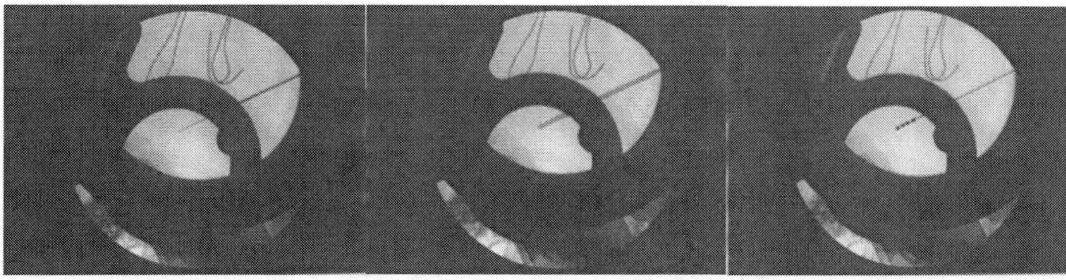

Figure 10. X-ray films. A) Semi-microelectrode. B) Lesion probe. C) DBS lead.

After verifying that this technique can be performed parallel paths of 1-3 mm between the semi-microelectrode and DBS lead, we chose to directly enter the DBS through a cannula (Figure 11). Since we do this method we have not seen any diversion of DBS lead over the semi-microelectrode.

Finally in the last 115 patients we devised a method to verify that DBS electrodes are well established. In the implantation of DBS lead we recorded neuronal activity through own DBS electrodes. This confirmed the good final position of DBS electrodes. The distal contact is located where the recording of cell activities and beneficial effects induced by stimulation are lost.

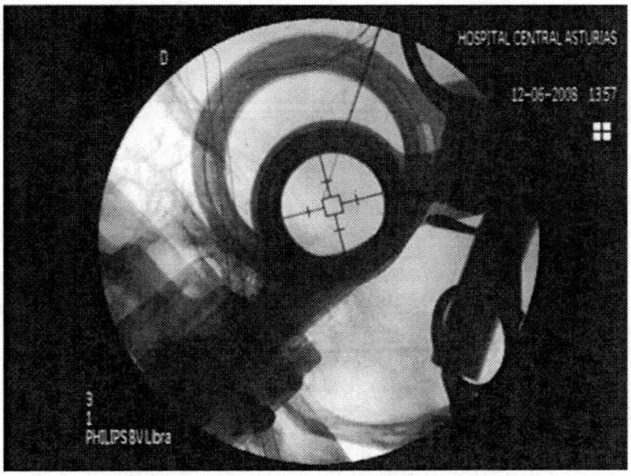

Figure 11. X-ray films. A) Semi-microelectrode. B) DBS lead with cannula.

Question Eight: When Is the Correct Moment for Radiological Control?

Immediately after surgery we performed a standard CT scan to exclude possible brain lesions (pneumoencephalus, haemorrhage).

Seventy-two hours after the operation, a new radiological control with a three-dimensional volumetric magnetic resonance was performed, with special focus on the CA-CP line and the position of the implanted DBS lead from that line because the final target position after semi-microelectrode recording must be deviated from the original anatomic coordinates [29]. We think that MRI is superior to CT in evaluating the possible shifting of electrodes during surgical placement because of the multiplanar capacities and because pins create significant artifactual distortion of CT imaging which can create a source of targeting error (Figure 12).

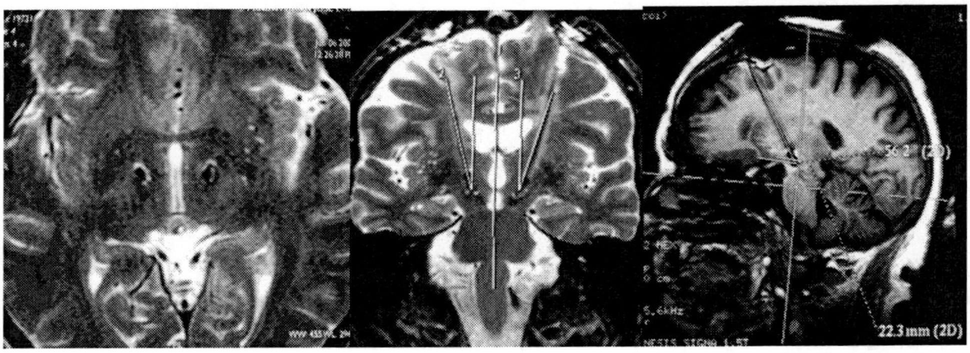

Figure 12. A) Axial T2-Weighted images. Measure X coordinate of electrodes with respect to third ventricle midline and Y coordinate with respect to intercommisural point (ICP). B) Coronal T2-Weighted images. Mesures β angle. C) Sagittal T2-Weighted images. Mesures α angle.

Although subcortical structure localization, using MRI or CT and a stereotactic head frame can have an accuracy of approximately 1 mm, discrepancies between the initial selected target and the DBS electrode position (electrophysiology based) are described [32, 56]. These discrepancies must be due to several factors including imaging distortion, mechanical inaccuracy of the stereotactic frame and brain shift. Many factors may contribute to cerebral shift, including gravitational force, loss of cerebral fluid, changes in pressure due to skull opening during the surgery, pneumocephalus, and forces due to insertion of the DBS lead. The number of microelectrode tracks may be a significant factor that can increase brain edema and increase the shift [13, 17]. Finally another factor that can affect the assessment of brain shift is the difference between the completely supine-positioned patient in the MRI scanner and the semi-seated position during surgery.

Normally, brain shift and pneumocephalus disappeared 72 hours after surgery [17]. Furthermore, the permanent DBS lead may vary ±1 mm, compared to the best localization of the semi-microelectrode due to potential movement during stylet removal [30, 31].

Since 2005, the numerical calculations of the specific absorption rate (SAR) [52] were taken into account and have always been below the regulatory limits in accordance with the Safety Guidelines (T2 SAR: 0.0056 W/kg; MPRAGE: 0.0034 W/kg.). Then we selected a specific MRI protocol with limited slices (five T2 slices), for post-operative electrode placement control. We followed the post-operative MRI image protocol below:

(1) Volumetric 3D MPRAGE in 1.5 mm sagittal slices was performed. The parameters were: 11.2/4,2/500 TR/TE/TI msec; flip angle 15°; 2 NEX; field of view, 28 x 21; section thickness, 2 mm; spacing 1.0; 116 number of sections, matrix, 256x192; and receive bandwidth, 7.8 KHz;

(2) Two sets of T2-weighted FR- FSE T2 images were performed at coronal and axial planes with the following parameters: 6000/114,2 msec TR/TE; number of sections acquired 5; section thickness, 3.0 mm; spacing 0.5; NEX 2; matrix, 320x256; field of view, 26x19,5; and receive bandwidth, 7.8 KHz.

On axial T2-Weighted images, at the AC-PC plane, we measured the X coordinate of the electrodes with respect to the third ventricle midline and the Y coordinate with respect to ICP. The Z coordinate is calculated at the plane crossing trough of the electrode tip, usually 1 or 2 slices inferior to the AC-PC plane (3-6 mm). On 3D MPRAGE reformatted oblique images, we measured the α angle with respect to the mid-coronal plane passing through the third ventricle and the β angle with respect to the AC-PC plane.

Before that appeared Specific Absorption rate recommendations (SAR) [52] we perform a 1.5-tesla MRI control on all operated patients (147 patients). All subjects were able to successfully complete the MR imaging examination. None the subjects complained of any abnormal sensations or discomfort caused by MR imaging with DBS electrodes in place.

Question Nine: What Are the Short-Term Complications in Deep Brain Stimulation Surgery?

Between June 1996 and December 2007, we operated on 207 patients; 183 PD, 16 tremors, 4 dystonias and 4 cluster headaches. A total of 387 DBS electrodes were implanted in the thalamus, internal pallidus, subthalamic nucleus (STN) and the hypothalamus.

We reviewed the complications in our Hospital between March 1998 and December 2004 [45]. One hundred and five consecutive PD patients underwent 223 STN DBS procedures. One hundred received bilateral and five unilateral STN DBS. The total number of implanted leads was 203. All DBS were implanted by the same surgeon (F.S.). Sixty one patients did not present any complications (58% of the patients), thirty seven presented one (35% of the patients) and seven patients presented one or more (7% of the patients).

Of the seven patients who presented two or more complications, two of them presented 3 complications and five of them presented 2 complications. In the two cases with 3 complications, one patient experienced bleeding, convulsions and a confusional state and the other patient presented convulsions, a confusional state and urinary tract infection. In the five patients who presented two complications, three presented bleeding and a confusional state and the other two presented an aborted procedure due to non identification of the STN with two additional procedures because of a misplaced lead, and an aborted procedure due to non identification of the STN and cardiac problems (this patient had a cardiac pacemaker), respectively.

The complications reviewed were aborted procedures, misplaced leads, intracranial haemorrhage, seizures, hardware complications and other complications.

An aborted procedure is a procedure in which the DBS lead could not be implanted in the STN. There were a total of 14 aborted procedures, which means 6.2% of all the procedures. Of the 14 aborted procedures, the STN could not be found in 11 of them; in one case, the stereotactic frame was disconnected during the surgery after implanting the first lead, the neurophysiologic recording system failed in one patient, disabling the left STN and the second lead implant, and finally, clinical changes were observed during the first procedure in another patient, which made us suspect the possibility of bleeding for which we cancelled surgery. After performing a CT, we observed a mild haematoma in the right thalamus. DBS leads were implanted afterwards in a second surgery in 12 of the 14 patients in which the lead could not be implanted in the first surgery. In spite of the sophisticated neuroimaging techniques, a difference of around 35% between the initial theoretical difference estimated by radiological sites and the final target localization was observed [50].

For us, a misplaced lead is any situation that required us to reposition the leads, due to bad positioning in the control MRI and a clinical response lower than 30% in the UPDRS (Part III) 6 months after surgery. The clinical improvement was below 30% in the UPDRS (Part III) in a total of 5 patients and the MRI indicated that the leads were not in the correct position. Four patients had unilateral misplacement and one patient had bilateral misplacement. Following repositioning of the lead, all patients presented a UPDRS (Part III) clinical improvement above 30% and the MRI indicated correct positioning of the lead. These cases represented 2.69% of all the procedures. The misplaced lead may be due to brain shift during the brain lead implant. When the brain regains its normal position after some time, the DBS electrode remains deeper in the brain due to its semi rigidity. This cerebral brain shift can be demonstrated during surgery when comparing the amount of physiological solution we can introduce into the cranial cavity in the first tract to the amount introduced when placing the lead.

Intracranial haemorrhage was present in 7 patients, representing 3.13% of the procedures. Two patients had cortical venous infarct with convulsions. One patient had a mild intraventricular haemorrhage without clinical symptoms. One patient had a mild thalamic haemorrhage associated with convulsions. Another had a small right frontal intracerebral haematoma with convulsions and a third patient developed an intracerebral haematoma throughout the lead trajectory which required emergency surgery in order to evacuate the haematoma, but which did not require lead explantation. As a sequela, a mild residual hemiparesis appeared. Another patient had a transitory intraoperative consciousness deterioration which forced us to cancel the procedure. CT was performed and a thalamic haematoma was seen. This case also appears with those described as aborted procedures.

Seizures affected a total of 11 patients out of 105, representing 4.9% of the procedures. Four patients presented bleeding and 8 did not have radiological findings in the post-operative routine CT scan. All seizures occurred within the first 24 hours after STN lead implant surgery and they improved with intravenous anticonvulsive treatment (phenytoin). The seizures did not reappear, and therefore, except for the patient who developed an intracerebral haematoma throughout the lead trajectory requiring emergency surgery, no patient required anticonvulsive treatment after discharge from the hospital. In the case of this last patient, despite the fact that he never had seizures, anticonvulsive treatment was not discontinued until 6 months after hospital discharge. This being due to the fact that up until the third month after discharge the electroencephalograms presented an irritable focus.

A total of 5 patients presented direct hardware-related complications, affecting 4.8% of all patients and 2.2% of the procedures. One month after surgery, a patient presented scarring and infection at the battery site, forcing explantation and antibiotic treatment. Three months later the battery was implanted without complications. Three months after DBS NST surgery, another patient presented scarring and infection at the lead/wire connection site, leading to removal of the whole DBS system and repositioning it 6 months later. The evaluation of the infectious episodes was performed based on clinical criteria (pain, heat and local tumefaction) and analytical values (leukocytosis and increased GSR). Another patient presented scarring at the wire trajectory one month after implantation, which resolved itself without surgical removal. Fourteen months after surgery, one patient had a lead fracture requiring replacement. Finally, during immediate post-operative lead placement, a patient had a cerebrospinal fluid leak through the burr hole ring and cap, requiring surgery.

A total of 13 patients presented complications different from those already mentioned, representing 5.4% of the procedures. These complications can be divided into minor complications (11 patients) and major complications such as worsening of cardiopathy in the patient with the cardiac pacemaker which made a new procedure in order to implant the second lead impossible, and a lower extremity deep venous thrombosis which required anticoagulant treatment for 6 months due to severe respiratory problems. The most frequent complications found in the abovementioned section on complications were confusional episodes. Even though we did not find a co- relationship between the number of sites, age and confusional episodes, it is likely that this symptomology, during immediate postoperative, may have a multifactor origin. This is a minor complication that disappears with time, and requires only vigilance during the first hours. On the other hand, all patients undergo in-dwelling urinary catheterization at the beginning of the intervention, in order to control their diuresis, and this could have influenced our two reported confusional episodes. Antibiotic treatment was started in the presence of clinical symptoms and pathological urinary sediment, without waiting for the result of the urine culture. In both cases the empirical treatment was proven to be sufficient for the treatment of confusion. We believe that the patient's in-dwelling urinary catheter is needed in order to maintain a correct and constant hydric balance during the long period of the surgery, despite the fact that surgery is performed with conscious patients.

References

[1] Albe-Fessard, DG, Arfel G. and Guiot G. Activités électriques characteristiques de quelques structures cérébrales chez l'homme. *Ann. Chir* 1963; 17:1185-1214.

[2] Benabid AL, Krack P, Benazzouz A, Limousin P, Koudsie A, Pollak P. Deep brain stimulation of the subthalamic nucleus for Parkinson´s disease: methodologic aspects and clinical criteria. *Neurology* 2000; 55(suppl 6): S40-S44.

[3] Benabid AL, Pollak P, Gervason C, Hoffmamm D, Gao DM, Hommel M, Perret JE, de Rougemont J. Long-term suppression of tremor by chronic stimulation of the ventral intermediate thalamic nucleus. *Lancet,* 1991; 337:403-406

[4] Burchiel K, Nguyen T, Coombs B, Suzumoski J. MRI distortion and stereotactic neurosurgery using the Cosman-Roberts-Wells and Leksell frames. Stereotac Funct *Neurosurg* 1996; 66:123-136.

[5] Campbell RL, Campbell JA, Heimburger R, Klasbeck JE, Mealey J. Ventriculography and myelography with absorbable radiopaque medium. *Radiology* 1964; 82:286-289.

[6] Cuny E, Guehl D, Burbaud P, Gross C, Dousset V, Rougier A. Lack of agreement between direct magnetic resonance imaging and statistical determination of a subthalamic target: role of electrophysiological guidance. *J Neurosurg* 2002; 97:591-597.

[7] Derosier C, Delegue G, Munier T, Pharaboz C, Cosnard G. IRM distortion géometrique de l´image et stéréotaxie. *J Radiol* 1991; 72:349-35.

[8] Fahn S. Concept and classification of dystonia. *Adv Neurol* 1988; 50:1-8.

[9] Fahn S, Elton RL, and the members of the Unified Parkinson's Disease Rating Scale. In: Fahn S, Marsden CD, Calne CB, Goldstein M, eds. *Recent Developments in Parkinson's Disease.* Vol. 2. Florham Park, NJ: MacMillan Healthcare Information; 1987. p 153-163, 293-304.

[10] Fernández-González F, Seijo F, Menéndez-Guisasola L, Salvador C, Roger RL, González-García FJ, Fernández-Martínez JM, Bulla B, Fernández-García C, González-González S, Galindo A. Identificación de las dianas esterotáxicas en la cirugía de la enfermedad de Parkinson. *Rev Neurol* 1999; 28:600-608.

[11] Fernández-González F, Seijo F, Salvador C, Menéndez-Guisasola, Lozano B, Valles C, Galindo A. Neurofisiología aplicada en el tratamiento con estimulación cerebral profunda del temblor severo de la esclerosis múltiple. *Rev Neurol* 2001; 32:559-567.

[12] Guerdes J, Hitchon P, Neerangun W, Torner J. Computed tomography versus magnetic resonance imaging in stereotactic localization. *Stereotact Funct Neurosurg* 1994; 63:124-129.

[13] Halpern CH, Danish SF, Baltuch GH, Jaggi JL. Brain shift during deep brain stimulation surgery for Parkinson´s disease. *Stereotact Funct Neurosurg* 2008;86:37-43.

[14] Hariz MI, Bergenheim T, Fodstard H. Comparison between ventriculographic and CT-guided determination of brain targets in functional stereotaxis. *Stereotact Funct Neurosurg (Abstract*) 1990; 54/55:240-241.

[15] Holtzheimer III PE, Roberts DW, Darcey TM. Magnetic resonance imaging versus computed tomography for target localization in functional stereotactic neurosurgery. *Neurosurgery* 1999; 45:290-298.

[16] Hubble JP, Busenbark KL, Wilkinson S, Pahwa R, Paulson GW, Lyons K, Koller WC: Effects of thalamic deep brain stimulation based on tremor type and diagnosis. *Mov Disord* 1997; 12:337-341.

[17] Khan MF, Mewes K, Gross R, Skrinjar O. Assessment of brain shift related to deep brain stimulation surgery. *Stereotac Funct Neurosurg* 2008; 86:44-53.

[18] Koike Y, Shima F, Nakamizo A, Miyagi Y. Direct localization of subthalamic nucleus supplemented by single-track electrophysiological guidance in deep brain stimulation lead implantation: techniques and clinical results. *Stereotact Funct Neurosurg* 2008; 86:173-178.

[19] Kondziolka D, Dempsey PK, Lunsford LD, Kostle JR, Dolan EJ, Kanal E, Tasker JJl. A comparison between magnetic resonante imaging and computed tomography for stereotactic coordinate determination. *Neurosurgery* 1992; 30:402-407.

[20] Krack P, Fraix V, Mendes A, Benabid AL and Pollack P. Postoperative Management of Subthalamic Nucleus Stimulation for Parkinson's disease Mov Disord 2002; 17:S188-197.

[21] Krauss JK, Akeyson EW, Giam P, Jankovic J. Propofol-induced dyskinesias in Parkinson´s disease. *Anesth Analg* 1996; 83:420-422.

[22] Krauss JK, King DE, Grossman RG: Alignment correction algorithm for transfomation of anterior comissure/posterior comissure based coordinates into frame coordinates in image-guided functional neurosurgery. *Neurosurgery* 1998; 42:806-811.

[23] Laitinen LV. Brain targets in surgery for Parkinson´s disease. *J Neurosurg* 1985; 62:349-351.

[24] Lang AE, Widner H. Deep brain stimulation for Parkinson´s disease: patient selection and evaluation. *Mov Disord* 2002; S3:S94-S101.

[25] Langston JW, Widner H, Gotees CG, Brooks D, Fahn S, Freeman T, Watts R. Core assessment program for intracerebral transplantations *Mov Disord* 1992; 7:2-13.

[26] Latchaw R, Lunsford L, Kennedy W. Reformatted imaging to define the intercommisural line for CT-guided stereotaxic functional neurosurgery. *A.J.N.R.* 1985; 6:429-433.

[27] Lee MW,De Salles AA, Frighetto L, Torres R, Behnke E, Bronstein JM. Deep brain stimulation in intraoperative MRI environment-Comparison of imaging techniques and electrode fixation methods. *Minim Invas Neurosurg* 2005; 48:1-6.

[28] Lehman R, Mezrich R, Sage J, Goldbe L. Peri and postoperative magnetic resonance imaging localization of pallidotomy. *Stereotact Funct Neurosurg* 1994; 62:61-70.

[29] Leone M, May A, Franzini A, Broggi G, Dodick D, Rapaport A, Goadsby P, Schoenen J, Bonavita V, Bussone G. Deep brain stimulation for intractable chronic cluster headache: proposals for patient selection. *Cephalalgia* 2004; 24:934-937.

[30] Litt B, Cranstoun. EEG and the anterior thalamic nucleus. *In:Deep brain stimulation and epilepsy*. Pp.171-185. Lüders HO Ed. Thomson Publishing Services. Andover, UK. 2004.

[31] Lozano AM, Hutchinson W, KissA, Tasker R, Dostrovsky J. Methods for microelectrode-guided posteroventral pallidotomy. *J Neurosurg* 1996; 84:194-202.

[32] Maciunas RJ, Galloway RL, Latimer JW. The application accuracy of stereotactic frames. *Neurosurg* Online 1994;35:682-695.

[33] Mandydur G, Morenski J, Kuniyoshi S, Iacomo R. Comparison of MRI and ventriculographic target acquisition for posteroventral pallidotomy. *Stereotact Funct Neurosurg* 1995; 65:54-59.

[34] Obwegeser A, Uitti RJ, Witte RJ, Lucas JA, Turk MF, Wharen RE. Quantitative and qualitative outcome measures after thalamic deep brain stimulation to treat disabling tremors. *Neurosurgery* 2001; 48:274-284.

[35] Ohye CH. and Narabayashi H. Activity of thalamic neurons and their receptive fields in different functional states in man. *In: Somjen GG editor Neurophysiology studies in man.* Amsterdam. Excerpta Med 1972; 23:79-84.

[36] Olivier A, Peters T, Bertrand G. Stereotactic system and apparatus for use with MRI, CT and DSA. *Appl Neurophysiol* 1985; 48:94-96.

[37] Pendfield W and Rasmussen T. *The cerebral cortex of man: A clinical study of localization and functions* The Macmillian Co., New York. 1957.

[38] Pralong E, Ghika J, Temperli P, Pollo C, Vingerhoets F and Villemure JG. Electrophysiological localization of the subthalamic nucleus in parkinsonian patients. *Neurosci Lett* (2002) 325:144-146.

[39] Riechert T. Development of human stereotactic surgery. *Confin Neurol* 1975; 37:399-409.

[40] Riechert T. *Stereotactic Brain Operations*. Bern; Hans Huber Publishers, 1980.

[41] Saint-Cyr JA, Hoque T, Pereira LC, Dostrosvsky JO, Hutchison WD, Mikulis DJ, Abosch A, Sime E, Lang AE, Lozano AM. Localization of clinically effective stimulating electrodes in the human subthalamic nucleus on magnetic resonance imaging. *J Neurosurg* 2002; 97:1152-1166.

[42] Schad L, Lott S, Schmitt F, Sturm V, Lorenz W. Correction of spatial distorsion in MR imaging: a prerequisite for accurate stereotaxy. *J Compt Assist Tomogr* 1987; 11:499-505.

[43] Schaltenbrand G, Wahren W. *Atlas for Stereotaxy of the Human Brain*. Stuttgart; Thieme, 1977.

[44] Schuurman PR, de Bie RM, Majoie CB, Speelman JD, Bosch DA. A prospective comparison between three-dimensional magnetic resonance imaging and ventriculography for target-coordinate determination in frame-based functional stereotactic neurosurgery. *J Neurosurg* 1999; 91:911-914.

[45] Seijo FJ, Alvarez-Vega MA, Gutiérrez JC, Fdez-Glez F, Lozano B. Complications in subthalamic nucleus stimulation surgery for treatment of Parkinson disease. Review of 272 procedures. *Acta Neurchirurgica*; 149:867-876.

[46] Shils JL, Taqliati M, Alterman RL. Intraoperative microelectrode recording equipment. What features are necessary? *Stereotact Funct Neurosurg* 2001; 77:101-107.

[47] Starr PA, Vitek JL, DeLong M, Bakay RA. Magnetic resonance imaging-based stereotactic localization of the globus pallidus and subthalamic nucleus. *Neurosurgery* 1999; 44:303-314.

[48] Starr PA, Vitek JL, DeLong M, Mewes K, Bakay AE. Pallidoty: theory and technique. *In: Techniques in Neurosurgery*, vol 5, nº 1:31-45. 1999. Lippincott Willians and Wilkins, Inc. Philadelphia.

[49] Talairach J, Tournoux P. *Co-planar Stereotaxic Atlas of the Human Brain*. Stuttgart; Thieme, 1988.

[50] Tasker RR. Deep brain stimulation is preferable to thalamotomy for tremor suppresision. *Surg Neurol* 1998; 49:145-154.

[51] Taveras JM, Word E. *Diagnostic Neuroradiology*. Vol 1. Baltimore; Williams & Wilkins 1976.

[52] Tremmel J (ed): Urgent device correction-change of safe limits for MRI procedures used with Medtronic Activa deep brain stimulation systems. *Medtronic*, 2005.

[53] Tsao K, Wilkinson S, Overman J, Koller WC, Batnitzky S, Gordon MA. Pallidotomy lesion locations: significance of microelectrode refinement. *Neurosurg* 1998; 43:506-513.

[54] Van Buren JM, Maccubbin DA. An outline atlas of the human basal ganglio with stimulation of anatomical variants. *J Neurosurg* 1962; 19:811-839.

[55] Williams D, Warwick R. *Functional Neuroanatomy of Man*. London; Churchill Livingstone, 1975.

[56] Yu C, Apuzzo M, Zee C, Petrovich Z. A phantom study of the geometric accuracy of computed tomographic and magnetic resonance imaging stereotactic localization with the Leksell stereotactic system. *Neurosurgery* 2001; 48:1092-1099.

[57] Yuan S, Zhang J, Gu M, Xu Y,Chen L, Yao Q, He Q. A new method to localize brain nuclei for surgery in extrapyramidal disease. *Stereotact Funct Neurosurg* 1995; 65:47-53.

[58] Zonenshanyn M, Rezai AR, Mogilner AY, Beric A, Sterio D, Nelly PJ. Comparison of anatomic and neurophysiological methods for subthalamic nucleus targeting. *Neurosurgery* 2000; 47:282-294.

In: Deep Brain Stimulation
Editors: Mark H. Rogers and Paul B. Anderson
ISBN 978-1-60692-895-0

Chapter II

Deep Brain Stimulation and Cortical Stimulation Methods: A Commentary on Established Applications and Expected Developments

Damianos E. Sakas*[*] *and Ioannis G. Panourias
Department of Neurosurgery, University of Athens Medical School,
Evangelismos Hospital, Athens, Greece

Abstract

Over the last twenty years, deep brain stimulation (DBS) has been increasingly accepted as an effective alternative treatment to the selective lesioning methods previously used in stereotactic and functional neurosurgery. This method, based on its reversibility and adaptability, has currently been used for the alleviation of medically-refractory cases of movement disorders, epilepsy, pain, and psychiatric diseases. In the present commentary, data comparing DBS with other brain stimulation methods such as electrical cortical stimulation (CS) and transcranial magnetic stimulation (TMS) are analyzed and the perspectives of the field are outlined. Progress in the related fields of neuromodulation, functional neuroprosthetic surgery, neuroinformatics, neurocomputation, and developments in neuroengineering that are expected to refine, enhance and widen the therapeutic applications of DBS are also discussed.

[*]Damianos E. Sakas, MD. Department of Neurosurgery, Evangelismos Hospital, 4 Marasli Street, 10676 Athens, Greece. Tel: +30 210 7201704 -5. Fax: +30 210 7249986. Email: sakasde@med.uoa.gr.

Introduction

Electricity and some of its various effects on the human body have been known since ancient times. The use of electrical stimulation, however, as a therapeutic tool has been limited. Traditionally, medicine has been applied by administration of pharmaceuticals and surgical interventions. Over the last 50 years, great progress in neurophysiology and neurosurgery made it possible to investigate the therapeutic potential of electrical brain stimulation. During the last two decades, the introduction of deep brain stimulation (DBS) and, to a lesser extent, of chronic electrical cortical stimulation (CS) transformed functional neurosurgery and neuroscience, in general. DBS offers superior clinical efficacy with fewer complications compared to the selective lesional procedures of conventional functional neurosurgery. More importantly, the success of DBS in improving outcome has signified the role of electricity in neurological disorders and the great benefits that can be derived by its modulation, thus creating a new field in medicine this of *selective focal electrotherapy* of the nervous system.

Therapeutic brain stimulation can be applied in networks which are located: a) in cortical or subcortical layers, b) in deep nuclei groups (relay nodes) or c) in a combination of both. DBS belongs to the domain of *operative neuromodulation* and particularly, to the field of *neural networks surgery* [45]; this field studies and applies advancements in neural networks research, digitised stereotactic brain imaging and implantable electrical or electronic devices in order to alter electrically the signal transmission in the nervous system, modulate neural networks and produce therapeutic effects.

In this article, we comment on the current state and future prospects of DBS of the human brain for the treatment of chronic medically-refractory neurological conditions such as Parkinson's disease, dystonia, tremor, epilepsy, pain, and psychiatric disorders. In certain specific applications, DBS is compared with CS with respect to their indications, benefits, advantages, and limitations as therapeutic tools. In addition, we comment on current limitations and future prospects of DBS and other brain stimulation methods and on expected scientific and technological advances and their implications for future therapeutic applications of DBS.

Parkinson's Disease

DBS has been acknowledged worldwide as the surgical treatment of choice for improving the incapacitating symptoms and the quality of life in patients with Parkinson's disease (PD). The efficacy of *subthalamic nucleus (STN)* DBS in alleviating the off-medication state of PD patients has been validated in prospective, randomized trials and meta-analysis studies [17, 23, 71, 75]. STN has gained general acceptance over *globus pallidus internal (GPi)* as the preferred target [16, 21] mainly because of easier targeting on MRI, longer effect of its stimulation, resulting to bigger reduction of required medication, and longer battery life due to lower stimulation settings required for the smaller in size STN compared to the GPi. Despite the undeniable benefit of DBS in PD, almost half of the patients are excluded from DBS therapy due to advanced age (>70 years), dementia, psychiatric comorbidity, poor response to levodopa, low score (<30-40) in the UPDRS part III or other contraindications.

The application of motor cortical stimulation (MCS) in PD has been limited but this may prove to be an efficacious alternative treatment modality, particularly, in patients presenting with marked laterality of symptoms and age >70 years. This number of patients will steadily increase, in the years to come, and will require, certainly, an alternative to DBS therapy. Nevertheless, there are patient categories that, currently, cannot be helped by either DBS or CS. These include patients with: a) unresponsive non-motor or levodopa-resistant symptoms, or b) parkinsonism due to multisystem atrophy or progressive supranuclear palsy. It is promising that TMS carries positive predictive value for MCS efficacy [4]. New predictive tests need to be developed that will be individualized for the specific method, i.e. DBS or CS, the age, and the stage of the disease. Future research in PD should explore the significance of new targets such as the peduculopontine nucleus (PPN), as well as the neuroprotective effect of DBS [51].

Dystonia

DBS of the *GPi* is currently the most effective treatment for medically-refractory primary dystonia and, particularly, cervical dystonia; improvements in mobility have been proven by randomized, sham stimulation-controlled trials and can approach the 70% mark [22, 24, 26, 32]. Recently, GPi DBS was also proved effective in treating truncal dystonia such as camptocephalia and camptocormia [47, 48]. Various investigators have tried other targets, such as the *thalamus* and *STN*; the reported results, however, although encouraging, are still scarce and contradictory [54]. The above suggests that GPi DBS will remain the mainstay of therapeutic electrical stimulation in dystonia in the foreseeable future. Following DBS, the phasic dystonic movements tend to improve soon after surgery but the response of tonic movements usually is delayed [25]. This difference should be studied further while taking seriously into consideration the observation that fixed dystonia responds much better to CS rather than to DBS [43]. Bidirectional interconnectivity between motor cortex and basal ganglia could explain why certain types of dystonia respond to electrical stimulation at either deep or cortical areas. CS may induce distant neuromodulatory activity either at the cortical and/or subcortical levels through orthodromic or antidromic effects [61]. It is very important to investigate further the therapeutic potential of modulating this interconnectivity. In addition, research in the future will likely continue to explore the mechanism of DBS action, the most appropriate programming settings for each specific type of dystonia, and alternative deep or cortical brain targets which, when stimulated, might have greater efficacy and fewer side effects compared to GPi DBS.

Tremor

DBS of the *ventral intermediate thalamic (VIM)* nucleus has resulted to great improvements in the control of essential tremor (ET), limb functionality, quality of life, and need for medication [27, 57]. VIM DBS has also controlled successfully multiple sclerosis-related tremor [73], Holmes tremor [42] and tremor associated with inherited cerebellar ataxia [50]. Unilateral VIM DBS controls effectively contralateral idiopathic and secondary tremor [10], but head, trunk and voice tremor are better suppressed by bilateral VIM DBS [59]. DBS of the subthalamic posteromedial white matter, i.e. *zona incerta (ZI)* has also suppressed markedly proximal tremor [33]. STN DBS has suppressed ET as well in patients with coexisting movement disorders such as PD [52]. It seems that distal limb tremor responds well to VIM DBS, whereas proximal limb tremor is better controlled by ZI DBS [34].

There are only few reports of successful application of CS in non-parkinsonian post-stroke distal rest and/or action tremor [4, 20, 35]. Noninvasive CS such as TMS has also not provided any clinical benefits in non-parkinsonian tremor [15]. Hence, it is quite doubtful that CS could represent an alternative to DBS treatment for ET. This may be attributed to the fact that the underlying pathophysiological dysfunction of ET affects the central portion of the corticospinal tracts rather than the cortex *per se* [9]. In addition, there is sufficient evidence on the involvement of the somatosensory thalamus and VIM nucleus in the integration of cortico-basal ganglia-spinal networks and the cerebello-thalamocortical system [62]. Currently, tremor appears to be the best indication of DBS and VIM DBS the "gold standard" in the treatment of medically-refractory tremor. Future progress may depend on understanding better the significance and the role of other nuclei such as ZI or STN.

Epilepsy

The promising results of DBS in animal epilepsy [67] and the experience gained in humans on DBS in movement disorders and, particularly, in dystonia, which frequently has a paroxysmal character similar to epilepsy, provided a solid scientific basis for conducting clinical trials of DBS in epilepsy. After the first reports of efficacy [63], several deep brain targets have been stimulated. Thalamus is a pivotal structure in epileptogenesis and two nuclei have been targeted for controlling seizures: the centromedian nucleus of the thalamus (CMT) and the anterior nucleus of the thalamus (ANT). In addition, STN and caudate nucleus have also been investigated. DBS of the aforementioned targets aims to modulate the abnormal cortical function by activating or inhibiting relay nodes which, although remote to the epileptogenic area, are critical epilepsy "gating mechanisms". Theoretically, DBS of the CMT or STN, which are relay nodes with extensive cortical afferent and efferent projections, should control generalized tonic/clonic seizures. Conversely, DBS of the ANT or hippocampus, which are integrated to the limbic system, is expected to control complex partial seizures [40]. SNr and STN are parts of the nigral control of the epilepsy system (NCES) [8]. High-frequency stimulation of the STN interrupts the normally exerted by STN inhibition on SNr; at this state, the SNr ceases inhibiting the Dorsal Midbrain Antiepileptic Zone (DMAZ) and the latter can exert its antieptileptic effects [5, 66].

Other areas that have been targeted by electrical stimulation are the cerebellum and hippocampus. Cerebellum, due to its thalamic projections, was first electrically stimulated in the 1970s [6], and more recently, a mean reduction of approximately 30% in motor seizures was reported [65]. However, the mumber of treated patients remains very small. A different approach involves the direct stimulation of the *epileptogenic zone per se* such as the hippocampus. Hippocampus has a pivotal role in the generation and propagation of temporal lobe seizures [37, 56], and its stimulation provided good or excellent control of temporal lobe seizures [64, 69].

Undoubtedly, epilepsy, particularly of the drug-resistant type, is a complex, multivariate, and global rather than localized phenomenon in the brain. It is, therefore, unlikely that DBS, in its current form to become ultimately the only solution to the problem of epilepsy. Alternative types of electrical stimulation will certainly play their role in modulating the mechanisms of epileptogenesis and the numerous epilepsy phenotypes. CS and TMS have evolved as alternative adjunctive therapies for epilepsies originating primarily at the cortical level. TMS decays with the square of the distance; therefore, TMS or CS, in general, are unlikely to have an impact on seizures originating in structures deeper than the cortical layers [70]. CS or TMS methods may have to be used in combination with DBS providing thus, a big hope for sufferers and a challenging field for further research and clinical work.

Current methods deliver stimulation in an "open-loop" arrangement, i.e. according to pre-programmed electrical parameters regardless of the patient's condition. A great leap forward is the development of intelligent "closed-loop" systems of "responsive stimulation" with integrated combined use of DBS and CS. These devices have incorporated software with seizure detection algorithms and deliver stimulation to the epileptogenic focus "on demand", i.e. once premonitory electroencephalographic (EEG) signs of imminent ictal activity are detected in order to suppress seizures before their clinical manifestation. To date, two such fully implantable systems, the RNS (Neuropace, Mountain View, CA) [13] and the Intercept^{TM} (Medtronic, Minneapolis, US), which is activated by the patient, whenever he feels that a seizure is likely to start (Medtronic's website, www.medtronics.com), have offered reductions in seizure frequency and are under clinical evaluation [55].

DBS or CS are promising methods for controlling intractable epilepsy. However, before either of them becomes an effective therapy, a few important issues that are described below should be addressed. Given the lack of homogeneity in the epileptic population, *patient selection* for DBS is a factor that can determine the outcome of treatment. DBS should be offered only in patients with well defined clinical, neuroimaging, anatomical, and genetic characteristics, and similar epileptic EEG activity. This will allow us to: a) evaluate objectively the efficacy of DBS or CS for each epileptic syndrome and b) identify the best candidates for DBS or CS. The determination of the *optimal stimulation parameters* for each epileptic syndrome will maximize the clinical benefits. This would prolong battery life and reduce the time spent in programming sessions. The *volume of stimulated cerebral tissue* around the electrode can affect the overall efficacy of either DBS or CS; this should become a subject of further intensive study. For instance, in the SNr, there are two different cell groups located very densely together, which have both reciprocal GABA projections [62].

Depending on which of the two is stimulated the effect of SNr stimulation on the DMAZ could be quite different. The *interaction of antiepileptic medication* with the electrical stimulation is another important issue that has not been investigated sufficiently. Notably, in most series, patients continue their drugs during DBS therapy. In addition, it has been found that CS, in the form of low-frequency TMS, combined with valproate acid induces epileptic activity. Obviously, well-controlled studies are needed to evaluate the antiepileptic effect of DBS or CS as monotherapy in order to validate DBS alone or combined with CS as powerful therapies for epilepsy.

Pain

The use of DBS in the management of intractable pain has been rather limited although pain was the first neurological condition on which DBS was applied. Wider application of DBS in pain management has been hindered by important limitations such as the heterogeneous nature of pain and the uncertainty regarding mechanisms and appropriate targets. Similarly to epilepsy, good patient selection is mandatory for the success of DBS. The existence of a known neuroanatomical basis of the pain is a factor that favors the success of DBS and the failure or resistance to conservative treatments and both spinal cord and peripheral nerve stimulation are important prerequisites. Compared to CS, another great limitation of DBS has been the lack of a noninvasive predictive test of efficacy. It is difficult to envisage how predictive tests of successful use of DBS in chronic pain could be developed in the foreseeable future since the DBS targets are small in size and deeply located in the brain and, at present, they can be investigated only by stereotactic approaches. In the coming years, all these factors are likely to restrict DBS for pain only in highly-specialized centers [7].

Compared to DBS, CS is likely to expand its role in pain. CS seems to have better prospects to become a more generalized method in the management of intractable pain, particularly in patients who have: a) profound laterality of painful symptoms, b) extensive representation of the painful area in the lateral cortical surface, or c) advanced age. Patients with trigeminopathic pain or arm deafferentation pain are more suitable for CS as compared to DBS [28]. Another important advantage of CS over DBS is the availability of a noninvasive highly positive predictor of potential efficacy of CS such as the TMS. Progress in DBS application in pain may come from a better understanding of the underlying mechanisms and advancements in brain functional imaging, and EEG source-localization of deep nuclei which become activated during the exacerbation of pain. Such advances may also help us in identifying more precisely the suitable candidates and the critical deep brain targets. Finally, in both DBS and CS, it is necessary to make the postoperative titration easier and the follow-up sessions less time-consuming for both practitioners and patients. Undoubtedly, this will be facilitated by the development of software-guided consensus stimulation protocols.

Psychiatric Disorders

Modern research indicates that the disorders of cognition or emotion can be understood as dysfunction of specific neuronal networks or circuits, which operate upon defined anatomical pathways and convey messages by neurotransmitters or sequences of electrical stimuli. The recognition that thought and emotion are rooted in the biology of the brain and that electrochemical abnormalities in the brain either genetic or acquired can give rise to cognitive or psychiatric symptoms has become a universally accepted notion in modern neuroscience. This fundamental concept leads to the conclusion that highly selective stimulation of the brain should be further investigated as an alternative therapy of intractable psychiatric disorders. In spite of this, neuromodulatory interventions in psychiatric disorders have remained in latency due to poor understanding of pathogenetic mechanisms, fear of potential irreversible side effects, debates over long-term efficacy, but, particularly, because of social criticism and hesitancy of the medical community based on the extensive, not well-founded and indiscriminate use of crude lesional methods in the 1950s [46].

Undoubtedly, the stigmatized past of lesional psychosurgery has influenced negatively patients and carers' attitude towards DBS applications in psychiatry. In spite of this, DBS practice has been guided by prior relevant lesioning experience and has shown promising results in treatment-refractory depression (TRD), in obsessive-compulsive disorder (OCD), and in Tourette's syndrome (TS). In addition, new targets for DBS in psychiatry have been discovered as a result of serendipity. Such an example is DBS of the ventral capsule/ventral striatum for OCD which provided pronounced antidepressant benefits [14]. With respect to depression, strong evidence on the potential role of DBS in the treatment of TRD came inadvertently from PD patients who developed severe depressive behavioural changes while undergoing DBS [60]. Remarkable improvement in mood and symptoms of anxiety and depression in patients who undergo STN DBS has also been reported [74]. This was attributed to inadvertent stimulation of areas such as ZI or SNr, which are parts of the limbic system, and has supported the assumption that DBS of relay nodes in the limbic system may prove beneficial in TRD. Various other targets have been investigated such as the inferior thalamic peduncle [19], ventral internal capsule/nucleus accumbens [49], and white matter in the subgenual cingulate gyrus (Cg25 area) with the latter target showning the best clinical results [30]. Brodman's area 24a (BA 24a) has also been proposed as a putative target for DBS in TRD [44]. Many investigators consider depression as the next major therapeutic application of DBS. Given that the population of depressed patients is far greater compared to that of patients suffering from movement disorders, the impact of DBS in depression is expected to be far greater than that in movement disorders.

In OCD, neuroimaging studies have demonstrated decreased volume or increased grey matter density in cortico-striatal-thalamic-cortical circuits, increased activity in orbitofrontal cortex, cingulate, and striatum at rest, as well as temporal dysfunction and amygdala involvement [41, 58, 76]. The targeted areas by DBS that have offered considerable reductions in the intensity of symptoms and substantial decreases in required medication include the anterior limb of the internal capsule and the ventral striatum/nucleus accumbens [14, 36, 53]. Apart from the IPG battery's short life expectancy and hypomania, DBS therapy has been well tolerated.

With respect to *TS,* imaging and physiological studies suggest that the disorder involves dysfunction in both the limbic and cortical-basal gaglia-thalamocortical circuitry, explaining thus the prevailing motor and non-motor symptoms of the disease. DBS of the medial intralaminar thalamic [68] and centromedian parafascicular nuclei [18], anterior limb of internal capsule [12] and GPi [1, 11] have shown high efficacy (>70%) in suppressing motor and vocal tics. Given that TS is a borderline condition among the traditionally divided domains of neurology and psychiatry, it is likely that DBS treatment will be accepted more easily for TS compared to OCD or depression. In our opinion, TS may prove to be the condition that will facilitate the acceptance of DBS for psychiatric disorders.

As research moves forward, certain important issues should be addressed before DBS becomes an effective therapeutic option for psychiatric disorders. Few of these issues are discussed below.

Neuropsychiatric disorders are diverse with regard to their clinical profile; symptoms of different psychiatric conditions may be present in the same patient, thus making diagnosis difficult. Pre- and postoperative assessments should be done by common evaluation rating scales in order that *patient selection* would be the best possible for DBS. This would ensure that data, produced by different groups, would be comparable and strong conclusions could be inferred. Other important issues are the *optimization of stimulation parameters* and the *delineation* of the *stimulation zone*. It is well known that DBS cannot stimulate a large volume of brain tissue. In current DBS practice in psychiatry, adjustments of stimulation parameters are largely guided by experience gained in movement disorders and short battery life has been a commonly reported problem. This implies either that high-intensity stimulation is needed in order to affect a large tissue volume and produce a clinical benefit or, alternatively, that our current delineation and targeting of the appropriate stimulation zones is suboptimal. These observations indicate that it is important to standardize and individualize the stimulation settings for each psychiatric illness. This will maximize clinical benefits, increase cost-effectiveness, and improve acceptance of DBS as a therapeutic tool by the referring physicians and psychiatrists, patient's relatives, and the patients themselves.

The *DBS-induced psychiatric effects* should be analyzed and studied. In PD patients, DBS has been associated with symptoms of anxiety, fear [38] and increased rates of suicide attempts [2]. Such observations, however, should not be extrapolated to DBS procedures for psychiatric disorders. The *interaction of DBS with medications* has not been studied adequately. Currently, only seriously debilitated and pharmacologically-resistant psychiatric patients are considered for DBS. DBS efficacy is usually evaluated without the medication being discontinued. Hence, the blindness of studies is doubtful and placebo effects are possible. Undeniably, it is important to evaluate the efficacy of DBS in earlier stages of intractable neuropsychiatric disorders and also the potential beneficial effects of DBS on illness progress. The *lack of animal models of psychiatric disorders* is a great hindrance to new developments in the field. In movement disorders, progress has been facilitated by reliable animal models where efficacy of DBS ensured a smooth and safe transition to human studies. This reality brings, again, to the spotlight the fact that a great limitation of DBS is the lack of a noninvasive predictor of its potential efficacy. Conversely, before any new potential application of CS, we can have some predicting evidence of possible efficacy by TMS or transcranial direct current stimulation (tDCS). This consideration suggests that a significant expansion of DBS therapy in neuropsychiatric disorders will be difficult in the foreseeable future. On the other hand, application of other methods of brain stimulation may be accepted more easily.

The best prospect for DBS in psychiatry may be found in progress in sophisticated structural and functional imaging methods. Advanced imaging may correlate disease-related brain activity and clinical improvement with effective DBS stimulation patterns, provide clarification of mechanisms of action and indicate new potential targets for DBS. The combination of advanced electrophysiological mapping with high-resolution imaging studies is expected to detect accurately deep targets or white matter bundles which may be critical structures in the treatment of psychiatric disorders. In conclusion, DBS is a viable and safe experimental treatment for intractable neuropsychiatric disorders and holds a great hope for the severe psychiatric patients. Its efficacy in OCD, TS and depression derives from reports of single cases or small series and it should be rigorously validated and replicated in big randomized controlled trials. Only further extensive and serious research and clinical work will prove that DBS is a reliable and powerful therapy for neuropsychiatric disorders. Such therapeutic developments should be transparent in their design and evolve only within a framework of serious scientific criteria. Finally, as we move forward, it is critical to safeguard human rights and keep high *ethical standards* in every step of exploring DBS in psychiatry.

Current General Limitations of DBS

The characteristics of minimal invasiveness, reversibility, and adjustability have rendered DBS to a safe and effective treatment for neurological and psychiatric disorders which are characterized by altered electrical conductivity. In order to foresee the future prospects of DBS, one has to review its established and emerging therapeutic uses, as well as to consider the technical problems and difficulties which, currently, hinder the potential future applications of DBS and are described below.

With respect to the *required resources*, DBS practice is based on expensive high-technology equipment including frame-based stereotaxis, sophisticated software for planning and monitoring, and, particularly, multidisciplinary personel teams consisting of neurosurgeons, neurophysiologists, movement disorder neurologists, pain therapists, psychiatrists, neuropsychologists, experienced technicians and specially-trained nurses. A wider application across the world cannot happen unless every interested hospital or health authority manages to fund the above resources and assemble the right team of specialists.

The *patient's preoperative clinical condition and evaluation* are other important variables. The patient should be mentally and physically able to undergo the preoperative clinical assessments and to attend the postoperative follow-up visits for titration of the stimulation. A significant proportion of sufferers are excluded because of advanced age (more than 70 years), medical co-morbidities, brain atrophy or cognitive and psychiatric impairment. There is a small risk (1-3%) of surgery-related complications (intracerebral hemorrhage, seizures, infection, neuropsychiatric and congitive effects). With respect to preoperative imaging evaluation, DBS is currently restricted by the imaging technology which is subject to spatial and geometrical distortions and the lack of reproducibility and uniformity among different imaging systems and devices. Thus, high accuracy becomes difficult and the comparison of data from different groups problematic.

It is generally accepted that the current DBS device, i.e. lead, wires and IPG, is susceptible and interferes with strong environmental magnetic fields. With respect to *electrode-tissue interactions*, our current understanding is limited, particularly regarding the long-term induced changes in the brain surrounding the electrode, the potential development of gliosis and how this can affect electrical conductivity and the efficacy of DBS, particularly in the long-term. Furthermore, in the coming years, it would be useful to work on the production of DBS electrodes with a high number of poles which could offer more somatotopically refined stimulation.

Although DBS has gained a protagonist role in the management of PD and other neurological disorders a comparison with CS leads to the conclusion that, currently, CS presents, in certain conditions, significant advantages over DBS. CS is less invasive in the cerebral tissue, carries a minimal perioperative risk of intracerebral hemorrhage and has a noninvasive preoperative predictive test in the form of either TMS or tDCS. Furthermore, CS does not require a stereotactic frame and, as being much less invasive, can be more acceptable by patients and referring physicians. Undoubtedly, with respect to both DBS and CS, the unsettled technical issues represent limitations; the process of elucidating these issues, however, will be associated with countless opportunities to gain new knowledge and offer great benefits to patients.

Scientific and Technological Advances: Implications for Future Prospects of Therapeutic DBS

The future of DBS will be influenced by developments in many important relevant areas. Some of them are described below.

1. Sophisticated batteries and electrodes

   In the future, IPGs will be smaller in size, miniaturized and contour-shaped to apply to the cranium or be inserted in a burr hole. Advanced chemistry will offer rechargeable batteries with more power in smaller size, extended life, and wireless connectivity to the electrodes. These devices may prove particularly helpful in patients with epilepsy or dystonia where electrode damage due to abrupt or violent movements is commonly encountered. The incorporation into the DBS electrodes of *microactuators* will enable precise permanent implantation after the initial temporary insertion, reducing thus considerably the operating time, as fine adjustments in the precise position of the electrode could be done more comfortably in the ward rather than in the operating theatre. The construction of ''*smart stimulators*'' with the capability for dynamic internal adjustments will also refine DBS practice [39].

2. Sophisticated graphics and programming software

The electrode implantation will be assisted by software programmes that combine magnetic resonance imaging, computed tomography, three-dimensional brain atlases and neurophysiological microelectrode recording data with the volume of brain tissue activated by DBS; such programmes have been evaluated in preliminary studies [31]. Developments in programming software are likely to optimize the pole selection after permanent implantation, individualize the stimulation parameters and maximize clinical efficacy [3]. The patient's dependence from the reference center and the need for follow-up visits will be minimized by programming the stimulation devices through remote access, telephone lines or via the internet.

3. Computational neuromodulation and computer models of neural networks.

New applications of DBS will be influenced by progress in computational neuromodulation which is a field of computational biology dedicated to the study of the biophysical and mathematical characteristics of the electrochemical modulation in the nervous system. All types of networks and neurons (motor, sensory, and interneurons) are subject to modulation. An area of expected developments that would have a great impact on DBS is the development of computer models of the bioelectrical and statistical aspects of neural recording and stimulation-induced recruitment. Neural computation and coding can be used to model, decipher and simulate the neural coding of biological neural systems. We could potentially alter the intrinsic properties of neurons, change their time-course, voltage-dependence and synaptic conductance and the strength of synaptic connections and, thus, reconfigure an anatomically defined network into a different functional circuit by altering the intrinsic properties or the synaptic strength of the neurons within the network. Hence, such intelligent implanted DBS devices could mimick the natural neuromodulation.

4. Microtechnology and nanotechnology systems

Our current implantable devices will improve and incorporate complex microsystems and sophisticated software. These will enable them to integrate information exchange between the device and the patient's brain. Microsystems technologies, microelectronics, and nanotechnologies promise us to develop cost-effective *advanced sensor and stimulation systems* and expand the therapeutic potential of both DBS and CS. The neurological disorders currently treated by DBS have as a common feature the altered electrical conductivity in certain areas of the cerebral tissue. These conditions could potentially be helped by nanomaterials such as *carbon nanofibers array* [72]. These can act as minimally traumatic CNS electrodes with increased accuracy of stimulation. Currently, such nanoelectrode arrays utilising aligned carbon nanofibers are under development at the NASA Ames Research Center. This technology holds a great promise that our ability to offer complex but precise patterns of stimulation would be enhanced making feasible to perform not only electrical microrecording but also electrochemical recording and stimulation [29]. These expected developments in micro- and nanotechnologies are likely to make feasible to link bi-directionally DBS with the human brain by "closed-loop" integrated monitoring and stimulating implantable systems, i.e. electrodes that monitor neuronal activity from multiple regions, generate ''network level'' representations of the brain and simultaneously stimulate. Promising work in epilepsy paves the road for Parkinson's disease. For instance, in PD patients, stimulation could be triggered by EMG signals elicited by patient's movement and detected by an advanced sensor being placed either in contact with the skin or embedded in muscles.

Conclusion

The methods of applying DBS and other electrical stimulation therapies are likely to improve and the indications of DBS are going to expand. The future of electrical brain stimulation will be influenced greatly by accumulating convincing evidence regarding efficacy, improved patient selection, increased awareness and understanding of current and new indications, and by developing reliable methods for assessing outcome. A more mature understanding of mechanisms of action will allow us to perform more effective and precise stimulation for each neurological or psychiatric condition, and predict more accurately the degree and duration of expected clinical benefits. Great advancements are likely to take place in the field of responsive DBS such as a closed-loop stimulation, triggered by the electrical changes that precede a seizure or an abnormal movement. Another great prospect is the integration of DBS with CS. Hence, investigators and clinical practitioners in this field should adopt a judicious but bold approach to those potential new applications of DBS and ensure a smooth transition from experimental evidence to clinical efficacy.

DBS, but similarly CS, are high-technology dependent fields that will be largely influenced by a shift away from the current dependence on pharmacological treatment and by the forthcoming advances in neuroengineering. Therapeutic electrical brain stimulation is an area of intersection, exchange and cross-fertilization of ideas from many disciplines. In this respect, a great breakthrough will be the integration of DBS and/or CS with processes of neuroplasticity, neural repair, and neuroprotection; this could have far-reaching consequences in modern neuroscience and the biomedical world, in general.

References

[1] Ackermans L., Temel Y, Cath D, et al. Deep brain stimulation in Tourette's syndrome: two targets? *Mov Disord* 2006;21:709-13.

[2] Burkhard PR, Vingerhoets FJ, Berney A, et al. Suicide after successful deep brain stimulation for movement disorders. *Neurology* 2004;63:2170-2.

[3] Butson CR, Noecker AM, Maks CB, McIntyre CC. StimExplorer: deep brain stimulation parameter selection software system. *Acta Neurochir Suppl* 2007;97(2):569-74.

[4] Canavero S, Bonicalzi V. Extradural cortical stimulation for movement disorders. *Acta Neurochir Suppl* 2007;97(2):223-32.

[5] Chabardes S, Kahane P, Minotti L, et al. Deep brain stimulation in epilepsy with particular reference to the subthalamic nucleus. *Epileptic Disord* 2002;4(suppl 3):S83–S93.

[6] Cooper IS, Amin I, Gilman S. The effect of chronic cerebellar stimulation upon epilepsy in man. *Trans Am Neurol Assoc* 1973;98:192-6.

[7] Cruccu G, Aziz TZ, Garcia-Larrea L, Hansson P, Jensena TS, Lefaucheur J-P, Simpson, Taylori RS. EFNS guidelines on neurostimulation therapy for neuropathic pain. *Eur J Neurol* 2007;14:952-70.

[8] Depaulis A, Moshe SL, "The basal ganglia and the epilepsies: translating experimental concepts to new therapies"*Epileptic Disord* (2002);4(Suppl. 3): pp. S7–8.

[9] Deuschl G, Elble RJ. The pathophysiology of essential tremor. *Neurology* 2000;54(11 Suppl 4):S14-S20.

[10] Deuschl G, Bain P. Deep brain stimulation for tremor [correction of trauma]: patient selection and evaluation. *Mov Disord* 2002;17(Suppl 3):S102-11.

[11] Diederich NJ, Kalteis K, Stamenkovic M, et al. Efficient internal pallidal stimulation in Gilles de la Tourette syndrome: a case report. *Mov Disord* 2005;20:1496-9.

[12] Flaherty AW, Willimas ZM, Amimovin R, et al. Deep brain stimulation of the anterior limb of internal capsule for the treatment of Tourette's syndrome: technical case report. *Neurosurgery* 2005;57(Suppl 4):E403.

[13] Fountas KN, Smith JR, Murro AM, Politsky J, Park YD, Jenkins PD. Implantation of a closed-loop stimulation in the management of medically refractory focal epilepsy: a technical note. *Stereotact Funct Neurosurg* 2005;83:153-8.

[14] Greenberg BD, Malone DA, Friehs GM, et al. Three-year outcomes in deep brain stimulation for highly resistant obsessive-compulsive disorder. *Neuropsychopharmacol* 2006;31:2384-2393.

[15] Hallett M. Transcranial Magnetic Stimulation: a primer. *Neuron* 2007;55:187-98.

[16] Halpern C, Urtig H, Jaggi J, Grossman M, Won M, Baltuch G. Deep brain stimulation in neurologic disorders. *Parkinsonims Relat Disord* 2007;13:1-16.

[17] Hamani C. Richter E, Schwalb JM, Lozano AM. Bilateral subthalmic nucleus stimulation for Parkinson's disease: a systematic review of clinical literature. *Neurosurgery* 2005;56:1313-21.

[18] Houeto JL, Karachi C, Mallet L, Pillon B, Yelnik J, Mesnage V et al. Tourette's syndrome and deep brain stimulation. *J Neurol Neurosurg* Psychiatr 2005;76:992-5.

[19] Jimenez F, Velasco F, Salin-Pascual R, Hernandez JA, Velasco M, Criales JL, Nicolini H. A patient with a resistant major depression disorder treated with deep brain stimulation in the inferior thalamic peduncle. *Neurosurgery* 2005;57:585-93.

[20] Katayama Y, Oshima H, Fukaya C, Kawamata T, Yamamoto T. Congrol of post-stroke movement disorders using chronic motor cortex stimulation. *Acta Neurochir Suppl* 2002;79:89-92.

[21] Kern DS, Kumar R. Deep brain stimulation. The Neurologist 2007;13:237-252.

[22] Kiss ZH, Doig-Beyaert K, Eliasziw M, et al. The Canadian multicentre study of deep brain stimulation for cervical dystonia. *Brain* 2007;130:2879-86.

[23] Kleiner-Fisman G. Herzog J, Fisman DN, et al. Subthalamic nucleus deep brain stimulation: summary and meta-analysis of outcomes. *Mov Disord* 2006;21(Suppl /14):S290-S304.

[24] Krauss JK, Pohle T, Weber S, Ozdoba C, Burgunder JM. Bilateral stimulation of globus pallidus internus for treatment of cervical dystonia. *Lancet* 1999;354:837-8.

[25] Krauss JK. Deep brain stimulation for dystonia in adults. Overview and developments. *Stereotact Funct Neurosurg*. 2002;78:168-82.

[26] Krauss JK, Loher TJ, Weigel R, Capelle HH, Weber S, Burgunder JM. Chronic stimulation of the globus pallidus internus for treatment of non-dYT1 generalized dystonia and choreoathetosis: 2-year follow up. *J Neurosurg*. 2003;98:785-92.

[27] Kumar R, Lozano AM, Sime E, Lang AE. Long-term follow-up of thalamic deep brain stimulation for essential and parkinsonian tremor. *Neurology* 2003;61:1601-04.

[28] Lazorthes Y, Sol JC, Roux FE, Verdie JC. Motor cortex stimulation for neuropathic pain. *Acta Neurochir Suppl* 2007;97(2):37-44.

[29] Li J, Andrews RJ. Trimodal nanoelectrode array for precise deep brain stimulation: prospects of a new technology based on carbon nanofiber arrays. *Acta Neurochir Suppl* 2007;97(2):537-46.

[30] Mayberg HS, Lozano AM, Voon V, et al. Deep brain stimulation for treatment-resistant depression. *Neuron* 2005;45:651-60.

[31] Miocinovic S, Noecker AM, Maks CB, Butson CR, McIntyre CC. Cicerone: stereotactic neurophysiological recording and deep brain stimulation electrode placement software system. *Acta Neurochir Suppl* 2007;97(2):569-74.

[32] Mueller J, Skogseid IM, Benecke R, , et al. Pallidal deep brain stimulation improves quality of life in segmental and generalized dystonia: results from a prospective, randomized sham-controlled trial. *Mov Disord.* 2008;23:131-4.

[33] Murata J, Kitagawa M, Uesugi H, Saitoh H, Kikuchi S, Tashiro K, Sawamura Y. Electrical stimulation of the posterior subthalamic area for the treatment of intractable proximal tremor. *J Neurosurg* 2003;99:708-15.

[34] Nandi D, Chir M, Liu X, et al. Electrophysiological confirmation of the zona incerta as a target for surgical treatment of disabling involuntary arm movements in multiple sclerosis: use of local field potentials. *J Clin Neurosci* 2002;9:64-8.

[35] Nguyen JP, Lefaucher JP, Le Guerinerl C, Eizenbaum JF, Nakano N, Carpentier et al. Motor cortex stimulation in the treatment of central and neuropathic pain. *Arch Med Res* 2000;31:263-5.

[36] Nuttin BJ, Gabriels LA, Cosyns PR. Long-term electrical capsular stimulation in patients with obsessive-compulsive disorder. *Neurosurg* 2003;52:1263-72.

[37] Oikawa H, Sasaki M, Tamakawa Y, Kamei A. The circuit of Papez in mesial temporal sclerosis: MRI. *Neuroradiology* 2001;43:205-10.

[38] Okun MS, Mann G, Foote KD, et al. Deep brain stimulation in the internal capsule and nucleus accumbens region: responses observed during active and sham programming. *J Neurol Neurosurg Psychiatry* 2007;78:310-4.

[39] Pancrazio JJ, Chen D, Fertig SJ, et al. Towards neurotechnology innovation: report from the 2005 Neural Interfaces Workshop. An NIH-sponsored event. *Neuromodulation* 2006;9:1-7.

[40] Pollo C, Villemure, J-G. Rationale, mechanisms of efficacy, anatomical targets and future prospects of electrical deep brain stimulation for epilepsy. *Acta Neurochir Suppl* 2007;97(2):311-20.

[41] Rauch SL, Baxter LR Jr. Neuroimaging in obsessive-compulsive disorder and related disorders. *In: Jenicke MA, Baer L, Minichiello WE, eds. Obsessive-compulsive disorders: practical management*, 3rd edn. St Louis, MI, USA: Mosby, 1998.

[42] Romanelli P, Bronte-Stewart H, Courtney T, Heit G. Possible necessity for deep brain stimulation of both the ventralis intermedius and subthalamic nuclei to resolve Holmes tremor. Case report. *J Neurosurg* 2003;99:566-71.

[43] Romito LM, Franzini A, Perani D, et al. Fixed dystonia unresponsive to pallidal stimulation improved by motor cortex stimulation. *Neurology* 2007;68:875-6.

[44] Sakas DE, Panourias IG. Rostral cingulate gyrus: A putative target for deep brain stimulation in treatment-refractory depression. *Med Hypothes* 2006;66:491-4.

[45] Sakas DE, Panourias IG, Simpson BA. An introduction to neural networks surgery, a field of neuromodulation which is based on advances in neural networks science and digitised brain imaging. *Acta Neurochir Suppl* 2007;97(2):3-13.

[46] Sakas DE, Panourias IG, Singounas E, Simpson BA. Neurosurgery for psychiatric disorders: from the excision of brain tissue to the chronic electrical stimulation of neural networks. *In: Sakas DE, Simpson BA, editors. Operative Neuromodulation: Neural networks surgery*. New York: Springer-Verlag; 2007. p. 365-74.

[47] Sakas DE, Panourias IG, Boviatsis ES et al. *Treatment of primary camptocormia* (dystonic bent spine or bent neck) by electrical stimulation of the globus pallidus internus: report of 3 cases. Abstract book, The 8th International Neuromodulation Society and the 11th Annual Meeting of the North American Neuromodulation Society, Acapulco, 2007, December 7-12.

[48] Sakas DE, Panourias IG, Boviatsis E, Themistocleous M, Stavrinou L, Gatzonis S. Treatment of idiopathic head-drop syndrome (camptocephalia) by bilateral chronic electrical stimulation of the globus pallidum internus. *J Neurosurg* 2008b [in press].

[49] Schlaepfer TE, Cohen MX, Frick C,et al. Deep brain stimulation to reward circuitry alleviates anhedonia in refractory major depression. *Neuropsychopharmacology* 2008;33:368-77.

[50] Schramm P, Scheihing M, Rasche D, Tronnier VM. Behr syndrome variant with tremor treated by VIM stimulation. *Acta Neurochir* (Wien) 2005;147:679-83.

[51] Simpson BA. The role of neruostimulation: the neurosurgical perspective. *J Pain Symptom Manage* 2006;31:S3-S5.

[52] Stover NP, Okun MS, Evatt ML, Raju DV, Bakay RA, Vitek JL. Stimulation of the subthalamic nucleus in a patient with Parkinson's disease and essential tremor. *Arch Neurol* 2005;62:141-3.

[53] Sturm V, Lenartz D, Koulousakis A, et al. The nucleus accumbens: a target for deep brain stimulation in obsessive-compulsive and anxiety disorders. *J Chem Neuroanat* 2003;26:293-9.

[54] Sun B, Chen S, Zhan S, Le W, Krahl SE. Subthalamic nucleus stimulation for primary dystonia and tardive dystonia. *Acta Neurochir Suppl* 2007;97:207-14.

[55] Sun FT, Morrell MJ, Wharen RE Jr. Responsive cortical stimulation for the treatment of epilepsy. *Neurotherapeutics* 2008;5:68-74.

[56] Swanson TH. The pathophysiology of human mesial temporal lobe epilepsy. *J Clin Neurophysiol* 1995;12:2-22.

[57] Sydow O, Thobois S, Alesch F, Speelman JD. Multicenter European study of thalamic stimulation in essential tremor: a six year follow-up. *J Neurol Neurosurg Psychiatr* 2003;74:1387-91.

[58] Szeszko PR, Robinson D, Alvir JMJ, et al. Orbital frontal and amygdala volume reductions in obsessive-compulsive disorder. *Arch Gen Psychiatry* 1999; 56**:** 913–19.

[59] Taha JM, Jansen MA, Favre J. Thalamic deep brain stimulation for the treatment of head, voice, and bilateral limb tremor. *J Neurosurg* 1999;91:68-72.

[60] Temel Y, Kessels A, Tan S, Topdag A, Boon P, Visser-Vandewalle V. Behavioural changes after bilateral subthalamic nucleus stimulation in advanced Parkinson's disease: A systematic review. *Parkinsonism Relat Disord* 2006;12:265-72.

[61] Tisch S, Rothwell JC, Limousin P, Hariz MI, Corcos DM. The physiological effects of pallidal deep brain stimulation in dystonia. *IEEE Trans Neural Syst Rehabil Eng* 2007;15:166-72.

[62] Utter AA, Basso MA. The basal ganglia: An overview of circuits and function. *Neurosci Biobehavior Rev 2008*;32:333–42.

[63] Velasco F, Velasco M, Jimenez F, et al. Predictors in the treatment of difficult-to-control seizures b electrical stimulation of the centromedian thalamic nucleus. *Neurosurgery* 2000;47:295-304.

[64] Velasco AL, Velasco M, Velasco F, et al. Sucabute and chronic electrical stimulation of the hippocampus on intractable temporal lobe seizures: preliminary report. *Arch Med Res* 2000;31:316-28.

[65] Velasco F, Carrillo-Ruiz JD, Brito F, Velasco M, Velasco AL, Marquez I, Davis R. Double-blind, randomized controlled pilot study of bilateral cerebellar stimulation for treatment of intractable motor seizures. *Epilepsia* 2005;46:1071-81.

[66] Veliskova J, Velsek L, Moshe SL. Subthalamic nucleus: a new anticonvulsant site in the brain. *Neuroreport* 1996;7:1786–1788.

[67] Vercueil L, Benazzouz A, Deransart C, Bressand K, Marescaux C, DepauLis A, Benabid A-L. High frequency stimulation of the subthalamic nucleus suppresses absence seizures in the rat: comparison with neurotoxic lesions. *Epilepsy Res* 1998;28:158-61.

[68] Visser-Vandewalle V, Temel Y, Boon P, et al. Chronic bilateral thalamic stimulation: a new therapeutic approach in intractable Tourette's syndrome. Report of three cases. *J Neurosurg* 2003;99:1094-1100.

[69] Vonck K, Boon P, Claeys P, Dedeurwaerdere S, Achten R, Van Roost D. Long-term deep brain stimulation for refractory lobe epilepsy. *Ann Neurol* 2005;52:556-65.

[70] Wagner T, Gangitano M, Romero R et al. Intracranial measurement of current densities induced by transcranial magnetic stimulation in the human brain. *Neurosci Lett* 2004;354:91-4.

[71] Weaver F. Follett K, Hur K, Ippolito D, Stern M. Deep brain stimulation in Parkinson's disease: a meta-analysis of patient outcomes. *J Neurosurg* 2005;103:956-67.

[72] Webster TJ, Waid MC, McKenzie JL, Price RL, Ejiofor JU. Nano-biotechnology: carbon nanofibers as improved nerual and orthopaedic implants. *Nanotechnology* 2004;15:48-54.

[73] Wishart HA, Roberts DW, Roth RM, et al. Chronic deep brain stimulation for the treatment of tremor in multiple sclerosis: review and case reports. *J Neurol Neurosurg Psychiatr* 2003;74:1392-7.

[74] Woods SP, Fields JA, Troster AI. Neuropsychological sequelae of subthalamic nucleus deep brain stimulation in Parkinson's disease: a critical review. *Neuropsychol Rev* 2002;12:111–6.

[75] Yu H, Neimat J. The treatment of movement disorders by deep brain stimulation. *Neurotherapeutics* 2008;5:26-36.

[76] Zungu-Dirwayi N, Hugo F, van Heerden BB, Stein DJ. Are musical obsessions a temporal lobe phenomenon? *J Neuropsychiatry Clin Neurosci* 1999; 11: 398–400.

In: Deep Brain Stimulation
Editors: Mark H. Rogers and Paul B. Anderson

ISBN 978-1-60692-895-0

Chapter III

Cortical Stimulation versus Deep Brain Stimulation in Neurological and Psychiatric Disorders: Current State and Future Prospects [*]

Damianos E. Sakas[†] and Ioannis G. Panourias
Department of Neurosurgery, University of Athens Medical School, Evangelismos Hospital, and P.S. Kokkalis Hellenic Center for Neurosurgical Research, Athens, Greece

Abstract

Therapeutic brain stimulation can be applied: a) in networks which are located in cortical and subcortical layers, b) in deep nuclei groups (relay nodes) or c) in combination. CS and DBS belong to the domain of *operative neuromodulation* and particularly to the field of *neural networks surgery* (Sakas et al 2007a), defined as the field that studies and applies advancements in neural networks research, digitized stereotactic brain imaging and implantable electrical or electronic devices in order to alter electrically the signal transmission in the nervous system, modulate neural networks and produce therapeutic effects.

Therapeutic brain stimulation methods are currently distinguished into two major categories: a) noninvasive and b) invasive. The *noninvasive* methods (rTMS, tDCS) stimulate electrically the brain cortex after applying electrical currents on the human scalp. The *invasive* methods require the surgical implantation of specially designed electrodes either in contact with the cortex of the brain, i.e., CS, or in deeply located selected targets, i.e., DBS. Instead of "*invasive*", the terms *implantable* or *by implantable*

---

[*] A version of this chapter was also published in *Text of Therapentic Cortical Stimulation*, edited by Sergio Canavero published by Nova Science Publishers, Inc. It was submitted for appropriate modification in an effort to encourage wider dissemination of research.

[†] Correspondence concerning this article should be addressed to Dr. Damianos E. Sakas, MD. E-mail: sakasde@med.uoa.gr.

devices" are much more appropriate, as they do not carry the negative association of a traumatic intervention that is implied by the term *invasive CS*. In this chapter, we describe and compare the current state and future prospects of DBS and CS in the fields of neurology and psychiatry.

Current Applications

1. Pain

DBS: The rationale for the use of DBS in chronic pain dates back to the 1950s and, to date, more than 1,300 patients have been offered such a treatment. However, many factors limited its use: insufficient understanding of the neural networks that convey the perception of pain, uncertainties about optimal brain targets, inconsistent efficacy, and the success of spinal cord stimulation and opioid infusion pumps. The US Food and Drug Administration, based on the results of two multicenter trials, withdrew permission to use DBS as a treatment for pain (Burchiel 2001). The method, however, still remains in practice in Canada, Europe and Asia, but the number of reported cases over the last decade is limited (Bartsch et al, 2008; Owen et al., 2006a and b; Rasche et al., 2006). Traditionally, the two most targeted areas for treatment of pain are: a) the sensory thalamus (Vc, ventrocaudalis) and b) the periaqueductal and periventricular gray (PAG and PVG). Most retrospective studies support the view that thalamic DBS has greater efficacy in neuropathic pain with 50-60% success rate (Levy et al., 1987; Bendok and Levy, 1998); mesencephalic DBS has proved more efficacious in nociceptive pain (including osteoarthritis and cancer (Rezai and Lozano, 2002) and the mixed-pain failed back surgery syndrome (Young and Rinaldi, 1997; Kumar et al., 1997) with 70% pain relief. However, DBS is poorly effective for central pain (Canavero and Bonicalzi 2007a,b), and contradictory results exist for phantom limb pain and postherpetic neuralgia (Owen et al 2006b; Rasche et al 2006). Recently, DBS of the posterior hypothalamic region has emerged as an effective treatment for otherwise medically-refractory cluster headache (CH) (Bartsch et al., 2008; Owen et al., 2007; Schoenen J et al., 2005; Starr et al., 2007), with half of the reported patients experiencing fair-to-excellent long-term relief in terms of frequency of pain attacks and severity of pain. The risk of intracerebral hemorrhage when bilaterally targeting such deeply-located structures remains a pervasive concern.

CS: MI ECS was introduced for the management of pain following the recognition that DBS of the sensory thalamic nuclei had offered disappointing long-term results. Initially, MI ECS was proposed as a treatment for central thalamic pain (chapter 9) and facial neurogenic pain (trigeminal neuropathy) (chapter 10). MI ECS has proved most effective for trigeminal neuropathic pain with about 60% of the sufferers reporting a fair to excellent long-term pain relief (chapter 10). MI ECS is also effective in about half of all reported patients with CPSP (chapter 9). In phantom limb and brachial plexus avulsion pain, MI ECS offers an average success rate of slightly above 40% (chapter 10). Sensory cortex stimulation may also afford analgesia (chapter 9) and should be explored further. The application of either motor or sensory CS by implantable systems is moving along with that of noninvasive cortical stimulation such as TMS or tDCS (chapter 8). Despite modest effects, analgesia is usually transient, and even with protracted sessions, it lasts no more than 1 month, at best. However, they may predict a positive outcome to ECS (Canavero and Bonicalzi, 2007a and b; chapter 8). The apparent superiority of tDCS over rTMS may pave the way to clinical application.

CS vs. DBS: Considerations, Limitations and Future Prospects

The small number of patients treated in randomized placebo-controlled clinical trials, the heterogeneous nature of pain disorders, the uncertainty regarding the appropriate target for each specific pain syndrome, the lack of universal stimulation protocols and systematic follow-up data, and DBS-associated complications (diplopia, seizures, nausea, paresthesia, and, above all, intracerebral hemorrhage) are all factors that are likely to hinder an expansion of DBS in pain therapy for the foreseeable future and restrict it only to a few highly-specialized centers (Cruccu et al., 2007).

Apparently, implantable CS devices offer the best alternative for the surgical treatment of intractable pain conditions. Apart from the aforementioned factors, other important criteria in selecting CS over DBS inlude: a) the profound laterality of painful symptoms, b) the extensive representation of the painful area in the lateral cortical surface, and c) advanced patient's age. Bilateral pain is not a contraindication for ECS: bilateral effects from unilateral stimulation have been reported. Yet, bilateral surgery should be offered with a word of caution. Another problem arises when the pain afflicts a body region, such as the leg, which is represented in the medial interhemispheric cortical surface in several patients. In this case, only the much more invasive subdural CS would be offered. This problem may become more complex if leg pain is bilateral; in such cases, the electrodes should be inserted in both aspects of the interhemispheric fissure which may not be an easy procedure in many patients. Undoubtedly, it is much easier to stimulate the lateral aspect of the cortex unilaterally rather than the interhemispheric surface bilaterally. Fortunately, there is evidence that unilateral CS can have bilatateral beneficial effects (Canavero et al., 2007b). Patients with trigeminal or arm neuropathic pains are especially suitable for ECS as compared to patients with bilateral leg pain. ECS appears to be a viable therapeutic option for drug-resistant central and trigeminal neuropathic pain. This is important, because neuropathic pain is a major concern for pain therapists due to its unresponsiveness to available drug and conservative treatments. Notably, the cut-off rate for success in pain relief is arbitrarily set at >50%; in the case of NP, however, pain improvement of 40% or even 30% has been sufficient to consider ECS effective. At this time, TMS or tDCS can be proposed as a preoperative test for selecting candidates for implantable CS procedures and possibly to alleviate painful conditions for a short period before a scheduled ECS procedure (chapter 8). A meta-analysis concluded that MI ECS appears to be more effective in alleviating chronic pain syndromes as compared to either MI rTMS or tDCS (Lima and Fregni, 2008). The availability of a noninvasive screening procedure for CS represents an important advantage of implantable (invasive) CS over DBS. Conversely, no drug-based or other test method has been developed that could predict the efficacy of DBS and, therefore, help us in selecting the right patients. DBS targets are small in size and deeply located in the brain and, at present, they can be investigated only by stereotactic approaches.

CS is likely to expand its role in pain management. Patient selection will be optimized by developing drug dissection protocols in order to identify "neurochemical signatures" portending a successful outcome and selecting stimulation targets on the basis of anomalies as seen in neuroimaging studies (Canavero and Bonicalzi 2007, chapter 9). For instance, SI cortex has been first targeted on the basis of theory and metabolic findings (Canavero and Bonicalzi 1995). The combination of anatomical, functional imaging, clinical, and intraoperative neurophysiological data (by keeping the patient awake during the procedure) will further improve target localization, together with confirmation by means of noninvasive stimulation. Securing the electrode in the predetermined position may reduce possible subsequent migration, with loss of effect. Software-guided stimulation protocols must be developed to facilitate postoperative titration and make the follow-up sessions less time-consuming and more comfortable for both practitioners and patients; moreover, it will probably eliminate the need of "intensive reprogramming" or surgical repositioning of the electrode in case of tolerance-like phenomena or loss of ECS efficacy over time. On the basis of the available published studies and evidence from noninvasive brain stimulation, CS by implantable devices will likely remain at the forefront of pain therapies in the foreseeable future, particularly as the mechanisms of action and clinical efficacy will be addressed and evaluated in large-scale randomized controlled trials.

2. Parkinson's Disesae

DBS: DBS has metamorphosed the treatment of PD by alleviating its troublesome symptoms and improving substantially the quality of life of sufferers. The reversibility, adjustability and programmability of DBS have favored it over the lesional procedures of the past. A change of rigidity is usually seen within 20-30 seconds with a maximum within 1 minute. Tremor can improve over weeks or months. Bradykinesia may respond after several hours or days and returns to baseline within up to 24 hours. The induction of dyskinesias with DBS in the short term predicts a favorable long-term outcome. Postoperatively, dopaminergic drugs may be reduced (about 50%) due to the additive effect; however, too rapid or too drastic a decrease in dopaminergic drugs carries the risk of unmasking apathy or depression or mania or psychosis or akinetic crisis. After optimization of parameters, levodopa may be gradually replaced with long-acting dopamine agonists. Postoperative dyskinesias or temporary worsening of PD due to drug reduction are possible. The thalamic *ventral intermediate (Vim) nucleus* was the first DBS target in the 1980s, with almost 90% of PD patients experiencing years-long control of their tremor (Benabid et al., 1996). The minimal effect of VIM DBS on rigidity and bradykinesia spurred researchers to explore alternative nuclei as potential targets. Animal studies showed that the *subthalamic nucleus (STN)* is an integral relay node in the cortical-basal ganglia-thalamocortical pathways. The efficacy of STN DBS has now been documented by numerous groups and validated in prospective, randomized trials. Long-term follow-up and meta-analysis studies have demonstrated sustained improvement in the Unified PD Rating Scale (UPDRS) motor subscores of tremor, rigidity, and akinesia in the off-medication state, but minimal improvement in the on-medication state (Kleiner-Fisman et al., 2006; Yu and Neimat, 2008). In prospective open-label trials, STN DBS offered a significant benefit on the quality of life, particularly in patients younger than 65 years (Derost et al., 2007; Deuschl et al., 2006; Krack et al., 2003). Bilateral STN DBS is considered the standard surgical therapy for medically-refractory PD; unilateral STN DBS is efficacious in highly asymmetric parkinsonism (Kern and Kumar, 2007). However, concerns regarding continuous ipsilateral deterioration of PD symptoms over time restrict unilateral STN DBS only to highly selected patients. Based on reports of efficacy of pallidotomy for PD, *globus pallidus internus (GPi)* emerged as a target for DBS. High-frequency stimulation of the GPi alleviates rigidity, tremor and bradykinesia in the off-medication state, substantially decreases disabling levodopa-induced dyskinesias in the on- and off-medication states and improves the quality of life (Deuschl et al., 2006; Wichmann and DeLong, 2006; Yu and Neimat, 2008). In contrast to patients who received STN DBS, those with GPi DBS are not able to substantially reduce their medications (Rodriguez-Oroz et al., 2005). *Peduculopontine nucleus (PPN)*, a relay node in the network connecting GPi and STN with the basal ganglia and the peripheral nervous system, has recently been proposed as a new target for DBS in PD. Clinical studies support its efficacy, particularly, for postural instability and akinesia in parkinsonism (Nandi et al., 2002a; Plaha and Gill, 2005). Similarly, DBS of the caudal *zona incerta (ZI)* has shown beneficial effects on parkinsonian tremor, rigidity and akinesia (Kitagawa et al., 2005; Plaha et al., 2005).

CS: Functional neuroimaging studies have shown that cortical areas such as the primary motor cortex and the supplementary motor area are hypo- or hyperactive in both early and late stages of PD (chapter 12). Canavero and collaborators first reported on the clinical benefits obtained from unilateral extradural MI ECS in three PD patients (Canavero and Paolotti, 2000; Canavero et al., 2002). UPDRS motor subscores (Part III) were decreased by 48% and the need for levodopa by 80%. Afterwards, the benefits of unilateral MI ECS in improving all parkinsonian symptoms (tremor, rigidity, bradykinesia, posture and gait disturbances, freezing) and reducing the required daily medications were confirmed in a large multicenter study (chapter 13 and 13b). The neurophysiologically documented prolonged modulatory activity of TMS on pathologically hyperactive or hypoactive areas of the human brain cortex has supported the assumption that TMS may also improve the motor components of PD (chapter 12).

CS vs. DBS: Considerations, Limitations and Future Prospects

DBS has been acknowledged worldwide as the surgical treatment of choice for improving the incapacitating symptoms and the quality of life in PD patients: in 2002, it received FDA's approval as a treatment option for PD. Bilateral STN or GPi DBS is effective in patients with severe medication-refractory tremor-dominant PD. DBS of the Vim is no longer recommended for PD (Kumar et al., 1999; Kern and Kumar, 2007; Krack et al., 2003). In spite of the absence of published blinded, randomized, controlled studies comparing the efficacy of DBS of the STN or GPi, the STN has gained general acceptance as the preferred target (Halpern et al., 2007; Kern and Kumar, 2007). The reasons for the supposed superiority of the STN over GPi DBS in PD include: easier targeting on MRI, longer stimulation effects of STN stimulation, larger reductions in medication, longer IPG battery life due to the lower intensity required for stimulating the smaller (as compared to GPi). Although longer follow-up data from randomized, controlled studies are needed to correlate the improvement induced by DBS with that due to medication, there is little doubt that DBS represents a breakthrough in the history of the treatment of PD. However, almost half of all PD sufferers are excluded from DBS mainly due to advanced age (>70 years), significant dementia or psychiatric comorbidity, poor response to levodopa, low scores (<30-40) in the UPDRS part III or other general contraindication to DBS. Non-motor and non-dopaminergic symptoms of PD respond poorly to DBS, but newer targets may boost DBS potential. DBS has been associated with neuropsychiatric untoward effects (e.g., dementia, apathy, anxiety, suicidal attempts) and cognitive undesired sequelae (e.g., a decline in lexical fluency and executive functions: Temel et al., 2006). There also exists a considerable risk of surgery- and hardware-related complications estimated to be 1-3% and up to 25%, respectively (Breit et al., 2004; Oh et al., 2002). A hint that DBS may slow the progression of Parkinson's disease remains unproven and, if DBS is not applied early in the course of PD, such evidence will not become available (Simpson, 2006a).

Due to the limited number of PD sufferers that have been treated by MI ECS so far, it is difficult to compare it to DBS. However, it seems that a considerable number of patients remain desperate and unrelieved. MI ECS appears to have some advantages over DBS in the treatment of PD: 1) it can alleviate all cardinal symptoms, but particularly the axial ones, 2) unilateral MI ECS induces beneficial effects bilaterally, 3) MI ECS is more suitable in elderly PD cases due to minimal surgery-related side effects and lower complication rates; moreover, the bilateral beneficial effects induced by unilateral MI ECS may delay the progressive deterioration of PD in the non-stimulated side, 4) MI ECS is more cost-effective because it does not require stereotactic equipment, and 5) MI ECS promises to potentially benefit almost half of the PD patients who have been excluded from DBS. Given that the number of PD sufferers aged >70 years will steadily increase, a considerable part of this patient population will require an alternative to DBS therapy; currently, CS appears the most likely option. A few caveats are in order: a) patients with levodopa-resistant parkinsonian symptoms are unlikely to respond to MI ECS, b) parkinsonism related to multisystem atrophy or progressive supranuclear palsy hardly benefits from MI ECS, and c) TMS-induced improvement of PD symptoms carries positive predictive value for MI ECS efficacy (Canavero 2007a). Nevertheless, a negative rTMS test does not predict failure of MI ECS (Cioni, et al., 2007). Future efforts should focus on exploring the potential efficacy of stimulation of premotor area and the neuroprotective potential of MI ECS (Canavero and Bonicalzi, 2007a).

3. Tremor

DBS: Tremor affects up to 2% of the general population worldwide, and can be essential (idiopathic) or associated with various conditions such as cerebellar dysfunction, multiple sclerosis, lesions of the brainstem (Holmes tremor) or head injury. Unilateral DBS has proved to be particularly effective in controlling contralateral idiopathic and secondary forms of tremor (Deuschl and Bain, 2002). Bilateral DBS has proved beneficial in head, trunk and voice tremor (Taha et al., 1999). Traditionally, based on the existing experience of lesional surgery, the *Vim thalamic nucleus* has been targeted. Long-term follow-up data of unilateral

Vim-DBS have documented the great improvement in essential tremor (ET) suppression, limb functionality, quality of life, and reduced need for medication (Kumar et al., 2003; Sydow et al., 2003). In 8 patients with ET, unilateral DBS of the posteromedial subthalamic white matter, i.e., *zona incerta* (ZI) suppressed contralateral proximal tremor by 81% for a mean follow-up of 22 months (Murata et al., 2003). STN DBS has suppressed ET in patients with coexisting movement disorders, such as PD (Stover et al 2005). It is generally accepted that distal limb tremor responds well to Vim DBS, whereas proximal limb tremor is better controlled by ZI DBS (Nandi et al, 2002b). In a systematic review of 78 patients with tremor secondary to multiple sclerosis, unilateral Vim DBS offered postoperative benefits in motor function and daily activities in 88% and 76% of sufferers, respectively (Wishart et al 2003). Vim DBS has also successfully controlled tremor associated with unusual pathological conditions such as Holmes tremor (Romanelli et al 2003) or inherited cerebellar ataxia (Schramm et al 2005).

CS: There are only few reports of successful CS application in non-parkinsonian tremor. MI ECS has shown the best efficacy in post-stroke distal rest and/or action tremor (Canavero and Bonicalzi, 2007a; Katayama et al., 2002). In most cases, it reduced tremor significantly when it was offered to alleviate coexisting pain or movement disorders. Otherwise, the results of MI ECS in the management of ET have been disappointing (chapter 13). Similarly, noninvasive cortical stimulation has not provided clinical benefits in non-parkinsonian tremor (Hallett, 2007).

CS vs. DBS: Considerations, Limitations and Future Prospects

Tremor has been part of the repertoire of stereotactic and functional surgery over the last fifty years. VIM DBS is the "gold standard" in the treatment of medically-refractory non-parkinsonian tremor with an efficacy up to 80% and long-lasting benefit for more than 7 years. MI ECS has not proved particularly effective in non-parkinsonian tremor, so far. This may be due to the pathophysiologic substrate of ET. Although recent reports support a cortical involvement (Raethjen et al., 2007), the role of the cortex in the generation of ET has not been elucidated. On the other hand, there is sufficient demonstration of the key role of the somatosensory thalamus, and the Vim nucleus in particular, in the integration of neural loops within both the cortico-basal ganglia-spinal networks and, also, the cerebello-thalamocortical system. These networks are essential in the pathogenesis of tremor and, therefore, have offered convincing support that Vim is the optimal target for alleviating tremulous conditions, regardless of the underlying cause. Yet, given MI ECS efficacy in relieving parkinsonian tremor (although less so than akinesia and rigidity), it is possible that its limited efficacy in non-parkinsonian tremor may be due to wrong targeting (other areas rather than MI should be stimulated), suboptimal stimulation protocols or electrode-related shortcomings. The development of new electrode arrays with a larger number of poles supported by multiple programming IPGs may enhance its efficacy in the future.

4. Dystonia

DBS: DBS is currently the most effective treatment for medically refractive dystonia. The main target used in primary dystonia (DYT1 gene positive) is the *Globus Pallidus internus (GPi)* and its efficacy has been shown in generalized dystonia, segmental dystonia, and complex cervical dystonia with movement scores typically improving by 75% (Kiss et al., 2007; Mueller et al., 2008; Krauss et al., 1999, 2003). Certain types of truncal dystonia (camptocephalia and camptocormia) are emerging as good candidates for pallidal DBS (Sakas et al., 2008b; Sakas et al., 2007c). DBS maintains marked long-term symptomatic and functional improvement in the majority of patients with dystonia. (Loher et al., 2008). Upon activating DBS, phasic dystonic movements tend to improve early after surgery, but the response of tonic movements to chronic stimulation may be delayed (Krauss et al., 2002). Other targets, such as the *thalamus* and *STN* have shown encouraging results, but the available data is still scarce and sometimes contradictory (Sun et al., 2007). In sum, GPi DBS is an established treatment for idiopathic dystonia, either generalized or segmental, and its efficacy has been proven by extensive experience and by randomized, sham stimulation-controlled trials. Future research will likely continue to address the most appropriate programming settings for various subpopulations of dystonia, the mechanism by which DBS affects this ailment, and the possibility of alternative brain targets that might have fewer associated side effects or greater efficacy than the GPi.

CS: CS has been reported to be effective in certain forms of fixed dystonia (chapter 13). The reports are only a few, but preliminary data implies that the mechanism of fixed dystonia is more corticalized than in primary torsion dystonia. Some task-specific forms of dystonia, such as writer's cramp or musician's cramp, may be related to maladaptive cortical plasticity as a result of overuse or improper use of the hand (Byl et al., 1996; Classen et al., 2003). Again, those focal forms of dystonia may be suitable candidates for CS. The optimal stimulation site remains to be elucidated. Based on results from rTMS on various forms of the disease, stimulation over the premotor cortex seems to yield better results than stimulation over the motor cortex (Murase et al., 2005). This may reflect both local and remote effects on distant, but connected sites (e.g., MI, the posterior parietal cortex and the basal ganglia). The assumption that stimulation over the premotor cortex may affect both the deep relay-nodes in the basal ganglia and the cortical sensory areas is in agreement with the known pathophysiology of dystonia, which involves the basal ganglia, MI and the somatosensory system in a diffuse sensory-motor processing dysfunction. Despite reports of invasive and non-invasive MI stimulation for fixed dystonia (chapter 13; Murase et al., 2005), it would be interesting to compare those effects with premotor cortex stimulation effects as well. Hence, even though MI ECS appears to have beneficial effects, it may be postulated that CS over the premotor cortex might be more effective.

CS vs. DBS: Considerations, Limitations and Future Prospects

Bidirectional interconnectivity between motor cortical areas and deep-seated structures, such as the basal ganglia, could explain why dystonia and other movement disorders respond to neuromodulation at multiple sites. CS may induce distant neuromodulatory effects either at the cortical and/or subcortical levels through orthodromic or antidromic effects, similarly to what is postulated as a possible mechanism of action of DBS (Tisch et al., 2007). The proven efficacy of GPi DBS and, to a lesser extent, STN DBS in treating a wide spectrum of dystonic phenotypes suggests that DBS will remain the mainstay of therapeutic neuromodulation of dystonia in the near future. CS should however be better assessed by, e.g., comparing unilateral versus bilateral stimulation of MI and non-primary motor areas in fixed rather than in torsion dystonia, and even combined with DBS. Initial experimental and clinical data suggest that the potential efficacy of CS should be explored in cases of fixed or unilateral focal segmental dystonia involving one arm and neck or part of the trunk or leg, in cases of unilateral secondary dystonia of a multisegmental character, especially with a normal MRI scan, where DBS is likely to be less effective. rTMS may provide a useful predictor of clinical outcome and help triaging those patients who are likely to respond to CS.

5. Epilepsy

DBS: 30% of epileptics are drug-resistant, due to either failure to respond to available antiepileptic drugs or medication-related adverse effects (Silanpää and Schmidt, 2006; Kwan and Brodie, 2000). Resective brain surgery of the epileptic focus can be effective in judiciously selected patients; unfortunately, up to 40% of sufferers are not eligible for such surgical treatment. Moreover, post-operatively, anticonvulsant agents cannot be discontinued, seizure remissions may occur and undesired neuropsychiatric sequelae often lessen the surgical success rate. Several brain areas have been targeted by DBS (Velasco et al., 2000a). The thalamus has been long considered a pivotal brain structure in the epileptogenic process and two thalamic nuclei have been targeted for suppressing intractable seizures: the *centromedian nucleus of the thalamus* (CMT) and the *anterior nucleus of the thalamus* (ANT). In addition, four other areas have been investigated: STN, cerebellum, caudate nucleus and hippocampus. The CMT has been considered a suitable DBS target on the assumption that it has an integrating role in the propagation of generalized seizures through its participation in an ascending brainstem-diencephalon-subcortical loop. CMT DBS has been successful in controlling mainly generalized tonic-clonic seizures and atypical absences (Velasco et al., 1993a; Velasco et al., 1993b; Velasco et al., 1995; Velasco et al., 2001) and, to a lesser degree, partial complex seizures (Fisher et al., 1992). The role of CMT DBS, although promising, remains moot and should be further evaluated by large scale randomized-controlled studies (Andrade et al., 2006; Fisher et al., 1992). The ANT, with its relatively small size, safe distance from vascular structures and documented anterograde projections to cortical, subcortical and limbic regions (Halpern et al., 2008) has been targeted for DBS. Bilateral ANT DBS reduced the frequency of partial complex seizures by approximately 50% in a small series and is being submitted to a controlled trial (Andrade et al., 2006; Hodaie et al., 2002; Kerrigan et al., 2004; Halpern et al., 2008). The STN has been also evaluated as a potential DBS target in drug-resistant epilepsy. In animal models, inhibition of the GABAergic neurons of the substantia nigra pars reticulata (SNr) reduces partial and generalized epileptic seizures (Iadarola and Gale 1982). Based on its excitatory effect on the nigral system, STN has been targeted in small, open-label prospective studies; notably, STN DBS reduced seizure frequency by 60-80% (Benabid et al., 2001; Chabardès et al., 2002; Handforth et al., 2006), but large trials are needed to confirm these initial results. In the early 1970s, the cerebellum, due to its thalamic projections, was electrically stimulated for suppressing seizures (Cooper et al., 1973) and Velasco et al., (2005) reported a mean reduction of approximately 30% in motor seizures in five patients. At present, less than 20 patients have been treated by cerebellar stimulation in controlled studies and less than five experienced a significant reduction in their generalized tonic/clonic seizures. Chronic electrical stimulation of the head of the caudate nucleus (HCN) is now being evaluated (Chkhenkeli and Chkhenkeli, 1997; Chkhenkeli et al., 2004). The reported suppression of seizures has been attributed to the hyperpolarization of cortical neurons, induced by activation of the HCN by low-frequency stimulation (4-8 Hz). DBS of the aforementioned targets aims to modulate the abnormal cortical function by activating or inhibiting relay nodes which, although distant from the epileptogenic area, are critical epilepsy "gating mechanisms". A different approach involves the direct stimulation of the epileptic zone per se. There is growing evidence that, in the years to come, stimulation of the amygdalohippocampal region will receive special attention. This technique may prove particularly helpful when the epileptogenic focus either involves eloquent brain areas or is not suitable for a resective procedure. The hippocampus, an integral component of Papez's circuit, plays a pivotal role in both the generation and propagation of temporal lobe seizures (Swanson, 1995; Oikawa et al 1994). Hippocampal stimulation provided excellent control of temporal lobe seizures in seven of 10 patients (Velasco et al., 2000b). Vonck et al. (2005) reported satisfactory suppression of seizures by bilateral amygdalohippocampal DBS; at 14-month follow-up, one of seven patients was free of complex partial seizures, five enjoyed a 20-50% reduction in seizure frequency and only one did not improve. Undeniably, results are still unconvincing for this target.

CS: Due to their intrinsic characteristics, CS and TMS are more likely to suppress seizures originating primarily in the cortex. Thus, if the epilepticogenic zone lies over the motor or speech area and a surgical excision is risky, CS could be an alternative method. In contrast, CS is unlikely to prove effective in cases with a deeply-located epileptogenic focus. The application of TMS to testing the mode of action and responsiveness to antiepileptic drugs (Macdonell et al 2002; Ziemann et al 1996) constituted the basis for the clinical evaluation of rTMS in epilepsy. Repetitive TMS provided promising, but unvalidated, results in a small number of patients suffering from complex partial seizures and temporal lobe epilepsy, focal cortical dysplasia or cortical myoclonus (chapter 18). Clearly, more work is needed. One issue with all commercially available DBS and CS devices is that the electrical stimulation is delivered in a pre-programmed manner with defined stimulation parameters (intensity, pulse width, frequency), mode of action (continuous versus cycling) and duration of stimulation, regardless of the subjects condition (so called *open-loop* stimulation). An important leap forward is the development of *closed-loop* stimulation systems. These devices have incorporated software with seizure detection algorithms and deliver stimulation to the epileptogenic focus "on demand", i.e., once premonitory electroencephalographic (EEG) signs of imminent ictal activity are detected, well before clinical manifestation. CS combined with depth monitoring of epileptic activity is the first closed-loop system to have entered a controlled trial (chapter 19). Another controlled trial is also underway in US to test ANT stimulation in partial-onset drug-resistant epilepsy; the patient can activate the neurostimulator (Intercept™, Medtronic, Minneapolis, US) when he/she feels the onset of seizure.

CS vs. DBS: Considerations, Limitations and Future Prospects

Complex partial seizures, atypical absences and generalized tonic/clonic seizures seem to be responsive to DBS. Theoretically, DBS of the CMT or STN, which are relay nodes with extensive cortical afferent and efferent projections, is likely to alleviate generalized seizures. In contrast, DBS of the ANT or hippocampus, which are functionally integrated into the limbic system, is expected to suppress partial seizures. Nevertheless, several critical issues should be addressed before either CS or DBS become effective therapeutic options for intractable epilepsy, such as a lack of homogeneity in the epileptic population. In clinical trials of CS or DBS, it is mandatory to include patients who have well defined anatomical, clinical, radiological and genetic characteristics, similar EEG activity in terms of intensity and frequency of spikes and also similar time elapsed since their last seizure. Standardized selection protocols based on proper phenotypical classification through video-EEG and neuroimaging studies should be developed, in order to help detect the appropriate candidates for CS or DBS, either as monotherapy or as an adjunct to other surgical treatments. At present, it remains unclear whether it is preferable to target the epileptogenic zone or the epileptogenic focus per se or whether subcortical epilepsy is best treated with DBS rather than CS. An important issue, therefore, is the definition of the optimal deep node or cortical zone to be targeted in each epileptic syndrome. H-coil TMS for depth (6 cm) stimulation may benefit some patients. Also, both high- (50 Hz) and low- (1 Hz) frequency CS of the epileptogenic zone can suppress epileptic activity and the impact of different stimulation parameters must be investigated (which applies to DBS too). In most series, patients continue their drugs during DBS therapy. It is important to evaluate the effect of DBS separately, but also compare it with that of the antiepileptic drugs. The synergistic or antagonistic actions of CS with antiepileptic drugs should also be studied. For instance, low-frequency TMS combined with valproate acid induces epileptic activity. Again, only well-conducted studies will answer these and other questions.

6. Psychiatric Disorders

DBS: Early neuropsychiatric DBS practice has been largely guided by prior relevant lesioning experience (Sakas et al., 2007b). Based on results of anterior capsulotomy and fMRI studies (Rauch et al 2006), DBS of the anterior limb of the internal capsule and the ventral striatum/nucleus accumbens (Nuttin et al., 2003; Sturm et al., 2003) has been brought to bear on treatment-refractory obsessive compulsive disorder (OCD) patients (30% of all cases: Picinelli et al., 1995). In one study, four of eight patients treated by DBS enjoyed a greater than 35% reduction in the intensity of their symptoms and a substantial decrease in medication (Greenberg et al 2006). Apart from the IPG battery's short life expectancy and hypomania, DBS therapy has been well tolerated. DBS of the medial intralaminar thalamic (Visser-Vandewalle et al., 2003) and centromedian parafascicular nuclei (Houeto et al., 2005), anterior limb of internal capsule (Flaherty et al., 2005) and GPi (Ackermans et al.,

2006; Diederich et al., 2005) has also shown high rates of efficacy (>70%) in suppressing drug-refractory motor and vocal tics in Tourette's syndrome, which are driven by dysfunctional limbic and cortico-basal gaglia-thalamo-cortical circuits. Patient selection guidelines (Mink et al., 2006) have been published. Severe behavioral changes may be induced in PD patients undergoing DBS (Temel et al., 2006) due, most probably, to inadvertent stimulation of parts of the limbic system such as ZI or SNr; this data supports the assumption that DBS of relay nodes of the limbic system may prove beneficial in treatment-resistant depression (TRD) (Fava, 2003). At present, DBS of the inferior thalamic peduncle (Jimenez et al., 2005), ventral internal capsule/nucleus accumbens (Schlaepfer et al., 2008), and particularly the white matter in the subgenual cingulate gyrus (Cg25 area) (Mayberg et al., 2005) have shown efficacy in depressed patients, with the latter target being now submitted to a controlled trial. Brodman's area 24a has also been proposed as a putative target for DBS in TRD (Sakas and Panourias, 2006). The superiority of Cg25 over the other targets may be due to its extensive connections to brain regions such as the brainstem, hypothalamus, insula, orbitofrontal, and cingulate cortex, which are all clearly implicated in the pathophysiology of depression (Marangell et al., 2007). Despite all these challenging data, DBS remains highly experimental for intractable neuropsychiatric disorders. These efficacy data need validation and replication in large randomized controlled trials in order to spare it the fate of ablative psychosurgery in the past.

CS: Noninvasive CS has been extensively tested and CS by implanted electrodes is now becoming reality. Over the last decade, the number of rTMS trials in psychiatric patients has steadily increased due to the high number of intractable or drug-intolerant psychiatric patients and the need to find alternatives to the rather brute-force approach of electroconvulsive therapy. The early promising results obtained from TMS of the dorsolateral prefrontal cortex (DLPFC) in intractable OCD were not replicated in other studies (chapter 17 and Sachdev et al 2007). Interestingly, in ten patients with comorbid OCD and TS, low-frequency rTMS of the supplementary motor area alleviated the symptoms and normalized overactive motor cortical regions (Mantovani et al., 2006; see also Munchau et al., 2002). Similar beneficial effect was shown in two other patients with TS and comorbid ADHD and MDD with an average improvement of 52%; this is highly comparable to that of approved behavioral or pharmacological treatments for TS (Mantovani et al 2007a). While low-frequency rTMS of the temporoparietal cortex has reduced hallucinations in schizophrenic patients (Aleman et al., 2007), high frequency rTMS of the left prefrontal (or bilateral prefrontal) cortices has provided equivocal results (Prikryl et al., 2007; chapter 17). DLPFC has been the most implicated area in the dysregulation of mood and the pathophysiology of depression. Antidepressant efficacy of high frequency rTMS of the left DLPFC has been repeatedly documented in randomized trials and meta-analyses (Fitzgerald, 2008; O'Reardon et al., 2007). Low frequency TMS of the right DLPFC has also been effective in TRD when offered either as a single TMS treatment (Isenberg et al., 2005) or combined with high-frequency rTMS of the left DLPFC (Fitzgerald et al., 2006). Efficacy of rTMS has also been reported in other comorbid or depressive conditions such as after stroke (Jorge et al., 2004), cerebrovascular disease-associated depression (Fabre et al., 2004), PD (chapter 12) or panic disorder (Mantovani et al., 2007b). tDCS of the left prefrontal region provided clinical benefits compared to sham stimulation in depressed patients (Boggio et al., 2007) and studies are underway to investigate the possible efficacy of tDCS in enhancing cognitive functions such as working memory, decision making and mood (Been et al., 2007). At this time, non-implantable CS should be viewed as a treatment for the acute state rather than a realistic long-term therapy for TRD. However, TMS/tDCS studies opened the way to implantable (invasive) CS. Certainly, this latter cannot be offered as easily as TMS or tDCS. Yet, implantable CS may prove more efficacious, because the electrodes are positioned very closely to the precise cortical area which has been indicated by functional imaging studies as the most appropriate to be stimulated. Given the high level of precision of implantable CS, we need to establish reliable criteria in order to select, among responders to TMS or tDCS, those who can expect the most benefit by implantable CS.

CS vs. DBS: Considerations, Limitations and Future Prospects

In the new era of brain stimulation, the application of CS or DBS in psychiatric disorders has advanced less compared to movement disorders or pain. Undeniably, the unfortunate past of ablative psychosurgery has influenced negatively physicians' attitude towards current brain stimulation efforts. DBS or CS experience in psychiatry is quite limited; therefore, definitive judgments on their clinical efficacy is impossible.

As research moves forward, a few important issues must be raised. The clinical profile of neuropsychiatric disorders is diverse and symptoms of different psychiatric conditions, i.e., TS, OCD and MDD, may coexist making accurate diagnosis debatable. The establishment of consensus guidelines in selecting candidates suitable for DBS therapy is highly recommended and has already become feasible in OCD and TS (OCD-DBS Collaborative Group, 2002; Mink et al., 2006). Additionally, keeping common evaluation rating scales during the patient selection process, plus preoperative and postoperative assessments ensures reliable comparative data from different centers and, hence, inference of strong conclusions. Reported TMS series include small cohorts of medically-refractory psychiatric patients at late stages of the disease. Most of the patients suffered from co-morbid conditions such as OCD and TS. In order to improve patient selection, the clinical benefits should be validated and replicated in patients with a clear psychiatric diagnosis who are enrolled in large-scale double-blind, sham-controlled studies. Hopefully, correlative studies between non-invasive and invasive stimulation will make response prediction feasible for implantable CS, similar to what is seen in chronic pain (chapter 8). This will spur the development of the field in a way that is not – apparently – possible for DBS. Compared to TMS or tDCS, implantable CS offers the opportunity to stimulate on a continuous or cyclical basis, without the patient having to return every month for therapy, and is better suited for sham-controlled studies. The development of the H-coil for TMS will make stimulation of, e.g., the orbitofrontal cortex feasible, while advanced imaging may reveal stimulation patterns of CS or DBS that can be correlated with disease-related activity and clinical improvement. High-resolution imaging needs to be combined with electrophysiological mapping in order to accurately detect cortical targets or white matter bundles which may be critical in mood performance. Advancements in cortical mapping are expected to clarify the precise cortical area that is stimulated and possibly indicate other potential targets for CS therapy. Although DBS cannot stimulate a large area of brain tissue, yet, deep structures such as the STN or thalamic nuclei can be precisely delineated by current neuro-monitoring methods and perhaps are more suitable for further exploration by DBS (Visser-Vandewalle et al 2003). New relay-nodes for DBS have been discovered rather fortuitously, e.g., DBS of the ventral capsule/ventral striatum for OCD provided prominent antidepressant effect (Greenberg et al., 2006). It should become a matter of priority, therefore, for investigation groups to provide detailed clinical and imaging information, as well as observations regarding target coordinates, lead location and clinical effectiveness; this will allow meaningful comparisons of targets and facilitate future developments. Short battery life is commonly reported in DBS studies for psychiatric disorders, implying either suboptimal targeting or that high-intensity stimulation is needed in order to produce a clinical effect. While adjustments of stimulation parameters are largely guided by experience gained in movement disorders, efforts should be directed to identifying stimulation settings individualized for each psychiatric illness in order to maximize the clinical benefits and improve acceptance of DBS as a therapeutic tool from both practitioners and patients. As research moves forward in the field, reported results should be comparable through common sets of stimulation parameters. With respect to TMS, further studies will clarify whether alternative stimulation paradigms such as theta burst stimulation (chapter 4) or priming stimulation (Iyer et al., 2003) will impact psychiatric disorders. Up to now, mostly seriously debilitated and drug-resistant psychiatric patients have been studied with TMS and DBS. In most series, efficacy of DBS is evaluated without discontinuing medications. This makes the "blindness" of studies doubtful and placebo effects possible. In the future, CS and DBS efficacy should be evaluated in the early stages of disease and in non-drug-resistant patients too and compared to patient cohorts treated only by medications. Since TMS may augment or hasten the clinical response of the patients to their medication (Fitzgerald, 2008), it would be interesting to explore possible effects of stimulation therapies on hastening the expected progress of psychiatric symptoms over time. Although DBS has been clearly associated with psychiatric symptoms such as anxiety, fear (Okun et al., 2007) and increased rates of suicide attempts (Burkhard et al., 2004) in movement disorders patients, caution should be exercised when extrapolating the above observations into psychiatry-oriented DBS practice: DBS is a safe and viable therapeutic option and should be further explored in psychiatry.

In sum, it should be clear for both practitioners and patients that invasive and noninvasive brain stimulation methods are still highly experimental and only much more work will establish them as powerful therapies for neuropsychiatric disorders. In this endeavor, it is critical to safeguard human rights and ethical rules as the future of the field is delineated. Therapeutic developments should evolve within a frame of evidence-based scientific knowledge, strict patient selection criteria and transparency in design and evaluation of clinical studies.

7. Stroke Rehabilitation

Stroke is a debilitating disorder: roughly half of all stroke victims have some degree of residual motor disability substantially affecting their daily activities, self-independence and overall quality of life (Hendricks et al., 2002). Functional recovery is mainly expected within a year after stroke; it may occur either spontaneously, possibly from partially or temporarily damaged cortical regions surrounding the stroke area, or by neurological reorganization of adjacent brain areas which take over the function of the irreversibly damaged areas. Physical therapy combined with peripheral nerve electrical stimulation is the only approved treatment for motor disability; unfortunately, many sufferers experience limited benefits at the end of the rehabilitation program.

DBS has been used to ameliorate stroke-induced movement disorders such as tremor; to the best of our knowledge, however, it has not yet been used as a therapeutic tool or an add-on treatment in stroke rehabilitation. DBS is exerted on well-defined deep "relay-nodes"; in the post-stroke state, however, no important deep targets implicated in the regeneration process and suitable for therapeutic stimulation have been recognized yet. The disease per se extensively damages cortical and white matter pathways rather than specific brain nuclei; our limited understanding of the mechanisms of neuroplasticity may account for the investigators' reluctance to offer DBS in stroke patients.

CS has been introduced in stroke rehabilitation on the basis of its efficacy in modulating neuroplasticity and enhancing motor performance (Hummel and Cohen, 2005). Extradural MI ECS has been reported to improve motor recovery after stroke (chapter 15); however, the invasive character of the method, the uncertainty regarding potential MI ECS interferences with the natural recovery processes and the overall high cost remain considerable limitations for its wider use as an adjunctive neurorehabilitation treatment. Moreover, in a phase III study enrolling 164 patients with chronic stroke, MI ECS plus rehabilitation therapy did not provide improved motor status as compared to rehabilitation therapy alone (Levy et al., 2008). Reasons can be adduced to explain such failure (chapter 15B).

CS by implantable devices grew out of TMS(<1Hz/inhibitory and >10Hz/excitatory) and tDCS (anodal/excitatory and cathodal/inhibitory) studies (chapter 14). The concept of "interhemispheric rivalry" in the motor areas between the stroke-injured and the non-injured hemisphere has been a key hypothesis in reported series (chapter 14 and Talleli and Rothwell 2006; but see Lotze et al., 2006). Motor impairments are supposed to be elicited by reduced output of the injured hemisphere and/or increased inhibitory activity of the non-injured hemisphere over the injured hemisphere. Both the stroke-affected and non-affected hemispheres have been stimulated variably in an effort to improve recovery from post-stroke motor impairments. Both TMS and tDCS have been offered in single or multiple sessions in order either to enhance the function of the injured hemisphere or to inhibit the non-injured hemisphere; the functional improvement ranged between 10-20% (Chapter 14 and Talelli and Rothwell 2006). Notably, TMS-induced improvements were also noted in stroke victims suffering from aphasia or visuospatial neglect (chapter 14).

CS vs. DBS: Considerations, Limitations and Future Prospects

DBS has been offered only in post-stroke tremor or hemiballism (Wichmann and Delong 2006) and thus the discussion can only be limited to CS. To date, TMS treatment has been offered only to small series of patients with subcortical lesions and rather mild motor impairment. To improve recovery by CS, it is important to define selection criteria to identify stroke patients most likely to benefit; several clinical parameters need to be defined including the somatic distribution and severity of the motor impairment and the type of brain lesion (cortical, subcortical or deep). It is mandatory to define, by means of randomized controlled studies, which type of intervention is more suitable for each type of stroke and each type of patient, taking into account the size and location of the lesion and the interval from stroke. The hand area has been the most targeted cortical region. The availability of tests evaluating hand performance, the accessibility of the hand cortical area, and the high incidence of residual hand motor deficits after stroke explain the above preference over other cortical regions. rTMS, however, has also provided moderate to good recovery of gait when the leg motor cortex was targeted (chapter 14). Clarification of whether stimulation of the ipsilesional, contralesional or both cerebral hemispheres provides the best recovery is mandatory. After stroke, functional magnetic resonance imaging (fMRI) can effectively locate the hand motor region or other brain regions with residual function and discriminate between the affected and non-affected brain areas which could offer better functional recovery when stimulated. An interesting feature is the feasibility of combining neuroimaging studies with TMS-induced motor-evoked potentials, in order to determine the degree of functional recovery and guide the stimulation dose (Cramer 2008). TMS is offered within the first year after stroke, but the best interval to stimulate the motor cortex remains unknown. rTMS has been tested in patients after the first year, after the conventional rehabilitation had been completed and the motor impairments were considered permanent; improvements in motor performance of paretic extremities were reported even five years after stroke (Mally and Dinya, 2008). TMS induced neuroregeneration in a Parkinsonian animal model (Arrias-Carrion et al., 2004); however, such a role in stroke remains speculative. It is important, therefore, to explore whether CS or DBS can influence processes such as synapse formation and outgrowth and, hence, could be used in neural regeneration and development. Future studies including larger series of patients with various degrees of severity of symptoms in both early and late stages of the disease are expected to clarify key interactions between CS efficacy and type of lesion, laterality of symptoms, time since stroke, stimulation algorithms, duration of stimulation, and stimulation combined with other forms of neurorehabilition.

One recent development might improve the prospects of this therapy, according to Canavero (personal communication). A recently developed neurochip (Jackson et al., 2006) creates an artificial connection between two sites in MI by using action potentials recorded on one electrode to trigger electrical stimuli delivered to another, in a chronically implanted array, over the long-term. Once configured, it operates autonomously. It can induce changes mediated by hebbian mechanisms by delivering stimuli within 50 ms (20 ms best) of recorded spikes. The linkage is explained by potentiation of horizontal pathways within MI and in cases of partial injury this could strengthen surviving projections between sites connected by the prosthesis.

At present, CS for neurorehabilitation should be considered as a highly experimental, but potentially effective method that holds great promise for functional improvement of otherwise treatment-refractory stroke sufferers. CS has the potential to address the multifaceted clinical profile of stroke that includes motor, sensory, cognitive and psychiatric impairments, and favor the rehabilitation outcome of various components of stroke.

Limits

Compared to other neurosurgical procedures, both CS and DBS, are minimally invasive and associated with low complication rates. The stimulation can be programmed to meet patient's needs or discontinued in case of undesirable effects or ineffectiveness. Yet, there is neither agreement on which targets should be stimulated in order to obtain maximum clinical benefit for each neurological or psychiatric disorder, nor sufficiently standardized stimulation protocols. These procedures have further limitations.

1. Resources and Personnel

Both DBS and CS require expensive high-technology equipment including frame-based stereotaxis or frameless neuronavigation, respectively, and multidisciplinary teams consisting of neurosurgeons, neurophysiologists, movement disorder neurologists, pain therapists, neuropsychologists, experienced technicians and specially-trained nurses. One key difference is that DBS for movement disorders requires the close collaboration of a neurologist-neurophysiologist during surgery, unless it is performed without microrecordings monitoring and intraoperative clinical testings. Conversely, in CS, the intraoperative collaboration of a neurologist is not usually necessary, unless meticulous awake mapping is considered essential for the success of the procedure. Both TMS and tDCS are dependent on high-technology equipment, advanced neuroimaging studies for identifying optimal targets, and experienced teams: although they may evolve into powerful predicting tools of efficacy of implantable CS, their therapeutic potential has not been elucidated yet.

2. Preoperative Evaluation

The application of DBS is restricted by certain technical limitations: a) current imaging technology is still subject to spatial and geometrical distortions and b) the reproducibility and uniformity among different imaging systems and devices varies considerably. This makes high accuracy problematic and the comparison of data from different groups very difficult. In CS, an important limitation is the difficulty in the precise identification of the cortical areas in the single individual, given the huge inter-subject variability. Various techniques have been used to ensure accurate cortical targeting including fMRI, TMS and PET fused with neuronavigation data and combined with intraoperative neurophysiological recordings (sensory and motor evoked potentials, bipolar extradural stimulation). FMRI, though, has limitations: 1) cerebral areas are variably activated depending on task performance and individual thresholding, 2) large draining veins, motion artifacts, and echo planar images compromise accuracy, 3) activation protocols are not yet standardized, 4) cortical activity is hard to detect within the fissures, and 5) often, the examination must be repeated due to lack of patient's cooperation. Intraoperative neurophysiological mapping too requires local anesthesia and a larger craniotomy and may not be well tolerated by chronic pain sufferers or elderly patients.

3. Electrode-tissue Interface

Deeply implanted DBS electrodes are in contact with the brain, i.e., there is a direct interface of the electrode with the neural tissue, which is not the case for extradural CS; however, alterations in the impedance due to the thickness of the underlying dura or cerebrospinal fluid (CSF) can affect the stimulation results (Manola and Holsheimer, 2007). Subdural CS, like DBS, is interfaced with neural tissue, but given its low overall efficacy and association with such complications as cortical lesions, bleeding, CSF leakage, seizures, secondary gliosis and scar tissue formation, it is rarely used. However, the interdural placement of the electrode (Sakas et al., 2008a) in a "patch-like" fashion might prove an effective alternative option to standard extradural and subdural cortical stimulation techniques.

4. Electrode Design and Stimulation Delivery

The stimulation of more extensive cortical zones by implanting multiple electrode arrays may improve clinical results. An important issue is whether the electrodes with a single array of stimulating poles should be replaced by electrodes with a double- or triple-array of stimulating poles. The three-array electrode (Lamitrode, ANS, Plano, Texas, US) may improve efficacy (figure 1), as it is supposed to deliver a better targeted "wedge-shaped" stimulation which, when necessary, can be offered in an alternating "sweeping" mode. It is also important to establish whether it is preferable to perform bipolar versus monopolar stimulation and what are the most effective electrical stimulation algorithms. The stimulation efficacy could also be affected by other parameters, such as the position of the electrode (perpendicular or parallel to the central sulcus) and the lack of precision in positioning or securing the electrode over the cortex.

5. Patient's Clinical Condition

DBS and CS call for mentally and physically able patients to undergo the demanding preoperative clinical assessments and to attend the postoperative follow-up sessions during the period of titration of the stimulation parameters. However, a considerable percentage of sufferers are excluded from DBS due to advanced age (usually more than 70 years), brain atrophy, cognitive impairment, psychiatric symptoms and medical co-morbidities. In DBS, there is a small (1-3%), but considerable risk of hardware- or surgery-related complications (intracerebral hemorrhage, seizures, infection), plus stimulation-related neuropsychiatric effects, such as apathy, hallucinations, cognitive dysfunction, decline in executive functions, depression, and even suicide attempts. CS is better tolerated because it is unilateral, does not involve penetration of brain tissue with all its associated risks (hematoma, contusion, parenchymal infection) and the risk of intracerebral hemorrhage is virtually non-existent; the risk of seizures is related to the stimulation parameters and usually controlled with changes in programming. In DBS, however, the risk of seizures may be related to the intraparenchymal presence of the electrode *per se* and, therefore, not easily corrected by better programming only.

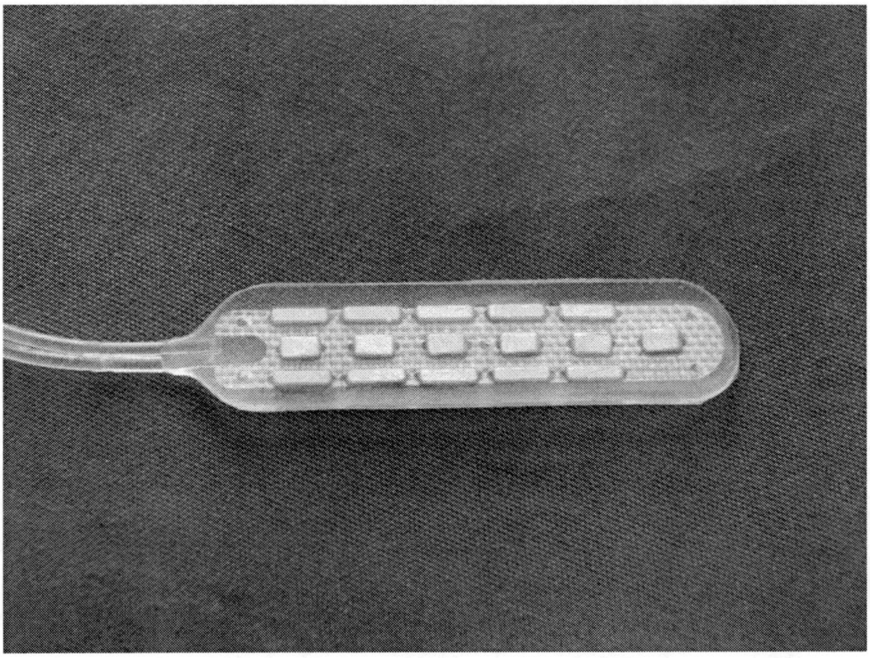

Figure 1. The three-array electrode (Lamitrode, ANS, Plano, Texas, US) offers the option of delivering "wedge-shaped" stimulation in an alternating "sweeping" mode. Such a stimulation type is expected to achieve a better targeted stimulation focus and maximize clinical benefits.

6. Device Features

Given the widespread appreciation of its unfulfilled potential, improvements and refinements in CS electrodes should be anticipated, whereas the more established and widespread use of the electrodes creates a lesser industrial incentive for development and refinement of the current quadripolar systems for DBS. Nevertheless, a higher number of poles would allow more refined stimulation. All current implantable devices for brain stimulation are susceptible to and interfere with magnetic environmental fields and they have not been cleared for safety in high-field (3-Tesla) MRI scanners. This is a problem that must be addressed by the device industry. As concerns the noninvasive technology, major shortcomings are the cost, the lack of portability of most machines that makes its routine use not easy, the patient's discomfort for certain stimulation algorithms and the difficulty to conduct blinded studies. tDCS has promise over tTMS, because the required equipment is less expensive, the technique is easier in application and maintenance, the stimulators can be battery-driven and are portable, the modulatory effect appears to last longer, and sham-stimulation is easily implemented as patients are unable to detect stimulation.

In Conclusion

a. Only well-structured and controlled clinical trials of rTMS and tDCS will verify their therapeutic potential and justify the enthusiasm generated by their introduction in clinical practice. At present, noninvasive brain stimulation methods have a strong potential for predicting a positive response to implantable CS and guide patient selection, timing of intervention and type of stimulation.
b. CS by implantable devices appears to be a promising and effective treatment modality for several neurological conditions. However, the clinical effectiveness of CS may wane over time and the long-term benefits may become less pronounced. There is a large inter-individual variability in terms of response to stimulation (in some cases leading to excitation, in others to inhibition, but a similar final result, e.g. analgesia). Moreover, some individuals on fMRI show pure SI activation during a motor task and in such patients SI must be engaged, not MI. This inconsistency of the effect and unpredictability of the outcome makes surgeons and neurologists hesitant to propose the procedure to patients. It is important to define -and possibly standardize- optimal cortical mapping, ideal targeting and protocols of programming in order for CS to become a first line treatment for neuropsychiatric disorders. Although DBS plays a starring role in the management of PD and other neurological disorders, implantable CS presents certain significant advantages, such as a lack of requirement for a stereotactic frame, close to nil risk of intracerebral hemorrhage, less invasiveness, better acceptability to both patients and neurologists, and the availability of a noninvasive preoperative predictive test.

Future Prospects

An exciting frontier is the development of the capability to artificially relay environmental sensory information by CS implants, i.e., relay of hearing or visual information, directly into the human brain. From a strict anatomical and surgical safety perspective, the cerebral cortex is likely to be a much more attractive implantation site compared to the brainstem, basal ganglia or other deep brain sites. However, one of the most difficult aspects of this work is the encoding of environmental sound or vision into parameters of electrical stimulation applicable to the cortex in order to convey the information. Research has shown that patients with profound auditory loss can discriminate between electrical stimuli based on the differences in the parameters of the stimulation current with the level of the electric current, being correlated to sound loudness and the frequency of the electric current to sound pitch. Following this discovery and taking advantage of the human's discriminatory ability, it became possible to design and build effective speech processors; these devices receive input from an external microphone and then electrically encode this acoustic information in a manner specifically designed to exploit the patient's ability to perceive differences in certain electrical stimulus parameters. On this basis, a *cortical auditory neural prosthesis* becomes possible (Howard et al., 2000). However, one of the most ambitious goals is the transmission of visual perception by cortical stimulation electrodes into the visual cortex of blind volunteers, i.e., a *cortical visual prosthesis* (chapter 22).

It is encouraging that the cerebral cortex seems to have the ability to adapt and to interpret in efficient manner electrical information that is applied in the right sequences and within a proper range of stimulation parameters by a large cortical-intracortical array. A relevant and important finding is that deaf patients do not appear to sustain deafferentation changes that would preclude the ''reactivation'' of normal auditory processing by the prosthetic stimulation device (Howard et al 2000) and a similar phenomenon could be expected to occur in the visual cortex and pathways of blind patients (chapter 22). A significant discovery that resulted from this research is that penetrating electrodes into the cerebral cortex are greatly superior in delivering more precisely the electrical stimulation compared to those electrodes that are placed in contact with the cortical surface. This opens the possibility of another field of therapeutic cortical stimulation namely *deep cortical* or *subcortical stimulation* (via an array of penetrating recording and stimulating electrodes), to be distinguished from both surface cortical stimulation (extradural or subdural) and DBS.

Computational neuromodulation is a field of computational biology dedicated to the study of the biophysical and mathematical characteristics of the electrochemical modulation in the nervous system. It is widely acknowledged that all types of networks and neurons (motor, sensory, and interneurons) are subject to modulation. Modulation may be induced in a circuit either extrinsically or intrinsically by circuit neurons or neural fibers (Fellous and Linster, 1998) or by artifical (manufactured) projecting systems or interfaces, including CS and DBS, with the aim to mimic "natural" neuromodulation. Given the complexity, convergence and divergence of neuromodulation in nature, the computational approach may provide a deeper understanding and the foundation for refined clinical applications. Areas amenable to computational analysis include synaptic drive, synaptic efficacy, and sensory encoding (Hille, 2001). With such approaches, altering the intrinsic properties of neurons, change their time-course, voltage-dependence and synaptic conductance and the strength of synaptic connections may become feasible. A single membrane current could be influenced and, depending on the conductance of the neuron membrane, a neuron brought across the boundaries of different behavior (Hille, 2001; Marder and Thirumalai, 2002). Furthermore, on the basis of current progress in computational biology, it is important to explore whether CS or DBS could be used in order: a) to offer a short synaptic input that can ''jump start'' a circuit, b) to influence the encoding of sensory information in spike trains, or c) to reconfigure an anatomically defined network into a different functional circuit by altering the intrinsic properties or the synaptic strength of the neurons within the network. Extrinsic modulation in particular (either natural or by implanted CS or DBS devices), could potentially be used to tune and configure whole networks and organize ensembles of circuits (Katz, 1995), in order to bias extensive networks or neurological systems into different functional outputs, in much the same way as changing parameters in a network model should bias or modify the output of the network (Marder and Tiramulai, 2002). Computer models of the bioelectrical and statistical aspects of neural recording and stimulation-induced recruitment can be used to model, and decipher neural coding. For instance, hippocampal functions can be replicated with a microchip implementation of the predictive mathematical models. Advances in this field hold the promise that individuals with damaged areas of the brain could be helped by CS based on such computational methods and that the use of neural interfaces could enhance normal or impaired neural function (Berger et al 2005).

CS and DBS may be further refined by developing electrodes that monitor neuronal activity from multiple regions, generate ‘‘network level’’ representations of the brain and simultaneously stimulate, i.e., “*closed-loop*” integrated monitoring and stimulating implantable systems. In these systems, the stimulation is activated “on demand” by intrinsic signals such as specific brain activity. Hence, these devices are capable of ‘‘*responsive neurostimulation*’’. A ‘‘closed loop’’ CS or DBS could be much more effective when it is activated by, i.e. it is responsive to, control signals derived from brain or body signals. Such technologies would be useful not only for epilepsy (chapter 19), but also for, e.g., Parkinson’s disease; research has shown that intended and self-timed movements are preceded by increased activity in the parietal cortex and sensorimotor putamen (Pancrazio et al., 2006). Patients will have an advanced sensor either in contact or embedded in muscles and stimulation will be triggered by EMG signals elicited by the patient’s movement. The possibility to offer effective intermittent stimulation would provide extended battery life. Responsive direct brain stimulation carries certain advantages over other methods as treatment is provided as needed, when needed, and for the time needed. The undesired effects of chronic stimulation are reduced, habituation is minimized, and, in epilepsy, the time of stimulation is the least necessary to suppress epileptiform activity; hence, the chances of potential failure due to reorganization of the epileptogenic circuitry are minimized. Temporal and spatial specificity, however, appear to play a pivotal role in the success of responsive stimulation. It is a high priority to develop sophisticated software that will allow early detection of epileptiform activity and enhance accuracy in lead or array implantation over the epileptogenic focus or zone. It is also important to develop seizure-prediction algorithms for each sufferer and stimulation devices able to drive several multicontact leads and arrays, and offer numerous combinations of cortical, subcortical or deep brain stimulation. Finally, all this technology should be incorporated into implantable, cosmetically acceptable devices in the most clinically effective fashion.

Numerous exciting developments in *neuroengineering* and *neurotechnology* are likely to influence the future applications of both CS and DBS. Future telemetric IPGs are expected to be smaller in size, more cosmetic, contour-shaped to apply to the cranium convexity or miniaturized to be implanted through a burr hole or small craniotomy. Batteries will be based on advanced chemistry offering more power in smaller size, will be rechargeable with extended life, and capable to be connected to the electrode(s) without extension wires. Such advancements may prove particular helpful in cases of cervical dystonia where hardware-related complications are commonly encountered. A great advance will be the incorporation into DBS electrodes of *microactuators* which will enable precise implantation after the initial insertion. This will reduce substantially the operating time, since fine adjustments for maximizing the clinical effect or minimizing untoward sequelae will be easier to carry out, at a later stage, rather than in the operating theatre. The construction of ‘‘*smart stimulators*’’ with the capability for dynamic internal adjustments will refine CS and DBS practice (Pancrazio et al 2006). Sophisticated software with advanced graphics for precise electrode insertion and for programming the stimulation in both CS and DBS procedures is expected to optimize pole selection after permanent implantation, individualize stimulation parameters and maximize clinical efficacy. Notably, such advanced software programs that combine MRI, CT, three-dimensional (3-D) brain atlases and neurophysiological microelectrode recording data with the volume of brain tissue activated by DBS have already been tested in preliminary studies (Miocinovic et al 2007; Butson et al 2007). Finally, the ability to program stimulation devices through remote access, telephone lines or via the Internet may render patients independent from the reference center and lessen the number of required follow-up visits. Sensitive, highly specific sensors which can be applied on the skin and detect physiological biosignals (e.g., changes in the heart rate, skin temperature, respiration rate, eyelid closure, EMG) are in development, and so are implantable chronic recording microelectrode arrays incorporating on board amplification, spike detection and wireless transmission of data and power (Pancrazio et al., 2006).

Finally, brain computer interfaces (BCI), defined as an electronic brain implant that translates the intention "to either communicate or move" into "communication or movement" through computer cursors, robotic devices or into actual movement of paralyzed limbs, represent the next opportunity to integrate CS and DBS into a larger clinical perspective. A BCI can detect changes in the user's brain activity and convert them into commands for a computer application. This is achieved through the application of signal processing techniques to the signals that the patient is still able to control. The key element in a BCI is a decoding algorithm that converts the main electrophysiological signal into an output that is suitable to control an external device. The interfaces rely on the natural adaptive ability of the human brain. The users have to learn to adapt their biological response, i.e., change the amplitude or frequency of the signal monitored. BCI technology will open new possibilities for severely disabled humans and offer systems that will deliver "communication or action" based on data derived from incorporated cortical monitoring and stimulation systems (Angelakis et al., 2007; Warwick et al., 2006). In this regard, the development of miniaturized, multi-functional, chronic neural implants *(BioMicroElectro-Mechanical Systems or Bio MEMS)* aims to obtain and control signals extracted from neuronal activity in order to enhance residual capabilities or perform actions such as moving a prosthetic arm with near natural performance. *Microelectrode arrays* are special types of micro-hardware constructed by using microfabrication and microelectronics by thin film-based planar and 3D-arrays of substrate microelectrodes. *Hybrid neural interfaces* or *cultured neural probes* can be coupled in vitro to populations of cultured neurons (Sanguineti et al 2003), where each electrode is covered and surrounded by a locally confined network of cultured neurons, obtained by chemical patterning of the substrate. These microsystems are designed to make connections and communicate with regenerating neurons and can be intended as hybrid neural information prosthetic transducers for stimulation and/or recording of neural activity in the brain or the spinal cord (Rutten et al., 2007).

Any neurological disorder that has altered electrical conductivity could potentially be helped by nanomaterials (Webster et al., 2004), which interact much more closely with cells than currently available materials. Carbon nanofibers can act as minimally traumatic CNS electrodes and carbon nanofibers arrays are expected to increase the accuracy of cerebral electrical stimulation. With such technology, our ability to offer complex, but precise patterns of stimulation may be enhanced; it will become possible to perform not only electrical microrecording, but also electrochemical recording and stimulation (Li and Andrews, 2007).

Neuromimetic or neuromorphic engineering, in which very large scale integration (VLSI) systems containing electronic analog circuits mimic the architecture and design of biological nervous systems in order to replicate their function, e.g., vision or hearing (Silver et al., 2007; Smith and Hamilton, 1999) may one day be integrated into CS or DBS.

Conclusion

Currently, the main indication of CS is central and trigeminal neuropathic pains. In the coming years, PD, dystonia, epilepsy, and psychiatric disorders are likely to become established indications for CS as well. Undoubtedly, CS will also play a starring role in neurorehabilitation, facing the great challenge of inducing movement in paretic extremities and releasing medically-refractory spasticity even years after stroke. The future of CS will be influenced greatly by increased awareness and understanding of existing indications and applications, improved case selection, introduction of new indications, more mature assessment of outcome and convincing evidence regarding efficacy (Simpson, 2006b). A deeper understanding of mechanisms of action will allow us to answer critical questions regarding type of stimulation (extradural, subdural or interdural), mode of stimulation (anodal or cathodal), specific sets of effective stimulation algorithms for each neurological or psychiatric condition, and prediction of degree and duration of expected clinical benefit. Certainly, the ability of unilateral CS to influence brain activity bilaterally, be it pain, PD or stroke, is a major advantage over DBS. Great advancements are likely to take place in the field of responsive CS, which will particularly impact young patients suffering from progressive disabling disease, such as epilepsy or dystonia. CS also holds the potential to enhance cognitive performances (Topper et al., 1998; Olivieri et al., 2001; Boroojerdi et al., 2001; Montes et al., 2002) and should be explored for dementia (Canavero S, personal communication). CS is a high-technology dependent field that will be largely influenced by forthcoming neuroengineering developments and a shift away from the current dependence on pharmacological treatment. A big challenge will be to integrate CS technology with relevant advancements in human neurobiology, neuroplasticity, and neural repair, as well as to explore the potential neuroprotective effects of CS. Current implantable CS devices may need to be redesigned in order to incorporate complex and intelligent miniaturized systems and sophisticated software which will enable them to integrate information exchange between the device and the patient's brain, while remaining cost-effective. Progress in microsystems technologies, microelectronics, nanotechnologies, and computer modelling software are likely to create new opportunities for developing advanced stimulation systems and for expanding the therapeutic potential of CS.

References

Ackermans L Temel Y, Cath D, et al. Deep brain stimulation in Tourette's syndrome: two targets? *Mov Disord* 2006;21:709-13.

Aleman A, Sommer IE, Kahn RS. Efficacy of slow repetitive transcranial magnetic stimulation in the treatment of resistant auditory hallucinations in schizophrenia: a meta-analysis. *J Clin Psychiatr* 2007;68:416-21.

Andrade DM, Zumsteg D, Hamani C, et al. Long-term follow-up of patients with thalamic deep brain stimulation for epilepsy. *Neurology* 2006;66:1571-3.

Angelakis E, Hatzis A, Panourias IG, Sakas DE. Brain computer interfaces: a reciprocal self-regulated neuromodulation. *Acta Neurochir Suppl* 2007;97(2):555-9.

Arrias-Carrion O, Verdugo-Diaz L, Feria-Velasco A. Neurogenesis in the subventricular zone following transcranial magnetic stimulation and nigrostriatal lesions. *J Neurosci Res* 2004;78:16-28.

Bartsch T, Pinsker MO, Rasche D, et al. Hypothalamic deep brain stimulation for cluster headache: experience from a new multicase series. *Cephalalgia* 2008;28:285-95.

Been G, Ngo TT, Miller SM, Fitzgerald PB. The use of t DCS and CVS as methods of noninvasive brain stimulation. *Brain Res Rev* 2007;56:346-61.

Benabid AL, Koudsie A, Benazzouz A, et al. Deep brain stimulation of the corpus luysi (subthalamic nucleus) and other targets in Parkinson's disease: extension to new indications such as dystonia and epilepsy. *J Neurol* 2001;248(Suppl 3):III37-47.

Benabid A-L, Pollak P, Gao D, et al. Chronic electrical stimulation of the ventralis intermedius nucleus of the thalamus as a treatment of movement disorders *J Neurosurg* 1996;84:203-14.

Bendok B, Levy RM. Brain stimulation for persistent pain management. In: Gildenberg PL, Tasker RR, editors. *Textbook of stereotactic and functional neurosurgery*. New York: McGraw Hill; 1998. p.1539.

Berger TW, Ahuja A, Courellis SH, Deadwyler SA, Erinjippurath G, Gerhardt GA et al. Restoring lost cognitive function. *IEEE Engl Med Biol Mag* 2005;24:30-44.

Boggio PS, Rigonatti SP, Ribeiro RB, et al. A randomized, double-blind clinical trial on the efficacy of cortical direct current stimulation for the treatment of major depression. *Int J Neuropsychopharmacol* 2007;11:173-83.

Boroojerdi B, Phipps M, Kopylev L, Wharton CM, Cohen LG, Grafman J. enhancing analogic reasoning with rTMS over the left prefrontal cortex. *Neurology* 2001; 56: 526-528

Breit S, Schultz JB, Benabid A-L. Deep brain stimulation. *Cell Tissue Res* 2004;318:275-8.

Burchiel K. Deep brain stimulation for chronic pain: the results of two multi-center trials and a structured review. *Pain Med* 2001;2:177.

Burkhard PR, Vingerhoets FJ, Berney A, et al. Suicide after successful deep brain stimulation for movement disorders. *Neurology* 2004;63:2170-2.

Butson CR, Noecker AM, Maks CB, McIntyre CC. StimExplorer: deep brain stimulation parameter selection software system. *Acta Neurochir Suppl* 2007;97(2):569-74.

Byl N, Wilson F, Merzenich M, Melnick M, Scott P, Oakes A, McKenzie A. Sensory dysfunction associated with repetitive strain injuries of tendinitis and focal hand dystonia: a comparative study. *J Orthop Sports Phys Ther* 1996;23:234-44.

Canavero S, Bonicalzi V. Cortical stimulation for central pain. *J Neurosurg* 1995;83:1117.

Canavero S and Paolotti R. Extradural motor cortex stimulation for advanced Parkinson's disease: case report. *Mov Disord* 2000;15:169-71.

Canavero S, Paolotti R, Bonicalzi V, et al. Extradural motor cortex stimulation for advanced Parkinson's disease: report of two cases. *J Neurosurg* 2002;97:1208-11.

Canavero S, Bonicalzi V. Extradural cortical stimulation for movement disorders. *Acta Neurochir Suppl* 2007a;97(2):223-32.

Canavero S, Bonicalzi V. Extradural cortical stimulation for central pain. *Acta Neurochir* Suppl 2007b;97(2):27-36

Canavero S, Bonicalzi V. *Central pain sindrome*. New York: Cambridge University Press, 2007

Canavero S, Bonicalzi V. Central pain sindrome: elucidation of genesis and treatment. *Exp Rev Neurother* 2007; 7: 1485-1497

Chabadres S, Kahane P, Minotti L, Koudsie A, Hirsch E, Benabid A-L. Deep brain stimulation in epilepsy with particular reference to the subthalamic nucleus. *Epileptic Disord* 2002;4 (Suppl 3): S83-S93.

Chkhenkeli SA, Chkhenkeli IS. Effects of therapeutic stimulation of nucleus caudatus on epileptic electrical activity of brain in patients with intractable epilepsy. *Stereotact Funct Neurosurg* 1997;69:221-4.

Chkhenkeli SA, Sramka M, Lortkipanidze GS, et al. Electrophysiological effects and clinical results of direct brain stimulation for intractable epilepsy. *Clin Neurol Neurosurg* 2004;106:318-29.

Cioni B, Meglio M, Perotti V, De Bonis P, Montano N. Neurophysiological aspects of chronic motor cortex stimulation. *Clin Neurophysiol* 2007;37:441-7.

Classen J. Focal hand dystonia-a disorder of neuroplasticity? *Brain* 2003;126:2571-2.

Cooper IS, Amin I, Gilman S. The effect of chronic cerebellar stimulation upon epilepsy in man. *Trans Am Neurol Assoc* 1973;98:192-6.

Cramer SC. Repairing the human brain after stroke. II. Restorative therapies. *Ann Neurol* 2008;63:549-60.

Cruccu G, Aziz TZ, Garcia-Larrea L, et al. EFNS guidelines on neurostimulation therapy for neuropathic pain. *Eur J Neurol* 2007;14:952-70.

Derost PP, Ouchchane L, Morand D, et al. Is DBS-STN appropriate to treat severe Parkinson's disease in an elderly population? *Neurology* 2007;68:267-271.

Deuschl G, Bain P. Deep brain stimulation for tremor [correction of trauma]: patient selection and evaluation. *Mov Disord* 2002;17(Suppl 3):S102-11.

Deuschl G, Schade-Brittinger C, Krack P, et al. A randomized trail of deep-brain stimulation for Parkinson's disease. *N Engl J Med* 2006;355:896-908.

Diederich NJ, Kalteis K, Stamenkovic M, et al. Efficient internal pallidal stimulation in Gilles de la Tourette syndrome: a case report. *Mov Disord* 2005;20:1496-9.

Fabre I, Galinowski A, Oppenheim C, et al. Antidepressant efficacy and cognitive effects of repetitive transcranial magnetic stimulation in vascular depression: an open trial. *Int J Ger Psychiatr* 2004;19:833-42.

Fava M. Diagnosis and definition of treatment-resistant depression. *Biol Psychiatry* 2003;53:649-59.

Fellous J-M, Linster C. Computational models of neuromodulation. *Neural Comput* 1998;10:771-85.

Fisher RS, Uematsu S, Krauss GL, et al. Placebo-controlled pilot study of centromedian thalamic stimulation in treatment of intractable seizures. *Epilepsy Res Suppl* 1992;5:217-29.

Fitzgerald PB, Benitez J, Brown T, et al. A double-blind sham controlled trial of repetitive transcranial magnetic stimulation in the treatment of refractory auditory hallucinations. *J Clin Psychopharmacol* 2005;25:358-62.

Fitzgerald PB, Benitez J, de Castella A, Daskalakis ZJ, Brown TL, Kulkarni J. A randomized, controlled trial of sequential bilateral repetitive transcranial magnetic stimulation for treatment-resistant depression. *Am J Psychiatr* 2006;163:88-94.

Fitzgerald P. Brain stimulation techniques for the treatment of depression and other psychiatric disorders. *Australasian Psychiatr* 2008;16:183-90.

Flaherty AW, Willimas ZM, Amimovin R, et al. Deep brain stimulation of the anterior limb of internal capsule for the treatment of Tourette's syndrome: technical case report. *Neurosurgery* 2005;57(Suppl 4):E403.

Greenberg BD, Malone DA, Friehs GM, et al. Three-year outcomes in deep brain stimulation for highly resistant obsessive-compulsive disorder. *Neuropsychopharmacol* 2006;31:2384-2393.

Hallett M. Transcranial Magnetic Stimulation: a primer. *Neuron* 2007;55:187-98.

Halpern C, Urtig H, Jaggi J, Grossman M, Won M, Baltuch G. Deep brain stimulation in neurologic disorders. *Parkinsonims Relat Disord* 2007;13:1-16.

Halpern C, Samadani U, Litt BB, Jaggi JL, Baltuch GH. Deep brain stimulation for epilepsy. *Neurotherapeutics* 2008;5:59-67.

Handforth A, DeSalles AA, Krahl SE. Deep brain stimulation of the subthalamic nucleus as adjunct treatment for refractory epilepsy. *Epilepsia* 2006;47:1239-41.

Hendricks HT, van Limbeek J, Geruts AC, Zwarts MJ. Motor recovery after stroke: a systematic review of the literature. *Arch Phys Med Rehab* 2002;11:1629-1637.

Hille B. *Ion channels of excitable membranes*. 3rd edition. Mass. Sinauer Associates Inc Sunderland, 2001.

Hodaie M, Wennberg RA, Dostrovsky JO, Lozano AM. Chronic anterior thalamus stimulation for intractable epilepsy. *Epilepsia* 2002;43:603-8.

Houeto JL, Karachi C, Mallet L, Pillon B, Yelnik J, Mesnage V et al. Tourette's syndrome and deep brain stimulation. *J Neurol Neurosurg Psychiatr* 2005;76:992-5.

Howard MA, Volkov IO, Noh D, Garell C, Abbas PJ, Rubinstein JT et al. Auditory cortex neural prosthetic devices. In: *Maciunas eds. Neural prostheses. Illinois: American Association of Neurological Surgeons Publications*, Park Ridge. 2000; p. 273-286.

Hummel FC, Cohen LG. Drivers of brain plasticity. *Curr Opin Neurol.* 2005a;18:667-74.

Iadarola MJ, Gale K. Substantia nigra in GABA-mediated anticonvulsant actions. *Adv Neurol* 1982;44:343-64.

Isenberg K, Down D, Pierce K, et al. Low frequency rTMS of the right frontal cortex is as effective as high frequency rTMS of the left frontal cortex for antidepressant-free, treatment-resistant depressed patients. *Ann Clin Psychiatr* 2005;17:153-9.

Iyer MB, Schleper N, Wassermann EM. Priming stimulation enhances the derpessant effect of low-frequency repetitive transcranial magnetic stimulation. *J Neurosci* 2003;23:10867-72.

Jackson A, Mavoori J, Fetz EE. Long-term motor cortex plasticity induced by an electronic neural implant. *Nature* 444 56-60 2006.

Jimenez F, Velasco F, Salin-Pascual R, Hernandez JA, Velasco M, Criales JL, Nicolini H. A patient with a resistant major depression disorder treated with deep brain stimulation in the inferior thalamic peduncle. *Neurosurgery* 2005;57:585-93.

Jorge RE, Robinson RG, Tateno K, et al. Repetitive transcranial magnetic stimulation as treatment of post-stroke depression: a preliminary study. *Biol Psychiatr* 2004;55:398-405.

Katayama Y, Oshima H, Fukaya C, Kawamata T, Yamamoto T. Congrol of post-stroke movement disorders using chronic motor cortex stimulation. *Acta Neurochir Suppl* 2002;79:89-92.

Katz PS. Ion channels of excitable membres. *Curr Opin Neurobiol* 1995;5:799-808.

Kern DS, Kumar R. Deep brain stimulation. *The Neurologist* 2007;13:237-252.

Kerrigan JF, Litt B, Fisher RS, et al. Electrical stimulation of the anterior nucleus of the thalamus for the treatment of intractable epilepsy. *Epilepsia* 2004;45:346-354.

Kiss ZH, Doig-Beyaert K, Eliasziw M, et al. The Canadian multicentre study of deep brain stimulation for cervical dystonia. *Brain* 2007;130:2879-86.

Kitagawa M, Murata J, Uesugi H, et al. Two-year follow-up of chronic stimulation of the posterior subthalamic white matter for tremor-dominant Parkinson's disease. *Neurosurgery* 2005;2005;56:281-9.

Kleiner-Fisman G. Herzog J, Fisman DN, et al. Subthalamic nucleus deep brain stimulation: summary and meta-analysis of outcomes. *Mov Disord* 2006;21(Suppl /14):S290-S304.

Krack P, Batir A, Van Blercom N, et al. Five-year follow-up of bilateral stimulation of the subthalamic nucleus in advanced Parkinson's disease. *N Engl J Med* 2003;349:1925-34.

Krauss JK, Pohle T, Weber S, Ozdoba C, Burgunder JM. Bilateral stimulation of globus pallidus internus for treatment of cervical dystonia. *Lancet* 1999;354:837-8.

Krauss JK. Deep brain stimulation for dystonia in adults. Overview and developments. *Stereotact Funct Neurosurg*. 2002;78:168-82.

Krauss JK, Loher TJ, Weigel R, Capelle HH, Weber S, Burgunder JM. Chronic stimulation of the globus pallidus internus for treatment of non-dYT1 generalized dystonia and choreoathetosis: 2-year follow up. *J Neurosurg*. 2003;98:785-92.

Kumar K, Toth C, Nath RK. Deep brain stimulation for intractable pain: a 15-year experience. *Neurosurgery* 1997;40:736-46.

Kumar R, Lozano AM, Sime E, et al. Comparative effects of unilateral and bilateral subthalamic nucleus deep brain stimulation. *Neurology* 1999;53:561-6.

Kumar R, Lozano AM, Sime E, Lang AE. Long-term follow-up of thalamic deep brain stimulation for essential and parkinsonian tremor. *Neurology* 2003;61:1601-04.

Kwan P, Brodie MJ. Early identification of refractory epilepsy. *N Engl J Med* 2000;342:314-9.

Levy RM, Lamb S, Adams JE. Treatment of chronic pain by deep brain stimulation: long-term follow-up and review of the literature. *Neurosurgery* 1987;21:885-93.

Levy R, Benson R, Winstein C, for the Everest Study Investigators. Cortical stimulation for upper-extremity hemiparesis from ischemic stroke: Everest Study primary endpoint results. *International Stroke Conference*, New Orleans, LA, February 20-22, 2008.

Li J, Andrews RJ. Trimodal nanoelectrode array for precise deep brain stimulation: prospects of a new technology based on carbon nanofiber arrays. *Acta Neurochir* Suppl 2007;97(2):537-46.

Lima MC, Fregni F. Motor cortex stimulation for chronic pain. Systematic review and meta-analysis of the literature. *Neurology* 2008;70:2329-37.

Loher TJ, Capelle HH, Kaelin-Lang A, et al. Deep brain stimulation for dystonia: outcome at long-term follow-up. *J Neurol* 2008; 255: 881-884

Lotze M, Markert J, Sauseng P, et al. The role of multiple contralesional motor areas for complex hand movements after internal capsular lesion. *J Neurosci* 2006;26:6096-6102.

Macdonell RA, Curatolo JM, Berkovic SF. Transcranial magnetic stimulation and epilepsy. *J Clin Neurophysiol* 2002;19:294-306.

Mally J, Dinya E. Recovery of motor disability and spasticity in post-stroke after repetitive transcranial magnetic stimulation (rTMS*). Brain Res Bull* 2008;75:388-95.

Manola L, Holsheimer J: Motor cortex stimulation: role of computer modelling. In: Sakas DE and Simpson B, editors. *Operative Neuromodulation: Neural Networks Surgery* (Vol. II). New York: Springer-Verlag; 2007, 497-503.

Mantovani A, Lisanby SH, Pieraccini F, Ulivelli M, Castrogiovanni P, Rossi S. Repetitive transcranial magnetic stimulation in the treatment of obsessive-compulsive disorder and Tourette's syndrome. *Int J Neuropsychopharmacol* 2006;9:95-100.

Mantovani A, Leckman JF, Grantz H, King RA, Sporn AL, Lisanby SH. Repetitive transcranial magnetic stimulation of the supplementary motor area in the treatment of Tourette's syndrome: report of two cases. *Clin Neurophysiol* 2007a;118:2314-5.

Mantovani A, Lisanby SH, Pieraccini F, Ulivelli M, Castrogiovanni P, Rossi S. Repetitive transcranial magnetic stimulation in the treatment of panic disorder with comorbid major depression. *J Affect Disord* 2007b;102:277-80.

Marangell LB, Martinez M, Jrdi RA, Zboyan H. Neurostimulation therapies in depression: a review of new modalities. *Acta Psychiatr Scand* 2007;116:174-81.

Marder E, Thiramulai V. Cellular, synaptic and network effects of neuromodulation. *Neural Netw* 2002;15:479-93.

Mayberg HS, Lozano AM, Voon V, et al. Deep brain stimulation for treatment-resistant depression. *Neuron* 2005;45:651-60.

Mink JW, Walkup J, Frey KA, et al. Patient selection and assessment recommendations for deep brain stimulation in Tourette syndrome. *Mov Disord* 2006;21:1831-8.

Miocinovic S, Noecker AM, Maks CB, Butson CR, McIntyre CC. Cicerone: stereotactic neurophysiological recording and deep brain stimulation electrode placement software system. *Acta Neurochir* Suppl 2007;97(2):569-74.

Montes C Mertens P Convers P Peyron R Sindou M Laurent B Mauguiere F Garcia-Larrea L Cognitive effects of precentral cortical stimulation for pain control: an ERP study, *Neurophysiol. Clin./Clin. Nurophysiol* 2002 ; 32 : 313-325

Mueller J, Skogseid IM, Benecke R, , et al. Pallidal deep brain stimulation improves quality of life in segmental and generalized dystonia: results from a prospective, randomized sham-controlled trial. *Mov Disord.* 2008;23:131-4.

Munchau A, Bloem BR, Thilo KV, Trimble MR, Rothwell JC, Robertson MM. Repetitive transcranial magnetic stimulation for Tourette syndrome. *Neurology* 2002;59:1789-91.

Murata J, Kitagawa M, Uesugi H, et al. Electrical stimulation of the posterior subthalamic area for the treatment of intractable proximal tremor. *J Neurosurg* 2003;99:708-15.

Murase N, Rothwell JC, Kaji R, et al. Subthreshold low-frequency repetitive transcranial magnetic stimulation over the premotor cortex modulates writer's cramp. *Brain* 2005;128:104-15.

Nandi D, Liu X, Winter JL, Aziz TZ, Stein JF. Deep brain stimulation of the peduculopontine region in the normal non-human primate. *J Clin Neurosci* 2002a;9:170-4.

Nandi D, Chir M, Liu X, et al. Electrophysiological confirmation of the zona incerta as a target for surgical treatment of disabling involuntary arm movements in multiple sclerosis: use of local field potentials. *J Clin Neurosci* 2002b;9:64-8.

Nuttin BJ, Gabriels LA, Cosyns PR. Long-term electrical capsular stimulation in patients with obsessive-compulsive disorder. *Neurosurg* 2003;52:1263-72.

OCD-DBS Collaborative Group. Deep brain stimulation for psychiatric disorders. *Neurosurgery* 2002;51:519.

Oh MY, Abosch A, Kim SH, Lang AE, Lozano AM. Long-term hardware-related complications of deep brain stimulation. *Neurosurgery* 2002;50:1268-74.

Oikawa H, Sasaki M, Tamakawa Y, Kamei A. The circuit of Papez in mesial temporal sclerosis: MRI. *Neuroradiology* 2001;43:205-10.

Okun MS, Mann G, Foote KD, et al. Deep brain stimulation in the internal capsule and nucleus accumbens region: responses observed during active and sham programming. *J Neurol Neurosurg Psychiatry* 2007;78:310-4.

Olivieri M, Turriziani P, Carlesimo Ga, et al. Parieto-frontal interactions in visual-object and visual-spatial working memory: evidence from trancranial magnetic stimulation. *Cereb Cortex* 2001; 11: 606-618

O'Reardon JP, Solvason B, Janicak PG, et al. Efficacy and safety of transcranial magnetic stimulation in the acute treatment of major depression: A multisite randomized controlled trial. *Biol Psychiatry* 2007;62:1208-16.

Owen SL, Green AL, Nandi D, Bittar RG, Wang S, Aziz TZ. Deep brain stimulation for neuropathic pain. *Neuromodulation* 2006a;9:100-6.

Owen SL, Green AL, Stein JF, et al. Deep brain stimulation for the alleviation of post-stroke neuropathic pain. *Pain* 2006b;120:202-6.

Owen SL, Green AL, Davies P, et al. Connectivity of an effective hypothalamic surgical target for cluster headache. *J Clin Neurosci* 2007;14:955-60.

Pancrazio JJ, Chen D, Fertig SJ, et al. Towards neurotechnology innovation: report from the 2005 Neural Interfaces Workshop. An NIH-sponsored event. *Neuromodulation* 2006;9:1-7.

Picinelli M, Pini S, Bellantuono C, Wilkinson G. Efficacy of drug treatment in obsessive compulsive disorder. A meta-analysis review. *Br J Psychiatry* 1995;166:424-43.

Plaha P, Gill SS. Bilateral deep brain stimulation of the pedunculopontine nucleus for Parkinson's disease. *Neuroreport* 2005;16:1883-87.

Prikryl R, Kasparek T, Skotakova S, Ustohal L Kucerova H, Ceskova E. Treatment of negative symptoms of schizophrenia using repetitive transcranial magnetic stimulation in a double-blind, randomized controlled study. *Schizophr Res* 2007;95:151-7.

Raethjen J, Govindan RB, Kopper F, Muthuraman M, Deuschl G. Cortical involvement in the generation of essential tremor. *J Neurophysiol* 2007;97:3219-28.

Rasche D, Rinaldi PC, Young RF, Tronnier VM. Deep brain stimulation for the treatment of various chronic pain syndromes. *Neurosurg Focus* 2006;21:E8

Rauch SL Dougherty DD, Malone D, et al. A functional neuroimaging investigation of deep brain stimulation in patients with obsessive-compulsive disorder. *J Neurosurg* 2006;104:558-65.

Rezai AR, Lozano AM. Deep brain stimulation for chronic pain. In: Burchiel KJ, ed. *Surgical management of pain*. New York: Thieme; 2002. p. 565-76.

Rodriguez-Oroz MC, Obeso JA, et al. Bilateral deep brain stimulation in Parkinson's disease: a multicentre study with 4 years follow-up. *Brain* 2005;128:2240-9.

Romanelli P, Bronte-Stewart H, Courtney T, Heit G. Possible necessity for deep brain stimulation of both the ventralis intermedius and subthalamic nuclei to resolve Holmes tremor. Case report. *J Neurosurg* 2003;99:566-71.

Rutten WLC, Ruardij TG, Marani E, Roelofsen BH. Neural networks on chemically patterned electrode arrays: towards a cultured probe. *Acta Neurochir Suppl* 2007;97(2):547-54.

Sachdev PS, Loo CK, Mitchell PB, McFarquhar TF, Malhi GS. Repetitive transcranial magnetic stimulation for the treatment obsessive-compulsive disorder. A double-blind controlled investigation. *Psychol Med* 2007;37:1645-9.

Sakas DE, Panourias IG. Rostral cingulate gyrus: A putative target for deep brain stimulation in treatment-refractory depression. *Med Hypothes* 2006;66:491-4.

Sakas DE, Panourias IG, Simpson BA. An introduction to neural networks surgery, a field of neuromodulation which is based on advances in neural networks science and digitised brain imaging. *Acta Neurochir* Suppl 2007a;97(2):3-13.

Sakas DE, Panourias IG, Singounas E, Simpson BA. Neurosurgery for psychiatric disorders: from the excision of brain tissue to the chronic electrical stimulation of neural networks. In: Sakas DE, Simpson BA, editors. *Operative Neuromodulation: Neural networks surgery*. New York: Springer-Verlag; 2007b, 365-74.

Sakas DE, Panourias IG, Boviatsis ES et al. Treatment of primary camptocormia (dystonic bent spine or bent neck) by electrical stimulation of the globus pallidus internus: report of 3 cases. Abstract book, *The 8th International Neuromodulation Society and the 11th Annual Meeting of the North American Neuromodulation Society, Acapulco*, 2007, December 7-12.

Sakas DE, Flaskas P, Panourias IG, Georgakoulias N. Cortical electrical stimulation by *interdural* ("patch-like") implantation of the electrodes: a new technique for increased efficacy and safety. *Neurosurgery* 2008a (under review)

Sakas DE, Panourias IG, Boviatsis E, Themistocleous M, Stavrinou L, Gatzonis S. Treatment of idiopathic head-drop syndrome (camptocephalia) by bilateral chronic electrical stimulation of the globus pallidum internus. *J Neurosurg* 2008b [in press].

Sanguineti V, Giugliano M, Grattarola M, Morasso P. Neuroengineering: from neural interfaces to biological computers. In: Riva G, Davide F, editors. *Communications throuhg virtual technology: identity community and technology in the internet age.* Amsterdam, IOS Press; 2003. p. 233-46.

Schlaepfer TE, Cohen MX, Frick C,et al. Deep brain stimulation to reward circuitry alleviates anhedonia in refractory major depression. *Neuropsychopharmacology* 2008 ; 33:368-77.

Schoenen J, Di Clemente L, Vandenheede M, et al. Hypothalamic stimulation in chronic cluster headache: a pilot study of efficacy and mode of action. *Brain* 2005;128:940-7.

Schramm P, Scheihing M, Rasche D, Tronnier VM. Behr syndrome variant with tremor treated by VIM stimulation. *Acta Neurochir* (Wien) 2005;147:679-83.

Silanpää M, Schmidt D. Natural history of treated childhood-onset epilepsy: prospective, long-term population-based study. *Brain* 2006;129:617-24.

Silver R, Boahen K, Grillner S, Kopell N, Olsen KL. Neurotech for neuroscience: unifying concepts, organizing principles, and emerging tools. *J Neurosci* 2007;27:11807-19.

Simpson BA. The role of neruostimulation: the neurosurgical perspective. *J Pain Symptom Manage* 2006a;31:S3-S5.

Simpson BA. Challenges for the 21st century: the future of electrical neuromodulation. *J Pain Symptom Manage* 2006b;31 (Suppl 4):S3-S5.

Smith LS, Hamilton A. Neuromorphic systems. Introduction. *Int J Neural Syst* 1999;9;371-3

Starr PA, Barbaro NM, Raskin NH, Ostrem JL. Chronic stimulation of the posterior hypothalamic region for cluster headache: technique and 1-year results in four patients. *J Neurosurg* 2007;106:999-1005.

Stover NP, Okun MS, Evatt ML, Raju DV, Bakay RA, Vitek JL. Stimulation of the subthalamic nucleus in a patient with Parkinson's disease and essential tremor. *Arch Neurol* 2005;62:141-3.

Sturm V, Lenartz D, Koulousakis A, et al. The nucleus accumbens: a target for deep brain stimulation in obsessive-compulsive and anxiety disorders. *J Chem Neuroanat* 2003;26:293-9.

Sun B, Chen S, Zhan S, Le W, Krahl SE. Subthalamic nucleus stimulation for primary dystonia and tardive dystonia. *Acta Neurochir* Suppl 2007;97:207-14.

Swanson TH. The pathophysiology of human mesial temporal lobe epilepsy. *J Clin Neurophysiol* 1995;12:2-22.

Sydow O, Thobois S, Alesch F, Speelman JD. Multicenter European study of thalamic stimulation in essential tremor: a six year follow-up. *J Neurol Neurosurg Psychiatr* 2003;74:1387-91.

Taha JM, Jansen MA, Favre J. Thalamic deep brain stimulation for the treatment of head, voice, and bilateral limb tremor. *J Neurosurg* 1999;91:68-72.

Talelli P, Rothwell J. Does brain stimulation after stroke have a future? *Curr Opin Neurol* 2006;19:543-50.

Temel Y, Kessels A, Tan S, Topdag A, Boon P, Visser-Vandewalle V. Behavioural changes after bilateral subthalamic nucleus stimulation in advanced Parkinson's disease: A systematic review. *Parkinsonism Relat Disord* 2006;12:265-72.

Tisch S, Rothwell JC, Limousin P, Hariz MI, Corcos DM. The physiological effects of pallidal deep brain stimulation in dystonia. *IEEE Trans Neural Syst Rehabil Eng* 2007;15:166-72.

Topper R, Mottaghy FM, Brugmann M, Noth J, Huber W. facilitation of picture naming by focal transcranial magnetic stimulation of wernicke's area. *Exp Brain Res* 1998; 121: 371-378

Velasco F, Velasco AL, Velasco G, Jimenez F. Effect of chronic electrical stimulation of the centromedian thalamic nuclei on various intractable seizures patterns: I. Clinical seizures and paroxysmal EEG activity. *Epilepsia* 1993a;34:1065-74.

Velasco F, Marquez I, Velasco G. Effect of chronic electrical stimulation of the centromedian thalamic nuclei on various intractable seizure patterns: II. Psychological performance and background EEG activity. *Acta Neurochir* Suppl 1993b;58:201-4.

Velasco M, Velasco AL, Jimenez F et al. Role of the centromedian thalamic nucleus in the genesis, propagation and arrest of epileptic activity. An electrophysiological study in man. *Epilepsia* 1995;36:63-71.

Velasco F, Velasco M, Jimenez F, et al. Predictors in the treatment of difficult-to-control seizures b electrical stimulation of the centromedian thalamic nucleus. *Neurosurgery* 2000a;47:295-304.

Velasco AL, Velasco M, Velasco F, et al. Sucabute and chronic electrical stimulation of the hippocampus on intractable temporal lobe seizures: preliminary report. *Arch Med Res* 2000b;31:316-28.

Velasco M, Velasco AL, Menez D, Rocha L. Centromedian-thalamic and hippocampal electrical stimulation for the control of intractable epileptic seizures. *Stereotactic Funct Neurosurg* 2001;77:223-7.

Velasco F, Carrillo-Ruiz JD, Brito F, et al. Double-blind, randomized controlled pilot study of bilateral cerebellar stimulation for treatment of intractable motor seizures. *Epilepsia* 2005;46:1071-81.

Visser-Vandewalle V, Temel Y, Boon P, et al. Chronic bilateral thalamic stimulation: a new therapeutic approach in intractable Tourette's syndrome. Report of three cases. *J Neurosurg* 2003;99:1094-1100.

Vonck K, Boon P, Claeys P, Dedeurwaerdere S, Achten R, Van Roost D. Long-term deep brain stimulation for refractory lobe epilepsy. *Ann Neurol* 2005;52:556-65.

Warwick K, Gasson MN, Spiers AJ. Therapeutic potential of computer to cerebral cortex implantable devices. *Acta Neurochir* Suppl 2007;97(2):529-35.

Weaver F. Follett K, Hur K, Ippolito D, Stern M. Deep brain stimulation in Parkinson's disease: a meta-analysis of patient outcomes. *J Neurosurg* 2005;103:956-67.

Webster TJ, Waid MC, McKenzie JL, Price RL, Ejiofor JU. Nano-biotechnology: carbon nanofibers as improved nerual and orthopaedic implants. *Nanotechnology* 2004;15:48-54.

Wichmann T, DeLong MR. Deep brain stimulation for neurologic and neuropsychiatric disorders. *Neuron* 2006;52:197-204.

Wishart HA, Roberts DW, Roth RM, et al. Chronic deep brain stimulation for the treatment of tremor in multiple sclerosis: review and case reports. *J Neurol Neurosurg Psychiatr* 2003;74:1392-7.

Young R, Rinaldi PC. Brain stimulation. In: North RB, Levy RM, editors. *Neurosurgical management of pain*. New York: Springer; 1997. p. 283-301.

Yu H, Neimat J. The treatment of movement disorders by deep brain stimulation. *Neurotherapeutics* 2008;5:26-36.

Ziemann U, Lonnecker S, Steinhoff BJ, Paulus W. Effects of antiepileptic drugs on motor cortex excitability in humans: transcranial magnetic stimulation study. *Ann Neurol* 1996;40:367-78.

In: Deep Brain Stimulation
Editors: Mark H. Rogers and Paul B. Anderson

ISBN 978-1-60692-895-0

Chapter IV

Invasive Cortical Stimulation for Parkinson's Disease and Movement Disorders[*]

B. Cioni*[†]*, A. R. Bentivoglio, C. De Simone, A. Fasano, C. Piano, D. Policicchio, V. Perotti and M. Meglio

Functional Neurosurgery, Anesthesiology, and Neurology, Università Cattolica, Roma, Italy

Abstract

Ever since the observation that motor cortex (MI) stimulation (MI ECS) could relieve some patients suffering post-stroke movement disorders (Katayama et al., 1997, 2002) and, above all, the successful introduction of MI ECS for the treatment of Parkinson's disease by Canavero in 1998 (Canavero and Paolotti 2000), extradural MI ECS has been employed for the treatment of several movement disorders. This chapter reviews this field.

[*] A version of this chapter was also published in *Text of Therapentic Cortical Stimulation*, edited by B. Cioni published by Nova Science Publishers, Inc. It was submitted for appropriate modification in an effort to encourage wider dissemination of research.

[†] Correspondence concerning this article should be addressed to: Dr. Beatrice Cioni, MD.E-mail: bcioni@rm.unicatt.it

Parkinson's Disease (PD) and Parkinsonism

A. Review of the Literature

A total of approximately 100 patients with Parkinson's disease have been treated by MI ECS.

1. The first report was that by Canavero and Paolotti (2000), who described the case of a 72 year old woman with advanced PD who showed a substantial improvement of all three cardinal parkinsonian symptoms following unilateral extradural MI ECS (electrode strip parallel to Rolandic fissure). In July 1998, a quadripolar electrode was positioned in the extradural space overlying the hand representation area of MI, contralateral to her worst clinical side. Chronic stimulation was delivered subthreshold for any movement or sensation, at 3V, 180 μs, 25Hz, 3+/0- setting, off during sleep. The clinical improvement was bilateral; she could stand without assistance, climb the stairs and walk for a short distance. The UPDRS III in On-Med condition decreased from 44 to 23 after 3 months. She had a moderate to severe PD-associated dementia and this aspect also improved. L-dopa was reduced by 80%. Importantly, after 3 months, the patient developed infection and was explanted. However, she lost benefit only gradually over several weeks, a sign of likely neuroplastic changes induced by stimulation. Upon reimplantation, she improved again. These results were confirmed in two further patients operated on in 2001 and 2002 (Canavero et al., 2002, 2003). Canavero also reported on a patient suffering multiple system atrophy-associated parkinsonism. Bilateral subthalamic deep brain stimulation was ineffective, but moderately responded to bilateral MI stimulation with the following parameters: 25-40 Hz, 90-180μs, 2-2.5V, bipolar stimulation (3+/0- or viceversa), continuously. Motor symptoms improved for about 9 months, while vegetative symptoms remained improved until death almost 3 years later (Canavero et al 2003).

2. Upon Canavero's urge, Pagni et al. (2003, 2005) implanted 5 new cases (in their 2005 publication, patients 5 and 6 were taken from Canavero's series). All of them were submitted to unilateral extradural MI ECS (electrode strip parallel to Rolandic fissure), opposite to the worst clinical side; chronic stimulation was delivered bipolarly at 2.5-6V, 150-180 μs, 25-40Hz, continuously; follow-up ranged from 4 months to 2.5 years. The patients were evaluated only in the On-Med state: global UPDRS decreased by 42-62%, UPDRS III (motor axis) by 32-83%. It was possible to decrease L-dopa by 11-33% in 3 cases and by 70-73% in 2 patients. The improvement was bilateral. One case had to be reimplanted due to misplacement. Interestingly, neuropsychological assessment (MMSE, 15 Rey's Words, Corsi block-tapping test, WAIS with revised digit span subtest and block design subtest, Prose Memory Test, Attention Matrices Test, Verbal Judgement Test, Arithmetic Judgement Test, SPM, Verbal Fluency, Token Test, MADRS, BPRS, QL-Index) of three of these patients at 1 year follow-up revealed stable cognitive functions, stability of mood disorders, disappearance of hallucinations (1 patient) and mildly improved quality of life in 2 of 3 patients (Munno et al 2007).

3. The Toronto's group (Kleiner-Fisman et al., 2003) reported on the efficacy of high-frequency *subdural* MI ECS (bipolar, or monopolar in 1 case) in 5 patients with Parkinsonism due to multiple systemic atrophy (MSA). Three patients reported subjective

improvement, although UPDRS scores did not change at 3 and 6 months. Thereafter, they (Strafella et al 2007) submitted 5 patients (age range 70-75)with advanced PD to unilateral subdural MI ECS (hand motor area, left in 3, right in 1). All had 30% motor improvement on levodopa and none met DBS criteria. One patient developed a cortical venous infarct and was excluded from study results. Multiple settings (5-185 Hz, 60-450 μs, 0.5-7V, monopolar and bipolar stimulation) were assessed immediately after surgery and after 1-2 weeks of stimulation. At 6 month follow-up, patients underwent double-blind evaluations randomized to stimulation on or off (for 2 weeks each), with and without medications (acute levodopa challenge); modified CAPIT and neuropsychological testing were performed and a PDQ-39 questionnaire was administered preoperatively and at 6 months. There were no acute improvements in akinesia, rigidity or gait function with stimulation. Tremor improved acutely in the patient with prominent tremor. The off drug UPDRS motor scores off- and on-stimulation (43 +/- 7.9 versus 39.5 +/-12.5) were not significantly different, nor the on-stim/on-med scores and preoperative on condition (18.7 +/- 8.6 versus 14.2 +/-2.2). Two patients worsened (more off time, less on), one was unchanged, one had some improvement with stimulation. These patients were also assessed with H2O PET at 6 months from surgical implantation following optimization of parameters (3-5V, 60-90 μs). Subjects were tested at rest and while performing a simple motor task with a joystick. Scanning was performed at 10 minutes intervals on stimulation off, 50 and 130 Hz stimulation. Joystick movement compared to rest while MI ECS was turned off augmented rCBF in the sensorimotor cortex (BA 4/3), lateral premotor cortex (BA6) and caudal supplementary motor cortex (SMA) contralateral to hand movement. During 50 Hz and 130 Hz stimulation, the same areas were activated when comparing joystick movement versus rest. However, these changes in rCBF were not significantly different when comparing across different stimulation settings (OFF vs 50 Hz vs 130 Hz); no significant movement-related rCBF changes were detected during MI ECS in other cortical areas such as the rostral SMA and dorsolateral prefrontal cortex. Motor performance during the joystick task did not change significantly across different stimulation frequencies, although a trend towards worsening was observed during 50 Hz stimulation. This study is ill-conceived. MI ECS has no acute clinical effects and the 10 minute intervals are simply inadequate.

4. Pagni, upon retiring in 2003, spearheaded a multicenter study to evaluate the efficacy of MI ECS in advanced PD, on behalf of the Italian Society of Neurosurgery.

The preliminary results of the multicenter study have been published (Bentivoglio et al 2005). Twenty-nine patients were treated. Initially, patients were submitted to a test period (1-2 weeks) before IPG implantation, but in the following cases the whole implant was made in a single session. All symptoms of PD (tremor, rigidity, motor dexterity, bradykinesia, posture and gait, freezing) were improved and L-dopa could be reduced. Best parameters were 2.5-6V, 150-180 (but also 90-120) μs, 25-40 (but also 60-80) Hz. In an "intention to treat analysis", after 6 months of MI ECS, the mean UPDRS III decreased by 21% in the off-med condition and by 34% in the on-med condition. At 1 year, the effect of MI ECS was less evident, with a decrease of UPDRS III of 13% and 21% respectively in the off and on-med conditions. Notably, the stimulation parameters differed in the various centers: monopolar or bipolar stimulation, 2-8V, 60-400 μs, 20-120Hz, continuously or only during day time. Some patients were unresponsive to MI ECS: many of these patients had MRI findings of leucoencephalopathy, white matter ischemic foci, cerebral atrophy, suggesting a diagnosis of Parkinsonism rather than true PD.

The long term results (up to 36 months) have been reported for 41 patients (Pagni et al 2008).

UPDRS evaluation was performed before implantation and after 3, 6,12, 24 and 36 months of MI ECS, both in the on-med and off-med conditions. Analysis of variance for repeated measures and Wilcoxon signed-rank paired samples test were used for statistical analysis. At 12, 24 and 36 months of follow up, significant decreases of global UPDRS off-med (by 21.9%, 14.6%, and 26.4%, respectively), of UPDRS III off-med (by 17.8%, 10.5% and 25.5%) of axial symptoms (subscores 27+28+29: by 19.9%, 16.2% and 21.3%), of UPDRS IV (by 37.7%, 18.1%, and 21.6%) and of UPDRS II off-med (by 27.6%, 21.3%, and 31.8% , respectively) were apparent. Drug therapy could be decreased by a mean of 20%. No major adverse event was encountered. Thus, MI ECS moderately improves motor symptoms (UPDRS III), decreases complications of therapy (UPDRS IV) and ameliorates activities of daily living (UPDRS II) in advanced PD. The clinical effect can be expected to last at least 3 years.

5. Benvenuti et al. (2006) submitted a 68 year old woman to MI ECS. Motor fluctuations uncontrolled by therapy, dyskinesias, depression and anxiety were severe. During MI ECS, UPDRS scores changed significantly (Activities of Daily Living: from 26 to 17; Motor: from 33 to 22; Complications of Therapy: from 13 to 7; Mentation: from 8 to 6). Dyskinesias and motor fluctuations were reduced and no longer disabling, rigidity was reduced bilaterally; standing, gait and motor performance were also improved. Levodopa was not reduced. Improvement was 35% on the UPDRS scale 8 weeks after surgery.

6. Verhagen et al. (2006) conducted a prospective multicenter study of 9 PD patients (H&Y OFF $\geq$ III) receiving extradural MI ECS (hand area) for 24 weeks. Stimulation effects were systematically explored at 20-127 Hz with constant pulse width (250 μs). At end of study, the UPDRS III score OFF medication was 42.13 +/- 13.78 compared to 38.78 +/- 8.08 at baseline. Three patients remained on stimulation 1 year later. Their UPDRS III scores at baseline, 24 and 52 weeks were 37, 30, 30; 29,37,20 and 29, 25 and 25. At 24 weeks "On Time Without Troublesome Dyskinesias" was 11.25 +/-2.10 hours, compared to 9.54 +/- 3.89 at baseline. PDQ-39 Total scores were 38.33+/-10.17 at 24 weeks compared to 43.62+/-8.33 at baseline. During programming, there were 2 fits. This study has limitations. The stimulation hardware was different from that used by all other groups, with a different waveform and current output, but, above all, only two contacts available spaced 31 mm apart corresponding to contacts 0 and 3 of the tetrapolar electrode commonly used for ECS. The 10 Hz band was not explored, and the pulse width was fixed at 250 μs. Finally, at least one patient was probably not PD (B Gliner, meeting communication, 2006).

7. Cilia et al. (2007) submitted to extradural MI ECS (hand area; electrode strip parallel to Rolandic fissure) 5 patients with PD who fulfilled CAPSIT criteria for DBS, with the exception of age >70 years (range 71-77). In particular, there were no vascular abnormalities or significant brain atrophy on MRI. Patients were assessed preoperatively and after 6 months of MI ECS of the left hemisphere, on and off medication, with stimulator on and 2 weeks later with stimulator off, by a blinded neurologist. Stimulation was monopolar (0-/3-/case +), 3-4V, 60 (40 in 1 patient) Hz, 180-210 μs, continuous (night and day). MI ECS determined a

reduction of daily OFF time (UPDRS item 39) in 3 patients, a mean L-DOPA reduction of 16% and a mean dopamine agonist reduction dosage of 49%, and a reduction of the Abnormal Involuntary Movements Scale (AIMS) of 19%. The off-med UPDRS II and UPDRS III scores did not vary, even if a trend towards improvement was shown in axial symptoms (items 14-28-29). On-Med UPDRS II and III scores values were unmodified. No behavior or mood changes were reported at 6 months. No immediate motor change was reported when stimulation was switched off, except for 1 patient who showed worsening gait. Fifteen days later, 3 patients complained of prolonged daily OFF time and freezing gait, and 2 patients with unchanged medication complained of an increase in dyskinesias as well. Four patients asked spontaneously to have the stimulator turned on again. In sum, "*4 of 5 patients reported subjective improvement involving mainly axial symptoms* (i.e., stability, posture and gait) *as well as a reduction in daily OFF time and dyskinesia*". Subjective clinical benefit was reported after a variable interval after switching on the stimulator (minutes to days). This study has a few limitations. Four out of 5 patients were monopolarly stimulated. Monopolar stimulation is not the same as bipolar stimulation. In fact, the best responder was the only one to receive bipolar stimulation (0-1-/2+3+): this was also the only akinetic-rigid dominant patient, whereas the remaining 4 were tremor dominant. These authors "*started from a frequency of 30 Hz and then slowly increased up to 60 Hz*". The 10-20 and 70-80 Hz bands were not explored, and these can be effective. In a follow-up paper (Cilia et al., 2008), these same authors reported on the same 5 patients, plus 1 (a 70 year old man), and studied them with Tc-99m cysteinate dimmer bicisate (ECD) SPECT off-medication with stimulator off and on. Patients were assessed preoperatively and 6 months after surgery, with both stimulator on and 2 weeks after switch-off by a blinded neurologist. All medications remained unchanged during the 2-week stim-off period. Parameters were assessed across different configurations (monopolar and bipolar, 0.5-5V, 60-210 μs, 20-120 Hz). Blinded evaluation in individual patients revealed clinical improvement of UPDRS II and III scores during stimulation compared to stim-off condition up to 40 and 20% respectively. UPDRS scores did not change significantly during bipolar stimulation (0-/3+) and 120 Hz. Clinical improvement occurred after several days to 4 weeks after stimulation parameters modifications. Objective motor benefit was observed mainly in axial symptoms (gait, stooped posture and postural instability). Subjective benefit was admitted by 4 of 6 patients, mainly in mobility and walking, associated with an increase in daily on-time (as if stimulation would delay wearing-off phenomenon). In two patients, battery exhausted about 12 months after implant: both experienced slow and progressive clinical deterioration, associated with an objective worsening of UPDRS III scores of 20% and 25% respectively, that reversed after battery replacement. ECD SPECT with a triple head camera and ultra high resolution collimators was conducted with stimulator on and 2 weeks after switching the stimulator off. At a statistical threshold of $p<0.001$, the authors found rCBF decrements in MI (BA4) and lateral premotor cortex (BA6) bilaterally (!), left dorsolateral prefrontal cortex (BA9) and right caudate head. Perfusion decrements occurred in BA19. At $p<0.01$, additional clusters were seen in right thalamus (stimulator was on left MI!), left caudate nucleus and right BA6. Significant perfusion increases were found in the right cerebellar lobe, and, with a less strict threshold, left BA18, left cerebellar lobe and vermis. Thus, effects were widespread and bilateral, paralleling clinical benefits.

8. Arle et al. (2008) applied extradural MI ECS (electrode strip parallel to Rolandic fissure) in 4 patients (bilateral in 3) aged 44-72. Three patients were eligible for DBS. All patients had at least 30% improvement in their UPDRS scores when taking L-Dopa. Programming was started within 24 hours of electrode implantation. Initially all contacts were checked in a monopolar setting at 130 Hz and 210 μs, with voltage slowly increased to 4V. Contacts 1 and 2 were left ON at 3V: if not tolerated, contact 3 or 0 alone was used. In all cases 2 contacts could be activated. Cathodal (not anodal) stimulation was used. If minimal benefit was noted during later sessions, more contacts were added to the monopolar configuration. In case of failure, contact 0 or 3 was placed in cathodal mode and the other 3 contacts set as the anode. Other investigated changes included PW 410 μs, 4V, 80Hz and 185Hz.

In the end, patient 1 was stimulated at 3.2 mA, 240 μs, 130 Hz, 0-/1-/2-/3off/case +; patient 2 at 3.5mA,210 μs, 130 Hz, left sided 0-/1-/2+/3+/case off and right sided 0off/1-/2-/3+/case off; patient 3 at 3.4 mA (left)/3.2 Amp (right), 210 μs, 100 Hz, left sided 0-/1-/2-/3off/case + and right sided 0-/1-/2-/3off/case +. Patient 4 was not detailed. One patient developed an infection and was explanted at 3 months: he had an improvement of about 50% over his baseline condition in dyskinesias, rigidity and tremor following unilateral implantation, but it significantly regressed upon device explantation. After reimplantation several months later, he achieved the same benefit. Two patients had a 20-30% reduction in medication requirements, but one needed 37% more. One patient had a return of dyskinesias after 3 months due to reduction of amplitude of stimulation following initial benefit: upon reincreasing the amplitude, dyskinesias were again controlled. Globally, there was a trend toward a significant difference in the UPDRS III scores between the baseline score and the scores at 1,3 and 6 months, but not at 12 months, possibly because of fewer data point observations available for analysis. At 1 month, there was a mean decrease in the UPDRS III score of 21(+/-13) points from baseline, at 3 months of 15(+/-11) points, at 6 months of 18(+/-16) points, but only of 9(+/-9) points at 1 year for the 2 patients with sufficient follow-up. More in detail, the UPDRS global scores during on-med/on-stim preoperatively, at 1,3,6 and 12 months in 3 patients (4th not available) were respectively: 46,52,47,51(12th month milestone not yet reached); 57,79,42,94,62; 53.5,23,32,54,37; during off-med and on-stim: 27,17,22,15 (12th month milestone not yet reached); 46,11,31,31,43; 41.5,12,10,5,25; 18,10,9,14 (12th month milestone not yet reached). The UPDRS III (motor) scores in on-med/on-stim in the same 3 patients were respectively: 19,26,25,23 (12th month milestone not yet reached); 32, 47,13,18,35; 24.5,12,18,27,5.

9. Seijo et al. (2009) submitted 6 patients not eligible for DBS to extradural unilateral MI ECS (contralateral to side of clinical onset). Five of six were akinetic-rigid, 1 had left hand tremor. Parameters adjustments were carried out during 1 week after initial implant. Optimal parameters were: *case 1*:3+/0-, 4.5V,450 μs, 30Hz; *case 2*:2+/1-,3V, 400 μs, 10 Hz; *case 3*: 3+/0-, 3.7V, 450 μs, 30 Hz; *case 4*: 3+/0-, 3.6V, 450 μs, 10 Hz; *case 5*: 3+/0-,3V, 330 μs, 25 Hz; *case 6*: 1-/2+, 3.6V,450 μs, 25 Hz. Follow-up was 1 year. In *case 1*, UPDRS III on-med/on-stim was 26 (but 42 off-med/on-stim), Hoehn&Yahr (H&Y) score was 2 and Schwab &England Daily Living Activities Scale (DLA) 90%. In *case 2*, they were 27 (vs 38), 3 and 80%: dyskinesias and freezing while walking were significantly decreased, with freezing restricted only to off-med periods. In *case 3*, they were 17 (vs 55), 2, 70%; levodopa was

decreased. In *case 4*, they were: 27 (vs 38), 2 and 90%: dyskinesias were reduced, though tremor was not. In *case 5*, they were 29 (vs 42), 2 and 80%: levodopa was reduced. In *case 6*, they were 26 (vs 42), 2 and 90%: levodopa was decreased. Globally, UPDRS III score improved in 2 patients (cases 1 and 4) comparing preoperative condition to on-med/on-stim conditions, but did not change in cases 2,3 and 5 or slightly worsened in case 6.

B. Personal Experience

In 2003, we started a prospective study to evaluate the efficacy of MI ECS in patients with advanced PD (Cioni et al., 2007; Cioni, 2007). The inclusion criteria were: idiopathic Parkinson disease (PDSBB criteria); at least 5 years disease's length; disease in the advanced state (UPDRS in off >/= 40/180; Hoehn and Yahrs >/= 3; motor complications: fluctuations and disabling dyskinesias); positive response to L-Dopa; DBS not accepted by the patient or contraindicated; patient's ability to give informed consent to the study. The exclusion criteria were: history of epilepsy or EEG epileptic activity; alcohol or drug abuse; mental deterioration; psychiatric symptoms; previous basal ganglia surgery; other major illness. Ten patients met the above mentioned criteria and were submitted to the implant of an epidural plate electrode over the motor cortex contralateral to the worst clinical side in 3 cases, and to a bilateral implant in the remaining 7 cases (Figures 1-2). Therapeutic stimulation during the first year was through the electrode contralateral to the worst clinical side; parameters were: 120μs, 80Hz, 3-6V (subthreshold for movements, and motor or sensory phenomena), delivered continuously through contacts 0 (anode) and 3 (cathode). After 12 months, in cases of bilateral implantation, stimulation was made bilateral (same parameters for the side ipsilateral to the worst clinical side). The clinical assessment before implant and at 1, 3, 6, 12, 18, 24, and 36 months included: UPDRS (Unified Parkinson Disease Rating Scale); finger tapping; walking time; PDQL (Parkinson Disease Quality of Life Scale); neuropsychological evaluation including MMSE (Mini Mental State Evaluation), behavioral assessment of mood and anxiety, tests for verbal short term memory, spatial short term memory, episodic verbal memory, non-verbal abstract reasoning, frontal executive functions and verbal fluency; EEG; oral medications and adverse events. The clinical motor evaluation was performed both in the off and in the on medication state and the motor assessment was videotaped. The "OFF" condition was achieved by withdrawing antiparkinsonian medications as follows: Levodopa for at least 12 hours, pergolide, pramipexole, ropinirole for at least 48 hours, cabergoline for at least 168 hours, apomorphine for at least 3 hours. The "ON" condition was achieved 60 minutes after administering a supra-threshold dose of standard levodopa, according to daily schedule. Cognitive and behavioral assessment were performed preoperatively and at 6, 12 and 18 months, in the on med status.

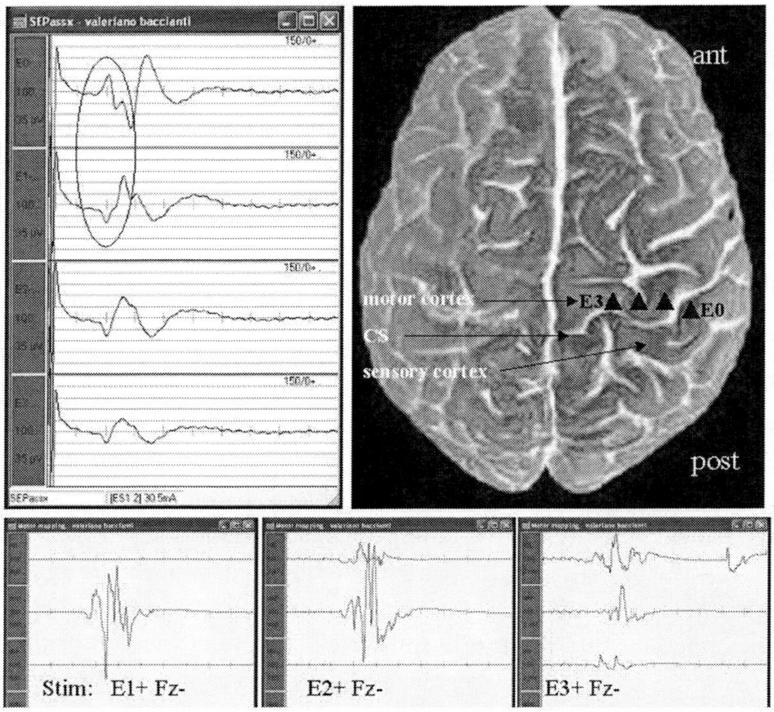

Figure 1. *Top right*: Central sulcus (CS) identification. Cortical median nerve SEPs (recording: E0, E1, E2, E3, referred to Fz) showing phase reversal between traces 1 and 2 (E0 and E1). *Bottom traces*: Motor cortex mapping, Recording from Biceps Brachii, Abductor Pollicis Brevis, Quadriceps after stimulation delivered through electrode E1, E2 and E3 (cathode) and 6 cm in front of Cz (anode). *Top left*: integrated anatomo-functional position of the quadripolar electrode.

A statistically (Wilcoxon's test and analysis of variance for repeated measures) significant improvement was present after 12 months of unilateral MI ECS, as of total UPDRS off-med, UPDRS II, UPDRS III off-med, subscore for axial symptoms (UPDRS III: items 27-31), UPDRS IV, PDQL. The effect of unilateral MI ECS was bilateral, with no significant difference between the two sides. It was evident after 1-2 weeks of stimulation, and in a case of accidental switching off of the stimulator the patient became aware of something going wrong after 2-3 weeks. After 1 year of unilateral stimulation, 7 patients needed bilateral MI ECS, the remaining 3 patients continued with unilateral stimulation. The statistical analysis at 24 and 36 months demonstrated a significant improvement in total UPDRS off-med, in UPDRS III off-med (by 20% compared to the preoperative score), in the subscore for axial symptoms, in UPDRS IV and in PDQL. Notably, in all the patients, the UPDRS III off med at 24 and 36 months was always lower than UPDRS III off med at preoperative evaluation. At 2 years, bilateral stimulation showed a trend towards greater benefit compared to unilateral stimulation, but a statistical analysis was not possible due to the small sample. Drug treatment could be decreased by 25%. No complication occurred; no adverse events, particularly no epileptic seizures nor EEG epileptic activity, were encountered. Cognitive assessment in the overall group of patients showed a significant postoperative improvement on the MMSE and on tasks of episodic verbal memory, but this most likely reflects a practice effect (Daniele et al., 2003). No significant postoperative decline was observed on any cognitive task, including those of phonological and semantic verbal fluency, whereas DBS patients show a significant decline on verbal fluency (Contarino et al., 2007). Unilateral stimulation of the left hemisphere showed a statistical trend towards a postoperative improvement of phonological verbal fluency, along with an increase of depressive symptoms. On the contrary, stimulation of the right hemisphere showed a trend towards a decrease of depression, and no effect on verbal fluency. We also assessed our patients with DAT scan (SPECT) in order to evaluate binding to the dopamine transporters before and after 6, 12 and 28 months of MI ECS, and IBZM-SPECT to evaluate activity of striatal postsynaptic D2 receptors, before and after 6 and 12 months of MI ECS. DAT-scans at 6 and 12 months showed an increase in the activity in both putamina, particularly on the side ipsilateral to the stimulation. Postsynaptic receptors activity was unmodified at 6 and 12 months.

Furthermore, we reported (Fasano et al., 2008) the case of a 72-year-old female patient affected by severe PD who underwent bilateral MI ECS. In baseline med-off condition the patient was unable to rise from a chair and to stand without assistance. Stimulation at 3 and 60 Hz failed to provide any improvement, whereas, when stimulating at 130 Hz, axial akinesia and walking improved consistently: the patient, in med-off condition, was able to rise from chair and to walk without assistance. The patient underwent two brain 99mTc-Ethylcysteinate Dimer-SPECT studies, which showed that the regional cerebral perfusion was significantly increased in the supplementary motor area during stimulation at 130 Hz. After five months, the benefit of MI ECS gradually disappeared.

We are now performing a controlled randomized study on the clinical usefulness of MI ECS in PD. The protocol has been published on *www.ClinicalTrials.gov (Identifier # NCT00637260)*. Another controlled study of 10 patients is on file (*Identifier # NCT00159172).*

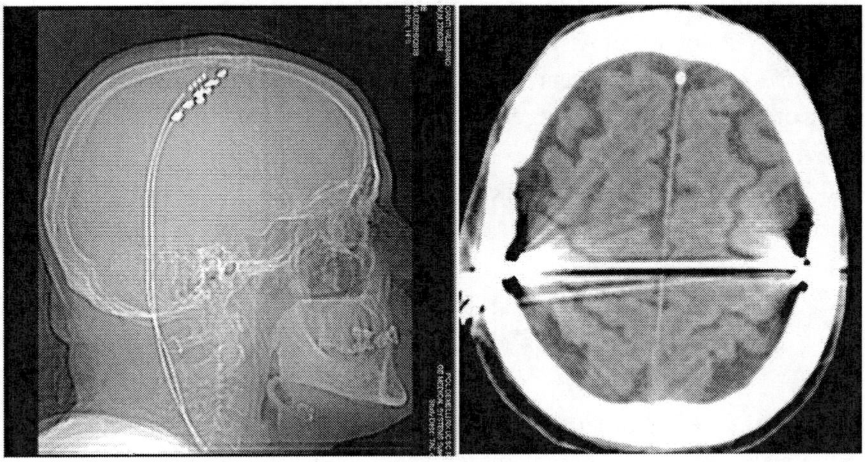

Figure 2. Skull X-rays and CT scan showing the position of the bilateral quadripolar strip electrode.

Pure Akinesia

Tani et al. (2007) presented a case of Levodopa-resistant akinesia, a DBS resistant motor disorder. After a positive trial of 10 Hz MI rTMS (500 pulses) (but negative trial of SMA rTMS), the patient underwent a bilateral implant of subdural electrodes over the motor cortex, close to the sagittal sinus. The best stimulation parameters were: 100Hz, 210μs, 1.8V, 1+/2- electrode setting, 30' on and 120' off (benefit lasted 3 hours). UPDRS decreased form 70 to 41 after 1 year and to 46 after 2 years; walking time (7 m) improved from 84.7 sec to 20sec at 1 year and 15 at 2 years, and so did step size; dysphagia also improved. Blinded switch-off resulted in deterioration within 48 hours. On the fourth day, the stimulator was reactivated and benefit was restored. A PET study showed a significant increase of rCBF in the left SMA (BA6) and right dorso-lateral prefrontal cortex (BA9) after 30' of bilateral MI ECS. Activation of SMA, involved in movement preparation and initiation, was one of the mechanisms hypothesized at the basis of MI ECS effects.

In our series of PD patients the best results were obtained on axial symptoms in patients with severe and unpredictable off periods. We submitted a patient with pure akinesia to bilateral MI ECS. There was a marked improvement of akinesia, posture, and gait; furthermore the patient showed a striking amelioration of verbal fluency.

Essential Tremor

Lyons et al. (2006) submitted to MI ECS (only two contacts available) two patients suffering essential tremor. The two burr-hole technique developed by Canavero was used (see chapter 2). They were evaluated with the Fahn-Tolosa-Marin Tremor Rating Scale at baseline and after 1 and 4 weeks of contralateral (to tremor) MI ECS. Patient 1 (75 year old man) received MI ECS at 30Hz, 3mA, 250 μs. His baseline score was 61, and 1 month after surgery it was 57. Patient 2 (60 year old man)'s stimulation parameters were 50Hz, 5 mA, 250 μs. His score was 47 before surgery and 43 1 month after MI ECS. In sum, MI ECS proved ineffective.

Arle and Shils (2008) reported 2 other patients with essential tremor treated by MI ECS with poor results.

Dystonia

Canavero et al. (2003) described the acute effects of MI ECS in a case of cervical dystonia previously treated with thalamotomy and, after recurrence, cervical rhizotomy, intrathecal baclofen and botulinum toxin. She developed painful dystonic paroxysms involving her right hemibody every 4 hours lasting about 30 min. MI ECS (MI thigh, chest and arm area) at 10 Hz, 450 μs and 1V controlled both pain and dystonia, except for the neck symptoms.

Franzini et al. (2003) reported on the efficacy of MI ECS (130 Hz) for central pain-associated "thalamic hand" in 2 of 3 patients. Two patients suffering intentional myoclonus were also relieved.

Romito et al. (2007) and Albanese et al. (2007) described a case of fixed dystonia unresponsive to pallidal stimulation, but improved by MI ECS. A right handed woman progressively developed a severe segmental dystonia with fixed elevation and anterorotation of the left shoulder, abduction of the upper limb, severe trunk involvement and fixed kyphoscoliosis. Gene mutations were absent. There was no evidence of a complex regional pain syndrome, no preceding trauma, and a complete psychological and psychiatric evaluation ruled out the diagnosis of psychogenic dystonia. The diagnosis was a distinct subtype of primary dystonia – primary fixed dystona. Pharmacological treatments failed as well as botulinum toxin. GPi DBS also failed. Stimulation of the right motor cortex (strip parallel to MI) started the day after implant (3.8V, 60 Hz, 60 μs, 0-/1+/2- setting) was followed by a gradual improvement and the dystonic postures and pain almost resolved after 6 months. The effect was still present at 22 months. A PET study was performed before and after 6 months of MI ECS showing significant hypometabolism in the cerebellum, more pronounced on the right, and no increase in cortical metabolism. Interestingly, PET during Gpi DBS showed significant CBF increases in SI/MI (more on the left) and SMA and ACC bilaterally.

Post-Stroke Movement Disorders

Tsubokawa et al. (1993) and Katayama et al. (1997, 2002) made the original observation that MI ECS can relieve post-stroke movement disorders. Katayama et al. (2002) analyzed the effects of MI ECS on post-stroke movement disorders in 50 patients: the purpose of MI ECS was to control pain in 42 cases and involuntary movements in 8 cases. Good control of involuntary movements was observed in 3 out of 3 patients with hemichoreo-athetosis, in 2 out of 2 cases with distal resting or action tremor and in 1 out of 3 patients with proximal postural tremor. High frequencies (50-125 Hz) seem to be necessary for these effects. Subjective improvement in motor performance was reported by 8 patients who had mild motor weakness; severe motor weakness did not respond. The same group (Katayama et al 2006) developed an on-demand type stimulation system which triggers MI ECS or DBS by detecting intrinsic signals of intention to move. They applied this kind of feed-forward control of involuntary movement in 6 cases in whom motor dysfunction was evident only when patients intended to move their body. On-demand stimulation provided satisfactory feed-forward control in 4 patients with postural tremor and 2 with motor weakness, when the activity of muscles involved in posturing or intention to move was fed into the system.

Nguyen et al (1998) reported a case of severe upper limb action tremor and facial pain following removal of an acoustic schwannoma completely controlled by bipolar MI ECS (1.8V, 60 μs, 50 Hz,cyclical mode) for 32 months.

Arle and Shils (2008) reported the effect of MI ECS in 4 cases of poststroke movement disorders associated with pain. In one case there was no benefit, while the others received varying degrees of benefit.

Our group submitted to MI ECS a patient with hemichorea who had a very good response to rTMS (Di Lazzaro et al., 2006). MI ECS proved inferior to rTMS.

Amyothophic Lateral Sclerosis

Sidoti and Agrillo (2006) published the results obtained by bilateral subdural MI ECS in 4 cases of amyotrophic lateral sclerosis (ALS). The motor hand area was targeted. The stimulating plate was parallel to the central sulcus. Stimulation parameters were 30 Hz, 60 μs, 4.5V, contacts 0 and 4 positive, contacts 3 and 7 negative and the rest off. Clinical evaluation included neurological examination and ALS Functional Rating Scale (ALSFRS). At two year follow up, 2 patients showed an arrest of the natural course of the illness during the first year and a slow worsening in the second year after surgery. In these 2 cases postoperative SPECT disclosed consistent complete recovery of flow disturbances. MI ECS was ineffective in the other two patients. A neuroprotective effect of MI ECS was speculated at least in a subgroup of ASL patients.

Di Lazzaro et al. (2006) investigated whether continuous theta burst TMS could have a beneficial effect on ALS. They performed a double blind placebo-controlled trial in 20 ALS patients. The patients submitted to active stimulation received TMS for five consecutive days every month for 6 consecutive months. The primary outcome was the rate of decline evaluated with the ALSFRS. The active group of patients showed a modest, but significant slowing of the deterioration rate.

On this basis we applied bilateral MI ECS in one patient with ALS. MI ECS was delivered at 3 and at 30 Hz. The rate of disease progression was not significantly affected.

Conclusions

In sum, extradural MI ECS may relieve all three main symptoms of PD (akinesia, rigidity, tremor) on both sides simultaneously, but results vary widely, ranging from positive to negative to mixed. Benefit on the various symptoms can vary too: some are improved, others are not, in the same patient.

Patients' population was not homogeneous in these studies, nor were parameters of stimulation or techniques of implantation (monopolar versus bipolar; low versus high frequency, extradural versus subdural, unilateral versus bilateral, continuous versus daily only, general versus local anaesthesia, burr hole versus craniotomy). Nonetheless, our personal data and published studies suggest that MI ECS can relieve all three major symptoms of PD (akinesia, rigidity, tremor) on both sides simultaneously, as well as other movement disorders. Axial symptoms, gait, akinesia and freezing are particularly improved.

The clinical effect of MI ECS cannot be compared with that of STN DBS due to the different inclusion criteria. DBS is usually contraindicated in patients submitted to MI ECS, because of age limits or the presence of MRI anatomical abnormalities (cerebral atrophy, white matter ischemic foci, etc.). However, STN DBS appears to be more effective on motor symptoms, whereas MI ECS seems to be more effective on axial symptoms (gait, posture).

Most dramatically, dyskinesias and painful dystonias are reduced (up to 90%) in almost all patients, well before reducing L-DOPA (a likely direct effect of stimulation). Clinical fluctuations too may be reduced. The complication and adverse events rates are lower for MI ECS, with no risk of intracerebral hemorrhage or infection (extradural approach only); verbal fluency is not impaired by MI ECS, and may even be improved. Hallucinations can occur sporadically and resolve with change of drug therapy and/or stimulation parameters.

Our DAT-Scan data also suggest that MI ECS may have a protective effect on putaminal degeneration, at least in the short term.

The clinical effects of MI ECS seem to decrease with time. This may be due to a placebo effect, and/or to the progressive nature of the disease; or it may reflect a true loss of effectiveness of the stimulation. Changing the parameters of stimulation may reverse this effect: for instance, changing the frequency or the intensity of stimulation according to the impedances (some fibrosis may develop between the electrode surface and the dura) may be useful (neurostimulators delivering impulses in current do not appear superior in this regard). With frequency up to 130Hz, fibers are more likely to be depolarized and excited (Fasano et al 2008). However, if the stimulation is maintained for long periods of time, some synapses may not follow the stimulus train and be blocked, with consequent inhibition. Specific frequencies may be necessary to impose specific patterns of activity, or to suppress abnormal rhythms, or time-protracted processes. Since stimulation is usually delivered continuously, the slight decline in the clinical benefit may be due to cortical habituation. If this is true, alternate stimulation (right side or left side) may be a solution. The clinical effect is long lasting, therefore a cyclic stimulation (only during daytime or even less) is feasible.

Not all the patients respond to MI ECS (7% non-responders in the Italian studies): this may be due to the rather large inclusion criteria, or to the different electrode position and different stimulation parameters. Most patients submitted to MI ECS up to now are older than 70, and cortical atrophy or micro-ischemic lesions may disrupt MI locally in some way in aged people, impairing MI ECS modulation in some cases. Younger patients must be included in future series.

The effect of rTMS may be predictive of the clinical outcome following MI ECS. However, the frequency and the duration of rTMS certainly differ from those used for MI ECS.

As regards the electrode position and stimulation parameters, the number of patients treated with MI ECS is still to low to allow statistical correlation analysis in order to identify prognostic factors.

The need for a bilateral implant has still to be demonstrated. Unilateral MI ECS improves motor performances bilaterally, but bilateral stimulation seems to add to such an improvement.

Finally, there is no place for subdural MI ECS: this can be burdened with fatal brain hemorrhage. If atrophy is found on imaging, the two burr hole technique introduced by Canavero is indicated to close the durocortical gap, even by adding a further silicone layer on the stimulating strip (Canavero S, personal communication).

In sum, MI ECS may be indicated in PD patients with prominent axial symptoms, gait disturbances and therapy complications. It is easy and safe and does away with the cumbersome and time-consuming procedure of DBS. A head-to-head controlled study with DBS is the only way to establish efficacy and safety of both MI ECS and DBS.

References

Albanese A, Romito LM, Piacentini S, Perani D, Carella F, Broggi G. Reply. *Neurology* 2007; 69: 1063

Arle JE, Apetauerova D, Zani J, et al. Motor cortex stimulation for Parkinson disease: 12 months follow up in 4 patients. *J Neurosurg* 2008; 109: 133-139

Arle JE, Shils J. Motor cortex stimulation for pain and movement disorders. *Neurotherapeutics* 2008; 5:37-49

Bentivoglio AR, Cavallo MA, Cioni B, et al. Motor cortex stimulation for movement disorders In: Meglio M (Ed) *Proceedings of the 14th Meeting of the World's Society for Stereotactic and Functional Neurosurgery*. Bologna: Medimond, 2005, pp 89-97

Benvenuti E, Cecchi F, Colombini A, Gori G. Extradural motor cortex stimulation as a method to treat advanced Parkinson's disease:new perspectives in geriatric medicine. *Aging Clin Exp Res* 2006; 18:347-348

Canavero S, Paolotti R. Extradural motor cortex stimulation for advanced Parkinson's disease. *Mov Disord* 2000; 15:169-171

Canavero S, Paolotti R, Bonicalzi V, et al. Extradural motor cortex stimulation for advanced Parkinson's disease: report of two cases. *J Neurosurg* 2002; 97:1208-1211

Canavero S, Bonicalzi V, Paolotti R, et al. Therapeutic extradural cortical stimulation for movement disorders: a review. *Neurol Res* 2003; 25: 118-122

Canavero S, Bonicalzi V. Cortical stimulation for parkinsonism. *Arch Neurol* 2004; 61: 606

Canavero S, Bonicalzi V. Extradural cortical stimulation for movement disorders. In: D Sakas, B Simpson, E Krames, eds. *Operative Neuromodulation*. II Neural Networks Surgery. Wien: Springer-Verlag, 2007, 223-232

Cilia R, Landi A, Vergari F, Sganzerla E, Pezzotti G, Antonini A. Extradural motor cortex stimulation in Parkinson's disease. *Mov Disord* 2007; 22:111-114

Cilia R, Marotta G, Landi A, et al. Cerebral activity modulation by extradural motor cortex stimulation in Parkinson's disease: a perfusion SPECT study. *Eur J Neurol* 2008; 15: 22-28

Cioni B. Motor cortex stimulation for Parkinson's disease. In: D Sakas, B Simpson, E Krames, eds. *Operative Neuromodulation*. II Neural Networks Surgery. Wien: Springer-Verlag, 2007, 233-238

Cioni B, Meglio M, Perotti V, DeBonis P, Montano N. Neurophysiological aspects of chronic motor cortex stimulation. *Clin Neurophysiol* 2007; 37:441-447

Contarino MF, Daniele A, Sibilia AH, et al. Cognitive outcome 5 years after bilateral chronic stimulation of the subthalamic nucleus in patients with Parkinson's disease. *J Neurol Neurosurg Psychiatry* 2007; 78:248-252

Daniele A, Albanese A, Contarino MF, et al. Cognitive and behavioural effects of chronic stimulation of the subthalamic nucleus in patients with Parkinson's disease *J Neurol Neurosurg Psychiatry* 2003; 74:175-182

Fasano A, Piano C, De Simone C, Cioni B, Meglio M, Bentivoglio AR. High frequency extradural motor cortex stimulation dramatically improves axial symptoms in a patient with Parkinson's disease. *Mov Disord* 2008; 23:1916-9.

Franzini A, Ferroli P, Dones I, Marras C, Broggi G. Chronic motor cortex stimulation for movement disorders: a promising perspective *Neurol Res* 2003; 25:123-126

Katayama Y, Fukaya C, Yamamoto T. Control of poststroke voluntary and involuntary movement disorders with deep brain or epidural cortical stimulation *Stereotact Funct Neurosurg* 1997; 69:73-79

Katayama Y, Oshima H, Fukaya C, Kawamata T, Yamamoto T. Control of post-stroke movement disorders using chronic motor cortex stimulation. *Acta Neurochir* 2002; 79(Suppl):89-92

Katayama Y, Kano T, Kobayashi K, Oshima H, Fukaia C, Yamamoto T. Feed-forward control of post-stroke movement disorders by on-demand type stimulation of the thalamus and motor cortex. *Acta Neurochir* Suppl 2006; 99:21-23

Kleiner-Fisman G, Fisman DN, Kahn FI, Sime E, Lozano A, Lang AE. Motor cortical stimulation for Parkinsonism in Multiple Systemic Atrophy. *Arch Neurol* 2003; 60:1554-1558

Lyons KE, Wilkinson SB, Pahwa R. Stimulation of the motor cortex for disabling essential tremor *Clin Neurol Neurosurg* 2006; 108:564-567

Munno D, Caporale S, Zullo G, et al. Neuropsychological assessment of patients with advanced Parkinson Disease submitted to extradural motor cortex stimulation. *Cog Behav Neuro*l 2007; 20: 1-6

Nguyen JP, Pollin B, Fève A, Geny C, Cesaro P. Improvement of action tremor by chronic cortical stimulation. *Mov Disord* 1998; 13:84-88

Pagni CA, Zeme S, Zenga F. Further experience with extradural motor cortex stimulation for treatment of advanced Parkinson's diseases. Report of 3 new cases *J Neurosurg Sci* 2003; 47:189-193

Pagni CA, Zeme S, Zenga F, Maina R.Extradural motor cortex stimulation in advanced Parkinson's disease: the Turin experience. *Neurosurg* 2005; 57 (ONS Suppl 3): ONS-402

Pagni CA, Albanese A, Bentivoglio A, Broggi G, Canavero S, Cioni B, et al. Results by motor cortex stimulation in treatment of focal dystonia, Parkinson's disease and post-ictal spasticity. The experience of the Italian Study Group of the Italian Neurosurgical Society. *Acta Neurochir Suppl*. 2008;101:13-21.

Romito LM, Franzini A, Perani D, et al. Fixed dystonia unresponsive to pallidal stimulation improved by motor cortex stimulation. *Neurology* 2007; 68:875-876

Strafella AP, Lozano AM, Lang AE, Ko J-H, Poon Y-Y, Moro E. Subdural motor cortex stimulation in Parkinson's disease does not modify movement-related rCBF pattern. *Mov Disorders* 2007; 22: 2113-2116

Seijo FJ, Gutierrez JC, Alvarez Vega M, Fernandez Gonzalez F, Lozano Aragonese B, Blazquez M. Therapeutic extradural cortical stimulation for Parkinson's disease: report of six cases and review of the literature. (*submitted*)

Sidoti C, Agrillo U. Chronic cortical stimulation for amyotrophic lateral sclerosis: a report of four consecutive operated cases after a 2-year follow up *Neurosurg* 2006; 58:E384

Tani N, Saitoh Y, Kishima H, et al. Motor cortex stimulation for levodopa-resistant akinesia: case report. *Mov Disorder* 2007; 22:1645-1649

Tsubokawa T, Katayama Y, Yamamoto T, Hirayama T, Koyama S. Chronic motor cortex stimulation in patients with thalamic pain. *J Neurosurg* 1993; 78:393-401

Verhagen Metman L, Pahwa R, Lyons K, et al. Motor cortex stimulation in Parkinson's disease: a pilot study. *Neurology* 2006 (suppl 2) 66: A47

In: Deep Brain Stimulation
Editors: Mark H. Rogers and Paul B. Anderson
ISBN 978-1-60692-895-0

Chapter V

Deep Brain Stimulation in Epilepsy: Experimental and Clinical Data*

M. Langlois[1], S. Saillet[1], B. Feddersen[5], L. Minotti[1, 2], L. Vercueil[1, 2], S Chabardès[1, 3], O. David[1], A. Depaulis[1] P. Kahane[1,2,4] and C. Deransart[† 1,2]

[1]Grenoble Institut des Neurosciences, INSERM U836-UJF-CEA,
[2]Neurology Department, and [3]Neurosurgery Department, Grenoble University Hospital,
[4]Institute for Children and adolescents with epilepsy – IDEE,
Hospices Civils de Lyon, France,
[5]Department of Neurology, Klinikum Grosshadern, University of Munich, Germany

1. Introduction

About 30% of epileptic patients do not respond to antiepileptic drugs (Kwan & Brodie, 2000), of whom only a minority can benefit from resective surgery. Such a therapeutic option is considered only in patients who suffer from focal seizures with an epileptogenic zone clearly identified and safely removable. Therefore, patients with seizures arising from eloquent cortices, or which are multifocal, bilateral, or generalized, represent a particular challenge to "new" or "alternative" therapies. For these patients, neurostimulation appears

* A version of this chapter was also published in *Recent Breakthroughs in Basal ganglia Research* , edited by Erwan Bezard published by Nova Science Publishers, Inc. It was submitted for appropriate modification in an effort to encourage wider dissemination of research.

† Corresponding author: Colin Deransart, Grenoble - Institut des Neurosciences, Centre de recherche Inserm U 836-UJF-CEA-CHU, Equipe 9: Dynamique des Réseaux Synchrones Epileptiques, Université Joseph Fourier - Faculté de Médecine, Domaine de la Merci, 38700 La Tronche, colin.deransart@ujf-grenoble.fr

with a great potential (Polkey et al., 2003; Theodore and Fisher, 2004). Different approaches to neurostimulation in epileptic patients now exist and depend on (i) the brain region which is targeted and (ii) the way the stimulation is applied (Oommen et al., 2005; Morrell, 2006; Theodore and Fisher, 2004; Vonck et al., 2007). The aim of neurostimulation in epilepsy is to reduce the probability of seizure occurrence and/or propagation, either by manipulating remote control systems (vagus nerve stimulation, deep brain stimulation), or by interfering with the epileptogenic zone itself (repetitive transcranial magnetic stimulation, cortical stimulation). In most cases, stimulation is delivered continuously or intermittently according to a scheduled protocol. In particular, new progress in biotechnology and EEG signal analysis now allows stimulation in response to detection of electrographic seizures (e.g., closed-loop stimulation). Here, we review the various experimental and clinical attempts that have been made to control epileptic seizures by the means of deep brain electrical stimulation.

2. Deep Brain Stimulation (DBS)

For more than two decades, stimulation of a number of deep brain targets has been shown to be feasible, safe, and effective in humans suffering from different forms of movement disorders. This has led to the development of deep brain stimulation (DBS) in an increasing number of neurological and non-neurological diseases, including epilepsy (Benabid et al., 2001). Although the cortex plays a crucial role in seizure generation, accumulating evidence has pointed to the role of subcortical structures in the clinical expression, propagation and control of epileptic seizures in humans (Semah, 2002; Vercueil and Hirsch, 2002). Based on experimental findings, DBS has been applied to a number of targets, including the cerebellum, different nuclei of the thalamus, and several structures of the basal ganglia system. Although encouraging, published results do not reach a definite conclusion and require further studies using animal models. Indeed, the study of the mechanisms of actions of such DBS on epileptic seizures is critical to understand the transitions between normal and paroxysmal activities of the epileptic networks.

2.1. Cerebellum

During the 1950s and 1960s, cortical cerebellar stimulation was shown to have antiepileptic properties on different animal models of seizures, mostly penicillin and cobalt foci in cats (Cooke and Snider, 1955; Dow et al., 1962; Mutani et al., 1969). Following this, and assuming cerebellar outflow is inhibitory in nearly all patients, Cooper and colleagues showed that seizures were modified or inhibited in 10 out of their 15 epileptic patients, without adverse effects (Cooper et al., 1973; 1976; 1978). These data raised the issue of distant modulation of cortical epileptogenicity by electrical currents. More especially, this study showed for the first time the feasibility and safety of a therapeutic stimulation technique in epileptic patients. Later, a large open study on 115 patients reported that 31 became seizure-free and 56 were significantly improved by stimulation of the cerebellum (Davis and Emmonds, 1992). Such promising results, however, were not confirmed in 3 controlled clinical trials involving 14 patients, of whom only 2 were improved (Krauss and Fisher, 1993; Van Buren et al., 1978; Wright et al., 1984). Additional animal studies conducted in monkeys with cortical focal seizures induced by alumina cream, or in kindled cats, did not confirm previous experimental findings (Ebner et al., 1980 ; Lockard et al., 1979 ; Majkowski et al., 1980) and the interest for cerebellar stimulation in epilepsy disappeared for many years. Recently, however, a double-blind, randomized controlled pilot study conducted in 5 patients suffering from intractable motor seizures has renewed the interest in such stimulation (Velasco et al., 2005). In this study, 10-Hz stimulations were applied to the upper medial surface of each cerebellar hemisphere, and parameters were adjusted to deliver a constant charge density of 2.0 microC/cm^2/phase. During the initial 3-month double-blind phase, seizures were significantly reduced when the patients were stimulated. Over the following 6-month open-label phase, where all the patients were stimulated, seizures were reduced by 41% (14-75%) and the difference was significant for tonic and tonic-clonic seizures. Effectiveness was maintained over 2 years and few complications occurred. Altogether, although cerebellar stimulation appears to possess antiepileptic effects in some patients and/or some forms of epilepsy, the rationale of such suppressive effects remains to be determined. No clinical studies targeting this structure are currently under progress.

2.2. Thalamus

Since the 1980s, different nuclei of the thalamus have been studied to understand the physiopathology of epilepsy because many interaction pathways exist between these nuclei and the cortex. Several thalamic targets have been stimulated to suppress seizures, mainly the anterior nucleus and the centromedian nucleus. There is limited proof from animal studies that stimulation of these structures can influence seizure threshold. However, there is clinical evidence that continuous stimulation of these targets in epileptic patients reduces seizure frequency and severity.

2.2.a. Anterior Thalamus (AN)

The anterior nucleus (AN) of the thalamus receives projections from the hippocampus via the fornix, the mamillary bodies and the mamillo-thalamic fascicle of Vicq d'Azir and has outputs to the cingulate cortex and, via the cingulum, to the entorhinal cortex and back to the hippocampus. It appears to be in close interaction with the circuit of Papez which is often involved in some forms of epilepsies (e.g., temporal lobe epilepsies). AN therefore is central in the network which underlies limbic seizures and, as such, represents an attractive target for DBS in epileptic patients. Cooper and his group, encouraged by their experience on cerebellar stimulation, were the first to direct their interest to this nucleus, based on the hypothesis that AN could act as a "pacemaker" for the cortex. They showed that bilateral chronic stimulation of AN in 6 epileptic patients resulted in 60% reduction of seizure frequency in 5 of them, as well as a decrease in EEG spikes (Cooper and Upton, 1985). Using an experimental approach, it was later shown that AN and mamillary bodies were involved in the genesis of pentylenetetrazol-induced seizures and were activated during ethosuximide-induced suppression of these seizures (Mirski and Ferrendelli, 1986a ; 1986b). In addition, the section of the mamillo-thalamic bundle prevented pentylenetetrazol-induced seizures in guinea pigs (Mirsky and Ferrendelli, 1984). Furthermore, it was reported that 100-Hz electrical stimulation of the mammilary nuclei and AN increased the seizure threshold of pentylenetetrazol in rats (Mirski and Fisher, 1994; Mirski et al., 1997). These anticonvulsant effects were dependent on the intensity of the stimulation rather than on its frequency. On the contrary, low-frequency AN stimulation tended to be proconvulsive (Mirski et al, 1997). More recently, high-frequency AN stimulation suppressed focal cortical and limbic seizures induced by intra-cortical or intra-amydaloid kainic acid injections, respectively (Takebayashi et al, 2007a and 2007b) and delayed both status epilepticus and seizures induced by pilocarpine although without complete suppression (Hamani et al., 2004, 2008). Finally, 100-Hz AN stimulation was found to *aggravate* recurrent seizures observed following status epilepticus produced by systemic kainic acid (Lado, 2006).

These experimental data gave weight to the need of re-assessing the effect of AN stimulation in epileptic patients, Four open-label trials were reported showing that seizure frequency was reduced from 20 to 92% and being statistically significant in 12 of the 18 patients (Hodaie et al., 2002 ; Kerrigan et al., 2004 ; Lim et al., 2007 ; Osorio et al., 2007). Two patients presented a complication (small frontal hemorrhage and extension erosion over the scalp), which did not result in major or permanent neurological deficit. A study showed that insertion of AN electrodes by itself could reduce seizures (Lim et al., 2007) and another one that the observed benefits did not differ between stimulation-on and stimulation-off periods (Hodaie et al., 2002), thus raising the issue of a lesional, placebo or carry-over effect. To address this question, a large multicenter prospective randomized trial of AN stimulation for partial and secondarily generalized seizures (Stimulation of the Anterior Nucleus of the Thalamus for Epilepsy or SANTE) is currently under investigation in North America. Whether AN stimulation could be more effective in temporal lobe epilepsy (Zumsteg et al., 2006) and whether other components of the circuit of Papez, namely the mamillary bodies and mamillo-thalamic tract (Duprez et al., 2005 ; van Rijckevorsel et al., 2005) are possible targets for DBS are important issues for clinical trials.

2.2.b. Centromedian Thalamus (CM)

In addition to the AN, attention was also directed towards one of the intralaminar nuclei of the thalamus, the centromedian nucleus (CM). This nucleus is part of the reticulothalamocortical system mediating cerebral cortex excitability (Jasper, 1991), and has been suggested to participate in the modulation of vigilance states (Velasco et al., 1979). Although experimental findings remain rare (Arduini and Lary Bounes, 1952), a first open-label study was conducted in 5 patients with bilateral CM stimulation at the end of the 1980s (Velasco et al., 1987). Initial results indicated an improvement of seizure frequency and EEG spiking over 3 months of chronic stimulation. Later, Velasco's group accumulated data in a cohort of 49 patients suffering from different forms of seizures and epilepsies (Velasco et al., 2001a ; 2002). Among these patients, 5 to 13 were followed over long-term follow-up studies (Velasco et al., 1993 ; 1995 ; 2000ab, 2006). Overall, the procedure was reported to be beneficial and generally well-tolerated, although a central nystagmus was induced in some cases (Taylor et al., 2000). A few patients were explanted because of repeated and multiple skin erosions (Velasco et al., 2006). It is interesting to note that a decrease of 80% of seizures were observed on average in patients with generalized tonic-clonic seizures and atypical absences of the Lennox-Gastaut syndrome, with a global improvement of patients in their ability scale scores (Velasco et al., 2006). By contrast, no improvements were found for either complex partial seizures or focal spikes in temporal regions. The best clinical results were seen when both electrodes contacts were located within the CM on both sides and when stimulation at 6-8 Hz and 60 Hz induced recruiting responses and regional DC shifts, respectively (Velasco et al., 2000a). Two hours of daily 130-Hz stimulation sessions (1-minute on, 4 minutes off), alternating the right and left CM were used. However, continuous bilateral stimulation led to faster and more significant results (Velasco et al. 2001b). As for AN stimulation, persistent antiepileptic effects were found 3 months or more after discontinuation of the stimulation (« off effect »), and possible plasticity which develops during the stimulation procedure was suggested (Velasco et al. 2001b). No such seizure suppression was found in a small placebo-controlled study conducted in 7 patients with mesial temporal lobe epilepsy. In this study, no statistically significant difference from the baseline in frequency of tonic-clonic seizures when the stimulator was on versus off (Fisher et al., 1992). In the open-label follow-up phase, however, 3 of 6 patients reported at least a 50% decrease in seizure frequency.

Up to now, very few animal studies have examined the role of the CM or of the parafascicular nucleus (PF) of the thalamus—which has similar connections—in the control of epileptic seizures. In a genetic model of absence epilepsy in the rat (GAERS), pharmacological activation of the PF was found to suppress spike-and-wave discharges (Nail-Boucherie et al., 2005). More recently, 130-Hz stimulation of this structure was reported to interrupt focal hippocampal seizures in a mouse model of mesiotemporal lobe epilepsy (Langlois et al., in preparation). Because of its unique location between cortical and limbic structures and the basal ganglia (see below), the CM/PF nuclei could well constitute an interesting target for DBS. More animal studies are clearly required to understand the role of this structure in the modulation of epileptic seizures.

2.3. Basal Ganglia

Since the beginning of the 1980s, experimental animal studies have suggested the existence of a “nigral control” of epileptic seizures (for review see Gale, 1995; Depaulis et al., 1994). Inhibition of the Substantia Nigra pars Reticulata (SNR) has potent anti-epileptic effects in different animal models of epilepsy (Deransart and Depaulis, 2002) and the GABAergic SNR output appears to be a critical relay in this control (Depaulis et al., 1990; Paz et al., 2005; 2007). Local manipulations of the basal ganglia that lead to an inhibition of the SNR neurons (e.g., activation of the striatum or pallidum, inhibition of the sub-thalamic nucleus) also had significant anti-epileptic effects (for review see Deransart and Depaulis, 2002), suggesting that different striato-nigral circuits are involved in the control of epileptic seizures. In humans, EEG, clinical and imaging data also support the involvement of the basal ganglia in the propagation and/or the control of epileptic discharges (Biraben et al., 2004; Bouilleret et al., 2008; Vercueil and Hirsch, 2002). Altogether, experimental and clinical data suggest a privileged role for the basal ganglia in the control of generation and/or spread of epileptic discharges in the cortex. Paradoxically, the therapeutic relevance of such findings was rarely considered until the 1990s.

2.3.a. Caudate Nucleus (CN)

Following experimental evidence that stimulation of the caudate nucleus (CN) has antiepileptic properties in different animal models of seizures (La Grutta et al., 1971, 1988; Mutani, 1969; Oakley and Ojemann, 1982 ; Psatta, 1983), Chkhenkeli and his group, as well as Sramka and colleagues, were the first to suggest the beneficial effect of striatal low-frequency stimulation (below 50 Hz) in epileptic patients (Chkhenkeli, 1978; Sramka et al., 1980). A decrease in focal and generalized discharges was observed in 57 patients bilaterally stimulated at low frequency (4–6Hz) in the CN (Chkhenkeli and Chkhenkeli, 1997). The study, however, was not controlled and the effects on seizures were not assessed. Interestingly, epileptic activity was worsened by stimulating the CN at higher frequency, a finding that was also reported in the aluminium-hydroxide monkey model of motor seizures (Oakley and Ojemann, 1982). Therefore, if one assumes that low-frequency stimulation is excitatory and high-frequency stimulation is inhibitory, these clinical data are in agreement with animal data (see Deransart and Depaulis, 2002). Indeed, activation of the striatum inhibits the SNR through GABAergic projections and therefore leads to seizure suppression (Deransart et al., 1998). Although further studies are needed, these results highlight the ability of the basal ganglia system to modulate cortical epileptogenicity.

2.3.b. Subthalamic Nucleus (STN)

In 1998, Vercueil et al. (1998) were the first to show that 130-Hz stimulation of the subthalamic nucleus (STN) could interrupt absence seizures in GAERS, a well-established genetic model of absence epilepsy (Danober et al., 1998; Marescaux et al. 1992). Since then, high-frequency stimulation of the subthalamic nucleus has been reported to protect against seizures induced by local kainate injection in the amygdala (Bressand et al., 1999; Loddenkemper et al., 2001; Usui et al., 2005) or by fluorothyl inhalation (Veliskova et al., 1996). This is in agreement with the antiepileptic effects reported after pharmacological inhibition of the STN on seizures induced by amygdala kindling (Deransart et al., 1998a), intravenous bicuculline or by its focal application into the anterior piriform cortex (Dybdal and Gale, 2000) and in GAERS (Deransart et al., 1996).

This led the group of Benabid at Grenoble University Hospital to perform the first STN stimulation in a 5-year-old girl with pharmacologically-resistant inoperable epilepsy caused by a focal centroparietal dysplasia (Benabid et al., 2002). Later, 11 additional patients suffering from different forms of epilepsy received high frequency STN stimulation at different institutions (Chabardès et al., 2002; Loddenkemper et al., 2001; Vesper et al., 2007). Overall, seizure occurrence was reduced by at least 50% in 7/12 cases, and the stimulation was well tolerated. Good responders suffered from very different epilepsy types including focal epilepsy, Dravet syndrome, Lennox-Gastaut syndrome and progressive myoclonic epilepsy. Surgical complications occurred in 2 patients, including infection of the generator in one, and a postimplantation subdural hematoma in another who later underwent surgical treatment, without sequelae (Chabardès et al., 2002). Bilateral stimulation appeared more effective than unilateral stimulation, in agreement with experimental data (Depaulis et al., 1994). However, whether it should be applied continuously or intermittently remains questionable (Chabardès et al., 2002). Furthermore, whether the optimal target in epileptic patients is the STN itself or, as is suggested in some patients, the SNR, remains an important issue (see below - Chabardès et al., 2002 ; Vesper et al., 2007). A double-blind cross-over multicentric study is in progress in France (STIMEP) and aims at evaluating the clinical effect of 130-Hz stimulation of the STN/SNR in patients with ring chromosome 20 epilepsy. These patients suffer from very long lasting epileptic seizures, evolving often into status epilepticus and are difficult to control with antiepileptic drugs. They exhibit a deficit of dopaminergic activity in the striatum as compared with normal subjects (Biraben et al., 2004), a finding which is in accordance with the critical role of striatal dopamine in the control of seizures (Deransart et al., 2000).

2.3.c. Substantia Nigra pars Reticulata (SNR)

In 1980, Gale and Iadarola were the first to correlate an increase of GABA in the SNR with antiepileptic effects (Gale and Iadarola, 1980). Later, they showed that the potentiation of the GABAergic neurotransmission within the SNR, by bilateral microinjections of GABAmimetic drugs, suppressed convulsions in various models of generalized seizures in the rat (Iadarola and Gale, 1982). The possibility that seizures are controlled by the SNR also emerged from pharmacological studies in GAERS showing that a bilateral inhibition of SNR suppresses cortical Spike-and-Waves discharges (SWDs) (Depaulis et al., 1988, 1989; Deransart et al., 1996, 1998, 2001). Since then, several studies have confirmed that inhibition of the SNR has a potent anti-epileptic effects in different animal models of epilepsy (Depaulis et al., 1994; Deransart and Depaulis, 2002; Paz et al.,2005; 2007).

In this context, it was shown that DBS applied to the SNR, also suppressed generalized convulsive seizures induced by fluorothyl inhalation (Velisek et al., 2002), amygdala-kindled seizures (Morimoto and Goddard,1987; Shi et al., 2006), absence seizures in GAERS (Feddersen et al., 2007) and also focal seizures in kainate treated mice (Deransart et al., 2004). In the model of generalized convulsive seizures induced by fluorothyl inhalation, bilateral and bipolar 130Hz SNR stimulation had anticonvulsivant effects in both adults and infant rats (Velisek et al., 2002). In amygdala-kindling, such stimulations were shown to induce a long lasting suppression of antiepileptogenesis (Shi et al., 2006). In GAERS, bilateral, bipolar, and monophasic SNR stimulations at a frequency of 60Hz and a pulse width of 60μs were defined as the optimal conditions to interrupt ongoing absence seizures without motor side effects (Feddersen et al., 2007). The threshold to interrupt epileptic seizures was lower using SNR stimulation compared to STN stimulation, using the same model and stimulation parameters. However, this last study showed that continuous stimulation fail to control the occurrence of seizures, in agreement with previous reports (Vercueil et al., 1998) and suggested that a refractory period of about 60 sec exists during which any stimulation is without effect. This study also showed that *continuous* stimulation of the SNR could even aggravate seizure occurrence. Adaptive stimulation may allow to alleviate this problem and to further specify the existence of a refractory period (see below).

3. Stimulation at Seizure Focus

Stimulating the epileptogenic cortex to interrupt epileptic seizures may appear paradoxical. Indeed, "stimulation" classically means "excitation" and the epilepsies are characterized by a pathological hyperexcitability and hypersynchrony of cortical neurons. The effects provoked by cortical stimulation, however, depend on the stimulation parameters used, the region which is stimulated, as well as the way that the stimulation is delivered (indirectly or directly). Furthermore, cortical stimulation is generally used to map functions in eloquent brain. It is known that cortical stimulation can evoke focal after-discharges that may evolve into clinical seizures. It has been shown that afterdischarges elicited by electrical stimulation via subdural electrodes can be interrupted by the application of brief bursts of 50-Hz electrical stimulation through subdural electrode contacts (Lesser et al. 1999). To date, a few studies have been conducted, including a limited number of patients, and therapeutic results are equivocal at best.

Several preclinical studies have found potential antiepileptic effects of brain stimulation in animal models. Notably, low-frequency (1 Hz) stimulation applied after kindling stimulation of the amygdala was found to inhibit the development of afterdischarges, an effect named *quenching* (Weiss et al., 1995). This quenching effect seems effective in adult as well as immature rats (Velisek et al., 2002). Interestingly, when applied immediately *before* the kindling stimulus, preemptive 1 Hz sine wave stimulation was also effective, thus suggesting some potential benefit for seizure prevention (Goodman et al., 2005). Other regions such as the hippocampus (Barbarosie and Avoli, 1997), the central piriform cortex (Yang et al., 2006; Zhu-ge et al., 2007) or the cerebral fastigial nucleus (Wang et al., 2008) may also appear as potentially effective targets for 1-Hz stimulation treatment of epilepsy. In general these data suggest that 1-Hz stimulation inhibits both acquisition and expression of kindling seizure by preventing afterdischarge generation and propagation in rat. Unexpectedly, such effects are also observed in the cerebral fastigial nucleus, suggesting that targets outside the limbic system may have a significant antiepileptic action.

In humans, both low- (1-Hz) and medium- (50 Hz) frequency stimulation have proven effective to reduce interictal epileptiform discharges (Kinoshita et al., 2005b; Yamamoto et al., 2002). Therapeutic stimulation, however, was applied at high frequency in almost all studies. The first attempt of therapeutic stimulation of temporal lobe structures was reported in 1980, in 3 patients, without clear benefit (Sramka et al., 1980). More recently, several investigators have tried continuous scheduled stimulation of epileptic foci, including hypothalamic hamartoma (Kahane et al., 2003), neocortical structures (Elisevich et al., 2006) and, mostly, mesio-temporal lobe (Tellez-Zenteno et al., 2006; Velasco et al., 2000c ; 2007; Vonck et al., 2002). The first pilot study of mesio-temporal lobe stimulation, conducted in 10 patients studied by intracranial electrodes before surgery, showed that stimulation stopped seizures and decreased the number of interictal EEG spikes in the 7 patients where the stimulated electrode was placed within the hippocampus or hippocampal gyrus (Velasco et al., 2000c). There were no side-effects on language and memory, and no histological damages were found in the stimulated tissue. Whether such an antiepileptic effect could be observed over a more prolonged stimulation procedure was later evaluated in a small open series conducted in 3 patients, all of whom exhibited more than 50% of seizure reduction after a mean follow-up of 5 months, without adverse events (Vonck et al., 2002).

Following this, 2 additional trials of hippocampal stimulation were conducted, leading to opposite results. In one double-blind study, the seizure outcome was significantly improved in all 9 patients over a long-term follow-up (Velasco et al., 2007), which showed more than 95% seizure reduction in the 5 patients with normal MRI, and 50-70% seizure reduction in the 4 patients who had hippocampal sclerosis. No adverse events were found but 3 patients were explanted after 2 years due to skin erosion in the trajectory system. It was suggested that beneficial effects of stimulation were associated with a high GABA tissue content and a low rate of cell loss (Cuellar-Herrera et al., 2004). By contrast, seizure frequency was reduced by only 15% in average in the 4 patients of the double-blind, multiple cross-over, randomized study of Tellez-Zenteno et al. (2006). Additionally, effects seemed to carry over into the off period, thus raising the issue of an implantation effect. Yet, no adverse events were found. Overall, stimulation of hippocampal foci shows beneficial trends, but whether the effect is significant, and of clear clinical relevance, remains debatable.

Currently, a randomized controlled trial of hippocampal stimulation for temporal lobe epilepsy (METTLE) is recruiting patients to determine whether unilateral hippocampal electrical stimulation is safe and more effective than simply implanting an electrode in the hippocampus without electrical stimulation, or treating with medical therapy alone. A prospective randomized controlled study of neurostimulation in the medial temporal lobe for patients with medically refractory medial temporal lobe epilepsy is also currently recruiting patients for a controlled randomized stimulation versus resection (CoRaStiR) study (www.clinicaltrials.gov).

4. Adaptative Stimulation

Continuous scheduled brain stimulation, whatever the target (DBS, cortical stimulation), has appeared to be safe and of potential benefit in treating medically intractable epilepsies (see above). Limited, but growing data suggests that responsive (seizure-triggered) stimulation might also be effective (Morrel, 2006). Such a strategy is distinct from continuous scheduled stimulation as it aims at blocking seizures when they occur, rather than at decreasing cortical excitability chronically. It is motivated by the reduction of power consumption, the paroxysmal nature of the seizures and the possible behavioural side-effects induced by chronic stimulations. Also, it has been suggested that continuous stimulations may aggravate seizures in animals (Feddersen et al., 2007). Seizure-triggered stimulation requires an implanted stimulating device coupled with real-time signal analysis techniques. Usually, a seizure detection algorithm allows the delivery of a stimulation to interrupt seizure prior to, or concomitantly to, the onset of clinical symptoms. A number of algorithms to detect seizures do exist (see for instance Osorio et al., 2002; Grewal and Gotman, 2005). The main stumbling block, as for continuous stimulation, is to find, ideally following an automatic search, optimal stimulation parameters to abort seizures. To our knowledge, existing literature about automatic seizure-triggered stimulation in animal models *in vivo* is rather limited. Using similar techniques as VNS therapy, Fanselow and colleagues have shown a reduction of pentylenetetrazole-induced seizure activity in awake rats by seizure-triggered trigeminal nerve stimulation (Fanselow et al., 2000). Interestingly, seizure-triggered stimulation was more effective than the stimulation protocol involving a fixed duty cycle, in terms of the percent seizure reduction per second of stimulation (up to 78%). Currently, a preliminary study in Grenoble (France) is testing a new technology based on stimulation combined to seizure-detection to interrupt absence seizures in GAERS (Saillet et al., submitted). This should allow to better determine the optimal target and parameters of stimulation required by such technology.

In humans, responsive stimulation can shorten or terminate electrically-elicited afterdischarges using brief bursts of 50-Hz electrical stimulation (Lesser et al., 1999), the effect being greater at primary sites than at adjacent electrodes (Motamedi et al., 2002). Preliminary trials of responsive stimulation, however, did not consistently use a similar paradigm (Kossof et al., 2004 ; Fountas et al., 2005 ; Osorio et al., 2005). The effects of responsive stimulation were first evaluated in 4 patients using an external neurostimulator, which proved effective at automatically detecting electrographic seizures, delivering targeted electrical stimuli, and altering or suppressing ictal discharges (Kossoff et al., 2004). Another feasibility study confirmed these results using a cranially implantable device in 8 patients (Fountas et al., 2005). Detection and stimulation were performed using electrodes placed over the seizure focus, and 7 of the 8 patients exhibited more than a 45% decrease in their seizure frequency, with a mean follow-up time of 9.2 months. In the third pilot study, conducted in 8 patients, stimulation was delivered either directly to the epileptogenic zone (local closed-loop, n=4), or indirectly through the anterior thalami (remote closed-loop, n=4), depending on whether the epileptogenic zone was single, or multiple (Osorio et al., 2005). On average, a 55.5% and 40.8% decrease of seizure frequency was observed in the local closed-loop group and in the remote closed-loop group, respectively. Overall, none of the 20 patients enrolled in these 3 pilot studies had adverse events. Although promising, this new therapy needs further evaluation and a multi-institutional prospective clinical trial is underway in the USA. The Responsive Neurostimulation System (RNS), sponsored by NeuroPace Inc., is designed to continuously monitor brain electrical activity from the electrodes and, after identifying the "signature" of a seizure's onset, deliver brief and mild electrical stimulation with the intention of suppressing the seizure. The purpose of the RNS System Pivotal Clinical Investigation is to assess the safety and to demonstrate that the RNS System is effective as an add-on (adjunctive) therapy in reducing the frequency of seizures in individuals with partial onset seizures that are refractory to two or more AED medications. Whether, in the near future, closed-loop stimulators will be able to react using seizure-prediction algorithms represents a particularly challenging issue.

5. Conclusions

Neurostimulation in non-surgically remediable epileptic patients represents an emerging treatment. It has the advantage of reversibility and adjustability, but remains palliative so that surgical resection remains the gold standard treatment of drug-resistant epilepsies whenever this option is possible. VNS is the only approved stimulation therapy for epilepsy so far and, as such, it is licensed in many countries as an adjunctive therapy. Other stimulation techniques must be considered experimental although several controlled studies are currently under investigation. Notably, results of direct brain stimulation, although encouraging, are not conclusive and further investigations are required to evaluate the real benefit of this emerging therapy, in as much as the risks of haemorrhage and infection, although low (around 5%), do exist. However, pathological examination in post-mortem studies and temporal lobe resection, in Parkinson's disease or epilepsy, suggest that chronic stimulation does not induce neural injury and can be delivered safely (Haberler et al., 2000; Pilitsis et al., 2008; Velasco et al., 2000c). In any case, seizure types or epileptic syndromes which may respond to stimulation should be identified, as well as the type of stimulation that is likely to be of potential efficacy depending on the patient's characteristics. This requires to improve our knowledge on the neural circuits in which seizures start and propagate, to better understand the precise mechanisms of the supposed effect of neurostimulation, and to search for optimal stimulation parameters. The development of experimental research in this field, as well as rigorous clinical evaluation, is essential for further improvements in clinical efficacy.

References

Akamatsu N, Fueta Y, Endo Y, Matsunaga K, Uozumi T, Tsuji S. Decreased susceptibility to pentylenetetrazole-inducded seizures after low frequency transcranial magnetic stimulaiton in the rat. *Neurosci Lett* 2001; 310:153-156.

Andy OJ, Jurko MF. Seizure control by mesothalamic reticular stimulation. *Clin Electroencephalography* 1986 ; 17 : 52-60.

Arduini D, Lary Bounes GC. Action de la stimulation électrique de la formation réticulaire du bulbe et des stimulations sensorielles sur les ondes strychniques. *Electroencephalogr Clin Neurophysiol* 1952; 4: 502-12.

Barbarosie M, Avoli M. CA3-driven hippocampal-entorhinal loop controls rather than sustains in vitro limbic seizures. *J Neurosci* 1997; 17 : 9308-9314.

Benabid AL, Koudsié A, Benazzouz A, Vercueil L, Fraix V, Chabardès S, Lebas JF, Pollak P. Deep brain stimulation of the corpus luysi (subthalamic nucleus) and other targets in Parkinson's disease. Extension to new indications such as dystonia and epilepsy. *J Neurol* 2001; 248 (suppl 3): III37-47.

Benabid AL, Minotti L, Koudsie A, de Saint Martin A, Hirsch E. Antiepileptic effect of high-frequency stimulation of the subthalamic nucleus (corpus luysi) in a case of medically intractable epilepsy caused by focal dysplasia: a 30-month follow-up: technical case report. *Neurosurgery* 2002; 50: 1385–1391.

Benazzouz A, Piallat B, Pollak P, Benabid AL. Responses of substantia nigra pars reticulata and glomus pallidus complex to high frequency stimulation of the subthalamic nucleus in rat: electrophysiological data. *Neurosci Lett* 1995; 189 : 77-80.

Biraben A, Semah F, Ribeiro MJ, Douaud G, Remy P, Depaulis A. PET evidence for a role of the basal ganglia in patients with ring chromosome 20 epilepsy. *Neurology* 2004; 63: 73-77.

Bouilleret V, Semah F, Chassoux F, Mantzaridez M, Biraben A, Trebossen R, Ribeiro MJ. Basal ganglia involvement in temporal lobe epilepsy: a functional and morphologic study. *Neurology* 2008; 70:177-184.

Brasil-Neto JP, de Arauja DP, Teixeira WA, Araujo VP, Boechat-Barros R. *Arq Neuropsiquiatr* 2004 ; 62 : 21-25.

Bressand K, Dematteis M, Kahane P, Benazzouz A, Benabid AL. Involvement of the subthalamic nucleus in the control of temporal lobe epilepsy: study by hight frequency stimulation in rats. *Soc Neurosci* 1999 25:1656.

Cantello R, Rossi S, Varrasi C, Ulivelli M, Civardi C, Bartalini S, Vatti G, Cincotta M, Borghoresi A, Zaccara G, Quartarone A, Crupi D, Langana A, Inghilleri M, Giallonardo AT, Berardelli A, Pacifici L, Ferreri F, Tombini M, Gilio F, Quarato P, Conte A, Manganotti P, Bongiovanni LG, Monaco F, Ferrante D, Rossini PM. Slow repetitive TMS for drug-reistant epilepsy : clinical and EEG findings of a placebo-controlled trial. *Epilepsia* 2007; 48: 366-374.

Chabardès S, Kahane P, Minotti L, Koudsie A, Hirsch E, Benabid A-L. Deep brain stimulation in epilepsy with particular reference to the subthalamic nucleus. *Epileptic disord* 2002; 4 (suppl 3): 83–93.

Chen R, Classen J, Gerloff C, Celnik P, Wassermann EM, Hallett M, Cohen LG. Depression of motor cortex excitability by low-frequency transcranial magnetic stimulation. *Neurology* 1997; 48: 1398-1403.

Chkhenkeli SA. The inhibitory influence of the nucleus caudatus electrostimulation on the human's amygdalar and hippocampal activity at temporal lobe epilepsy. *Bull Georgian Acad Sci* 1978; 4/6: 406-11.

Chkhenkeli SA, Chkhenkeli IS. Effects of therapeutic stimulation of nucleus caudatus on epileptic electrical activity of brain in patients with intractable epilepsy. *Stereotact Funct Neurosurg* 1997; 69: 221-224.

Cooke PM, Snider RS. Some cerebellar influences on electrically-induced cerebral seizures. *Epilepsia* 1955; 4: 19-28.

Cooper I. *Cerebellar stimulation in man.* New York: Raven Press, 1978: 1–212.

Cooper IS, Upton ARM. The effect of chronic stimulation of cerebellum and thalamus upon neurophysiology and neurochemistry of cerebral cortex. In: Lazorthes Y, Upton ARM, eds. *Neurostimulation: an overview.* New York: Futura, 1985: 207-211.

Cooper IS, Amin I, Riklan M, Waltz JM, Poon TP. Chronic cerebellar stimulation in epilepsy. Clinical and anatomical studies. *Arch Neurol* 1976; 33: 559-70.

Cooper IS, Amin I, Gilman S. The effect of chronic cerebellar stimulation upon epilepsy in man. *Trans Am Neurol Assoc* 1973; 98: 192-6.

Cuellar-Herrera M, Velasco M, Velasco F, Velasco AL, Jimenez F, Orozco S, Briones M, Rocha L. Evaluation of GABA system and cell damage in parahippocampus of patients with temporal lobe epilepsy showing antiepileptic effects after subacute electrical stimulation. *Epilepsia* 2004; 45: 459-466.

Danober L, Deransart C, Depaulis A, Vergnes M, Marescaux C. Pathophysiological mechanisms of genetic absence epilepsy in rat. *Prog Neurobiol* 1998; 55: 27-57.

Davis R, Emmonds SE. Cerebellar stimulation for seizure control: 17-year study. *Stereotact Funct Neurosurg* 1992; 58: 200–208.

Depaulis A, Vergnes M, Depaulis A. Endogenous control of epilepsy: the nigral inhibitory system. *Prog Neurobiol* 1994; 42: 33-52.

Deransart C, Depaulis A. The control of seizures by the basal ganglia? A review of experimental data. *Epileptic Disord* 2002; 4 (suppl 3): S61-S72.

Deransart C, Marescaux C, Depaulis A. Involvement of nigral glutamatergic inputs in the control of seizures in a genetic model of absence epilepsy in the rat. *Neuroscience* 1996; 71: 721-728.

Deransart C, Lê BT, Marescaux C, Depaulis A. Role of the subthalamo-nigral input in the control of amygdale-kindled seizures in rat. *Brain Res* 1998a; 807: 78-83.

Deransart C, Riban V, Lê BT, Marescaux C, Depaulis A. Dopamine in the nucleus accumbens modulates seizures in a genetic model of absence epilepsy in the rat. *Neuroscience* 2000; 100: 335-344.

Deransart C, Depaulis A (2004) Le concept de contrôle nigral des épilepsies s'applique-t-il aux épilepsies partielles pharmacorésistantes? *Epilepsies* 16(2) 75-82.

Dow RS, Ferandez-Guardiola A, Manni E. The influence of the cerebellum on experimental epilepsy. *Electroencephalogr Clin Neurophysiol* 1962; 14: 383-398.

Duprez TP, Serieh BA, Raftopoulos C. Absence of memory dysfunction after bilateral mammillary body and mammillothalamic tract electrode implantation: preliminary experience in three patients. *AJNR Am J Neuroradiol* 2005; 26: 195-197.

Ebner TJ, Bantli H, Bloedel JR. Effects of cerebellar stimulation on unitary activity within a chronic epileptic focus in a primate. *Electroencephalogr Clin Neurophysiol* 1980; 49: 585-599.

Elisevich K, Jenrow K, Schuh L, Smith B. Long-term electrical stimulation-induced inhibition of partial epilepsy. Case report. *J Neurosurg* 2006; 105: 894-897.

Fanselow EE, Reid AP, Nicolelis MA. Reduction of pentylenetetrazole-induced seizure activity in awake rats by seizure-triggered trigeminal nerve stimulation. *J Neurosci.* 2000; 20(21):8160-8.

Feddersen B, Vercueil L, Noachtar S, David O, Depaulis A, Deransart C. Controlling seizures is not controlling epilepsy: a parametric study of deep brain stimulation for epilepsy. *Neurobiol Dis* 2007; 27: 292-300.

Feger J, Robledo P. The effects of activation or inhibition of the subthalamic nucleus on the metabolic and electrophysiological activities within the pallidal complex and the substantia nigra in the rat. *Eur J Neurosci* 1991; 3: 947-952.

Fisher RS, Uematsu S, Krauss GL, Cysyk B, McPherson R, Lesser RP, Gordon B, Schwerdt P, Rise M. Placebo-controlled pilot study of centromedian thalamic stimulation in treatment of intractable seizures. *Epilepsia* 1992; 33: 841-851.

Fountas KN, Smith JR, Murro AM, Politsky J, Park YD, Jenkins PD. Implantation of a closed-loop stimulation in the management of medically refractory focal epilepsy: a technical note. *Stereotact Funct Neurosurg* 2005; 83: 153-158.

Fregni F, Otachi PT, Do Valle A, Boggio PS, Thut G, Rigonatti SP, Pascual-Leone A, Valente KD. A randomized clinical trial of repetitive transcranial magnetic stimulation in patients with refractory epilepsy. *Ann Neurol* 2006; 60: 447-455.

Gale K, Iadarola MJ. Seizure protection and increased nerve-terminal GABA: delayed effects of GABA transaminase inhibition. *Science* 1980; 208: 288-291.

Goodman JH, Berger RE, Tcheng TK. Preemptive low-frequency stimulation decreases the incidence of amygdala-kindled seizures. *Epilepsia* 2005; 46: 1-7.

Grewal S, Gotman J. An automatic warning system for epileptic seizures recorded on intracerebral EEGs. *Clin Neurophysiol.* 2005;116(10):2460-72.

Haberler C, Alesch F, Mazal PR, Pilz P, Jellinger K, Pinter MM, Hainfellner JA, Budka H. No tissue damage by chronic deep brain stimulation in Parkinson's disease. *Ann Neurol* 2000; 48: 372-376.

Hamani C, Ewerton FI, Bonilha SM, Ballester G, Mello LE, Lozano AM. Bilateral anterior thalamic nucleus lesions and high-frequency stimulation are protective against pilocarpine-induced seizures and status epilepticus. *Neurosurgery* 2004; 54:191-195.

Hamani C, Hodaie M, Chiang J, del Campo M, Andrade DM, Sherman D, Mirski M, Mello LE, Lozano AM. Deep brain stimulation of the anterior nucleus of the thalamus: effects of electrical stimulation on pilocarpine-induced seizures and status epilepticus. *Epilepsy Res.* 2008 Feb;78(2-3):117-23

Hodaie M, Wennberg RA, Dostrovsky JO, Lozano AM. Chronic anterior thalamus stimulation for intractable epilepsy. *Epilepsia* 2002; 43: 603-608.

Iadarola MJ, Gale K. Substantia nigra: site of anticonvulsant activity mediated by gammaaminobutyric acid. *Science* 1982; 218 : 1237-1240.

Jasper H. Current evaluation of the concepts of centrencephalic and cortico-reticular seizures. *Electroencephalogr Clin Neurophysiol* 1991; 78: 2-11.

Jennum P, Klitgaard H. Repetitive transcranial magnetic stimulations of the rat. Effect of acute and chronic stimulations on pentylenetetrazole-induced clonic seizures. *Epilepsy Res* 1996; 23: 115-122.

Joo EY, Han SJ, Chung S-H, Cho J-W, Seo DW, Hong SB. Antiepileptic effects of low frequency repetitive transcranial magnetic stimulation by different stimulation durations and locations. *Clinical Neurophysiology* 2007; 118 : 702-708.

Kahane P, Ryvlin P, Hoffmann D, Minotti L, Benabid AL. From hypothalamic hamartoma to cortex: what can be learnt from depth recordings and stimulation? *Epileptic Disord* 2003; 5: 205-217.

Kerrigan JF, Litt B, Fisher RS, Cranstoun S, French JA, Blum DE, Dichter M, Shetter A, Baltuch G, Jaggi J, Krone S, Brodie MA, Rise M, Graves N. Electrical stimulation of the anterior nucleus of the thalamus for the treatment of intractable epilepsy. *Epilepsia* 2004; 45: 346-354.

Kinoshita M, Ikeda A, Begum T, Yamamoto J, Hitomi T, Shibasaki H. Low-frequency repetitive transcranial magnetic stimulation for seizure suppression in patients with extratemporal lobe epilepsy – a pilot study. *Seizure* 2005a; 14: 387-392.

Kinoshita M, Ikeda A, Matsuhashi M, Matsumoto R, Hitomi T, Begum T, Usui K, Takayama M, Mikuni N, Miyamoto S, Hashimoto N, Shibasaki H. Electric cortical stimulation suppresses epileptic and background activities in neocortical epilepsy and mesial temporal lobe epilepsy. *Clin Neurophysiol* 2005b; 116: 1291-1299.

Kobayashi M, Pascual-Leone A. Transcranial magnetic stimulation in neurology. *Lancet Neurol* 2003; 2: 145-156.

Kossoff EH, Ritzl EK, Politsky JM, Murro AM, Smith JR, Duckrow RB, Spencer DD, Bergey GK. Effect of an external responsive neurostimulator on seizures and electrographic discharges during subdural electrode monitoring. *Epilepsia* 2004; 45: 1560-1567.

Krauss GL, Fisher RS. Cerebellar and thalamic stimulation for epilepsy. *Adv Neurol* 1993; 63: 231–245.

Kwan P, Brodie M. Early identification of refractory epilepsy. *N Engl J Med* 2000; 342: 314-319.

Lado FA. Chronic bilateral stimulation of the anterior thalamus of kainate-treated rats increases seizure frequency. *Epilepsia* 2006; 47: 27-32.

La Grutta V, Amato G, Zagami MT. The importance of the caudate nucleus in the control of convulsive activity in the amygdaloid complex and the temporal cortex of the cat. *Electroencephalogr Clin Neurophysiol* 1971; 31: 57-69.

La Grutta V, Sabatino M, Gravante G, Morici G, Ferraro G, La Grutta G. A study of caudate inhibition on an epileptic focus in the cat hippocampus. *Arch Int Physiol Biochim* 1988; 96: 113–120.

Lesser RP, Kim SH, Beyderman L, Miglioretti DL, Webber WR, Bare M, Cysyk B, Krauss G, Gordon B. Brief bursts of pulse stimulation terminate afterdischarges caused by cortical stimulation. *Neurology* 1999; 53: 2073-2081.

Lim SN, Lee ST, Tsai YT, Chen IA, Tu PH, Chen JL, Chang HW, Su YC, Wu T. Electrical stimulation of the anterior nucleus of the thalamus for intractable epilepsy : a long term follow-up study. *Epilepsia* 2007; 48: 342-347.

Lockard JS, Ojemann GA, Congdon WC, DuCharme LL. Cerebellar stimulation in alumina-gel monkey model: inverse relationship between clinical seizures and EEG interictal bursts. *Epilepsia* 1979; 20: 223-234.

Loddenkemper T, Pan A, Neme S, Baker KB, Rezai AR, Dinner DS, Montgomery EB Jr, Lüders HO. Deep brain stimulation in epilepsy. *J Clin Neurophysiol* 2001; 18: 514-532.

Majkowski J, Karliński A, Klimowicz-Młodzik I. Effect of cerebellar stimulation of hippocampal epileptic discharges in kindling preparation. *Monogr Neural Sci* 1980; 5: 40-45.

Marescaux C, Vergnes M, Depaulis A. Genetic absence epilepsy in rats from strasbourg. *J Neural Transm Suppl* 1992; 35: 37-69.

Menkes DL, Gruenthal M. Slow-frequency repetitive transcranial magnetic stimulation in a patient withfocal cortical dysplasia. *Epilepsia* 2000; 4:240–42

Mirski MA, Ferrendelli JA. Interruption of the mammillothalamic tract prevents seizures in guinea pigs. *Science* 1984; 226: 72-74.

Mirski MA, Ferrendelli JA. Anterior thalamic mediation of generalized pentylenetetrazol seizures. *Brain Res* 1986a; 399: 212-223.

Mirski MA, Ferrendelli JA. Selective metabolic activation of the mammillary bodies and their connections during ethosuximide-induced suppression of pentylenetetrazol seizures. *Epilepsia* 1986b; 27: 194-203.

Mirski MA, Fisher RS. Electrical stimulation of the mammillary nuclei increases seizure threshold to pentylenetetrazol in rats. *Epilepsia* 1994; 35: 1309-1316.

Mirski MA, Rossell LA, Terry JB, Fisher RS. Anticonvulsant effect of anterior thalamic high frequency electrical stimulation in the rat. *Epilepsy Res* 1997; 28: 89-100.

Misawa S, Kuwabara S, Shibuya K, Mamada K, Hattori T. Low-frequency transcranial magnetic stimulation for epilepsia partialis continua due to cortical dysplasia. *J Neurol Sci* 2005; 234: 37-39.

Morrell M. Brain stimulation for epilepsy : can scheduled or responsive neurostimulation stop seizures? *Curr Opin Neurol* 2006; 19: 164-168.

Motamedi GK, Lesser RP, Miglioretti DL, Mizuno-Matsumoto Y, Gordon B, Webber WR, Jackson DC, Sepkuty JP, Crone NE. Optimizing parameters for terminating cortical afterdischarges with pulse stimulation. *Epilepsia* 2002; 43: 836-846.

Mutani R. Experimental evidence for the existence of an extrarhinencephalic control of the activity of the cobalt rhinencephalic epileptogenic focus, part 1: the role played by the caudate nucleus. *Epilepsia* 1969; 10: 337–350.

Mutani R, Bergamini L, Doriguzzi T. Experimental evidence for the existence of an extrarhinencephalic control of the activity of the cobalt rhinencephalic epileptogenic focus. Part 2. Effects of the paleocerebellar stimulation. *Epilepsia* 1969; 10: 351-362.

Nail-Boucherie K, Lê-Pham BT, Gobaille S, Maitre M, Aunis D, Depaulis A. Evidence for a role of the parafascicular nucleus of the thalamus in the control of epileptic seizures by the superior colliculus. *Epilepsia* 2005; 46: 141-145.

Nanobashvili Z, Chachua T, Nanobashvili A, Bilanishvili I, Lindvall O, Kokaia Z. Suppression of limbic motor seizures by electrical stimulation in thalamic reticular nucleus. *Exp Neurol* 2003; 181: 224-230.

Oakley JC, Ojemann GA. Effects of chronic stimulation of the caudate nucleus on a preexisting alumina seizure focus. Exp Neurol 1982; 75:360–67.

Oommen J, Morrell M, Fisher RS. Experimental electrical stimulation for epilepsy. *Curr Treat Options Neurol* 2005 ; 7 : 261-271.

Osorio I, Frei MG, Giftakis J, Peters T, Ingram J, Turnbull M, Herzog M, Rise MT, Schaffner S, Wennberg RA, Walczak TS, Risinger MW, Ajmone-Marsan C. Performance reassessment of a real-time seizure-detection algorithm on long ECoG series. *Epilepsia.* 2002;43(12):1522-35.

Osorio I, Frein MG, Sunderam S, Giftakis J, Bhavaraju NC, Schaffner SF, Wilkinson SB. Automated seizure abatement in humans using electrical stimulation. *Ann Neurol* 2005; 57: 258-268

Osorio I, Overman J, Giftakis J, Wilkinson SB. High frequency thalamic stimulation for inoperable mesial temporal epilepsy. *Epilepsia* 2007; 48: 1561-1571.

Paz JT, Deniau JM, Charpier S. Rhythmic Bursting in the Cortico-Subthalamo-Pallidal Network during Spontaneous Genetically Determined Spike and Wave Discharges. *J Neurosci* 2005; 25: 2092-2101.

Paz JT, Chavez M, Saillet S, Deniau JM, Charpier S. Activity of ventral medial thalamic neurons during absence seizures and modulation of cortical paroxysms by the nigrothalamic pathway. *J Neurosci* 2007; 27: 929-941.

Pilitsis JG, Chu Y, Kordower J, Bergen CD, Cochran EJ, Bakay RA. Postmortem study of deep brain stimulation of the anterior thalamus: case report. *Neurosurgery* 2008; 62: 530-532.

Polkey CE. Alternative surgical procedures ti help drug-resistant epilepsy – a review. *Epileptic Disord* 2003; 5 : 63-75.

Psatta DM. Control of chronic experimental focal epilepsy by feedback caudatum stimulations. *Epilepsia* 1983; 24: 444-454.

Rotenberg A, Muller P, Birnbaum D, Harrington M, Riviello JJ, Pascual-Leone A, Jensen FE. Seizure suppression by EEG-guided repetitive transcranial magnetic stimulation in the rat. *Clin Neurophysiol* 2008; 119:2697-2702.

Saillet S, Charvet G, Gharbi S, Depaulis A, Guillemaud R, David O. Closed loop control of seizures in a rat model of absence epilepsy using the BioMEATM system. *IEEE Neural Eng*. Submitted

Santiago-Rodriguez E, Cardenas-Morales L, Harmony T, Fernandez-Bouzas A, Porras-Kattz E, Hernandez A. Repetitive transcranial magnetic stimulation decreases the number of seizures in patients with focal neocortical epilepsy. *Seizure* 2008 ; may 19 [Epub ahead of print].

Semah F. PET imaging in epilepsy: basal ganglia and thalamic involvement. *Epileptic Disord* 2002; 4 (suppl 3): S55-S60.

Shi LH, Luo F, Woodward D, Chang JY. Deepbrain stimulation of the substantia nigra pars reticulata exerts long lasting suppression of amygdale-kindled seizures. *Brain Res* 2006; 1090 (1): 202-207.

Sramka M, Fritz G, Gajdosova D, Nadvornik P. Central stimulation treatment of epilepsy. *Acta Neurochir Suppl* 1980; 30: 183-187.

Takebayashi S, Hashizume K, Tanaka T, Hodozuka A. The effect of electrical stimulation and lesioning of the anterior thalamic nucleus on kainic acid-induced focal cortical seizure status in rats. *Epilepsia*. 2007**a** Feb;48(2):348-58.

Takebayashi S, Hashizume K, Tanaka T, Hodozuka A. Anti-convulsant effect of electrical stimulation and lesioning of the anterior thalamic nucleus on kainic acid-induced focal limbic seizure in rats. *Epilepsy Res*. 2007**b** May;74(2-3):163-70.

Tassinari CA, Cincotta M, Zaccara G, Michelucci R.Transcranial magnetic stimulation and epilepsy. *Clin Neurophysiol* 2003; 114: 777-798.

Taylor RB, Wennberg RA, Lozano AM, Sharpe JA. Central nystagmus induced by deep-brain stimulation for epilepsy. *Epilepsia* 2000; 41: 1637-1641.

Tellez-Zenteno JF, McLachlan RS, Parrent A, Kubu CS, Wiebe S. Hippocampal electrical stimulation in mesial temporal lobe epilepsy. *Neurology* 2006; 66: 1490-1494.

Tergau F, Naumann U, Paulus W, Steinhoff BJ. Low-frequency repetitive transcranial magnetic stimulation improves intractable epilepsy. *Lancet* 1999; 353: 2209.

Theodore WH, Fisher RS. Brain stimulation for epilepsy. *Lancet Neurol* 2004; 3: 111-118.

Theodore WH, Hunter K, Chen R, et al. Transcranial magnetic stimulation for the treatment of seizures: a controlled study. *Neurology* 2002; 59: 560-562.

Usui N, Maesawa S, Kajita Y, Endo O, Takebayashi S, Yoshida J. Suppression of secondary generalization of limbic seizures by stimulation of subthalamic nucleus in rat. *J Neurosurg* 2005; 102 (6): 1122-1129.

Van Buren JM, Wood JH, Oakley J, Hambrecht F. Preliminary evaluation of cerebellar stimulation by double blind stimulation and biological criteria in the treatment of epilepsy. *J Neurosurg* 1978; 48: 407-16.

van Rijckevorsel K, Abu Serieh B, de Tourtchaninoff M, Raftopoulos C. Deep EEG recordings of the mammillary body in epilepsy patients. *Epilepsia* 2005; 46: 781-785.

Velasco F, Velasco M, Cepeda C, Munoz H. Wakefulness-sleep modulation of thalamic multiple unit activity and EEG in man. *Electroencephalogr Clin Neurophysiol* 1979; 47: 597-606.

Velasco F, Velasco M, Ogarrio C, Fanghanel G. Electrical stimulation of the centromedian thalamic nucleus in the treatment of convulsives seizures: a preliminary report. *Epilepsia* 1987; 28: 421-430.

Velasco F, Velasco M, Velasco AL, Jimenez F. Effect of chronic electrical stimulation of the centromedian thalamic nuclei on various intractable seizure patterns, I: clinical seizures and paroxysmal EEG activity. *Epilepsia* 1993; 34: 1052-1064.

Velasco F, Velasco M, Velasco AL, Jimenez F, Marquez I, Rise M. Electrical stimulation of the centromedian thalamic nucleus in control of seizures : long term studies. *Epilepsia* 1995; 36: 63-71.

Velasco F, Velasco M, Jimenez F, Velasco AL, Brto F, Rise M, Carrillo-Ruiz JD. Predictors in the treatment of difficult to control seizures by electrical stimulation of the centromedian thalamic nucleus. *Neurosurgery* 2000a ; 47: 295-305.

Velasco M, Velasco F, Velasco AL, Jimenez F, Brito F, Marquez I. Acute and chronic electrical stimulation of the centromedian thalamic nucleus: modulation of reticulo-cortical systems and predictor factors for generalized seizure control. *Arch Med Res* 2000b; 31:304-315.

Velasco M, Velasco F, Velasco AL, Boleaga B, Jimenez F, Brito F, Marquez I. Subacute electrical stimulation of the hippocampus blocks intractable temporal lobe seizures and paroxysmal EEG activities. *Epilepsia* 2000c; 41: 158-169.

Velasco F, Velasco M, Jimenez F, Velasco AL, Marquez I. Stimulation of the central median thalamic nucleus for epilepsy. *Stereotact Funct Neurosurg* 2001a; 77: 228–232.

Velasco M, Velasco F, Velasco AL. Centromedian-thalamic and hippocampal electrical stimulation for the control of intractable epileptic seizures. *J Clin Neurophysiol* 2001b; 18: 495-513.

Velasco F, Velasco M, Jimenez F, Velasco AL, Rojas B. Centromedian nucleus stimulation for epilepsy. Clinical, electroencephalographic, and behavioral observations. *Thalamus & Related systems* 2002 ; 1: 387-398.

Velasco F, Carrillo-Ruiz JD, Brto F, Velasco M, Velasco A.L., Marquez I, Davis R. double-blind, randomized controlled pilot study of bilateral cerebellar stimulation for treatment of intractable motor seizures. *Epilepsia* 2005; 46: 1071-1081.

Velasco AL, Velasco F, Jimenez F, Velasco M, Casro G, Carrillo-Ruiz JD, Fanghanel G, Boleaga B. Neuromodulation of the centromedian thalamic nuclei in the treatment of generalized seizures and the improvement of the quality of life in patients with Lennox-Gastaut syndrome. *Epilepsia* 2006; 47: 1203-1212.

Velasco AL, Velasco F, Velasco M, Trejo D, Castro G, Carrillo-Ruiz JD. Electrical stimulation of the hippocampal epileptic foci for seizure control : a double-blind, long-term follow-up study. *Epilepsia* 2007; 48: 1895-1903.

Velisek L, Veliskova J, Moshe S L. Electrical stimulation of substantia nigra pars reticulate is anticonvulsant in adult and young male rats. *Exp Neurol* 2002; 173 (1): 145-152.

Velisek L, Velsikova J, Stanton PK. Low-frequency stimulation of the kindling focus delays basolateral amygdala kindling in immature rats. *Neurosci Lett* 2002 ; 326 ; 61-63.

Veliskova J, Claudio OI, Galanopoulou AS, Kyrozis A, Lado FA, Ravizza T, Velisek L, Moshe SL. Developmental espects of the basal ganglia and therapeutic perspectives. *Epileptic Disord* 4 2002; Suppl 3: S73-82.

Vercueil L, Hirsch E. Seizures and the basal ganglia: a review of the clinical data. *Epileptic Disord* 2002; 4 (suppl 3): S47-S54.

Vercueil L., Benazzouz A., Deransart C., Bressand K., Marescaux C., Depaulis A., Benabid A.L. High-frequency stimulation of the sub-thalamic nucleus suppresses absence seizures in the rat: comparison with neurotoxic lesions. *Epilepsy Res* 1998; 31: 39-46.

Vesper J, Steinhoff B, Rona S, Wille C, Bilic S, Nikkhah G, Ostertag C. Chronic high-frequency deep brain stimulation of the STN/SNr for progressive myoclonic epilepsy. *Epilepsia* 2007; 48: 1984-1989.

Vonck K, Boon P, Achten E, De Reuck J, Caemaert J. Long-term amygdalohippocampal stimulation for refractory temporal lobe epilepsy. *Ann Neurol* 2002; 52: 556-565.

Vonck K, Boon P, Van Roost D. Anatomical and physiological basis and mechanism of action of neurostimulation for epilepsy. *Acta Neurochir* 2007; 97 (suppl): 321-328.

Wang S, Wu DC, Ding MP, Li Q, Zhuge ZB, Zhang SH, Chen Z. Low-frequency stimulation of cerebellar fastigial nucleus inhibits amygdaloid kindling acquisition in sprague-dawley rats. *Neurobiol Dis* 2008; 29 (1): 52_58.

Wassermann EM, Lisanby SH. Therapeutic application of repetitive transcranial magnetic stimulation: a review. *Clin Neurophysiol* 2001; 112: 1367-1377.

Weiss SRB, Li XL, Rosen JB, Li H, Heynen T, Post RM. Quenching : inhibition of the development and expression of amygdala kindled seizures with low frequency stimulation. *Neuroreport* 1995; 4: 2171-2176.

Wright GD, Mc Lellan DL, Brice JG. A double-blind trial of chronic cerebellar stimulation in twelve patients with severe epilepsy. *J Neurol Neurosurg Psychiatry* 1984; 47: 769-74.

Yamamoto J, Ikeda A, Satow T, Takeshita K, Takayama M, Matsuhashi M, Matsumoto R, Ohara S, Mikuni N, Takahashi J, Miyamoto S, Taki W, Hashimoto N, Rothwell JC, Shibasaki H. Low-frequency electric cortical stimulation has an inhibitory effect on cortical focus in mesial temporal lobe epilepsy. *Epilepsia* 2002 ; 43 : 491-495.

Yang LX, Jin CL, Zhu-Ge ZB, Wang S, Wei EQ, Bruce IC, Chen Z. Unilateral low-frequency stimulation of central piriform delays seizure development induced by amygdaloid-kindled in rats. *Neuroscience* 2006; 138: 1089-1096.

Zhu-Ge ZB, Zhu YY, Wu DC, Wang S, Liu LY, Hu WW, Chen Z. Unilateral low-frequency stimulation of central piriform cortex inhibits amygdaloid-kindled seizures in Sprague-Dawley rats. *Neuroscience* 2007; 146: 901-906.

Zumsteg D, Lozano AM, Wennberg RA. Mesial temporal inhibition in a patient with deep brain stimulation of the anterior thalamus for epilepsy. *Epilepsia* 2006; 47: 1958-1962.

In: Deep Brain Stimulation
Editors: Mark H. Rogers and Paul B. Anderson
ISBN 978-1-60692-895-0

Chapter VI

Psychosurgery of Obsessive-Compulsive Disorder: A New Indication for Deep Brain Stimulation?*

Dominique Guehl, Abdelhamid Benazzouz, Bernard Bioulac and Pierre Burbaud
Service de Neurophysiologie Clinique, Université Victor Segalen Bordeaux 2, CNRS UMR 5543, Centre Hospitalier Pellegrin, Place Amélie-Raba Léon, 33076 Bordeaux, France

Emmanuel Cuny and Alain Rougier
Service de Neurochirurgie, Université Victor Segalen Bordeaux 2, Centre Hospitalier Pellegrin, Place Amélie-Raba Léon, 33076 Bordeaux, France

Jean Tignol
Service de Psychiatrie d'Adultes, Université Victor Segalen Bordeaux 2, Centre Hospitalier Charles Perrens, Centre Carreire, 121 rue de la Béchade, 33076 Bordeaux, France

Bruno Aouizerate
Service de Psychiatrie d'Adultes, Université Victor Segalen Bordeaux 2, Centre Hospitalier Charles Perrens, Centre Carreire, 121 rue de la Béchade, 33076 Bordeaux, France
Service de Neurophysiologie Clinique, Université Victor Segalen Bordeaux 2, CNRS UMR 5543, Centre Hospitalier Pellegrin, Place Amélie-Raba Léon, 33076 Bordeaux, France

* A version of this chapter was also published in *Recent Breakthroughs in Basal ganglia Research* , edited by Erwan Bezard published by Nova Science Publishers, Inc. It was submitted for appropriate modification in an effort to encourage wider dissemination of research

Abstract

Obsessive-compulsive disorder (OCD) is a relatively common psychiatric condition with an estimated lifetime prevalence of 2–3% of the general population. It is generally characterized by a chronic course leading to a profound impairment in psychosocial functioning and quality of life. Although its pathophysiology is still far from resolved, an ample body of literature suggests the role of an overactivity in the frontal-subcortical loops originating in the orbitofrontal cortex and the anterior cingulate cortex, respectively. Today, the well-established efficacy of antidepressants, acting preferentially by blocking serotonin reuptake, in addition to psychological treatments, have considerably changed the poor prognosis of the illness. However, both conventional therapeutic approaches failed to substantially alleviate obsessive-compulsive symptoms in 20–30% of cases. From these considerations, several surgical strategies have been successfully proposed for treating the resistant forms of OCD, including anterior capsulotomy, anterior cingulotomy, subcaudate tractotomy and limbic leucotomy. They have been performed in order to interrupt the orbitofrontal and anterior cingulate loops at either cortical or subcortical level, which have been found as disrupted in OCD. Despite these lesion-producing techniques have relatively low incidence of serious complications or undesirable effects, deep brain stimulation, as a reversible procedure, has recently been introduced in the field of OCD, primarily targeting the limb part of the internal capsule or the ventral caudate nucleus. It has been shown to be of promising benefit that should be considered with caution and confirmed by further research in this area.

Introduction

Obsessive-compulsive disorder (OCD) is a relatively common anxiety disorder that affects 2 to 3% of the general population (Robins et al., 1984; Karno et al., 1988). According to this estimated lifetime prevalence rate, OCD is the fourth most frequent psychiatric condition following the phobias, substance abuse and major depression. OCD, which is characterized by recurrent intrusive thoughts and repetitive, time-consuming behaviors, is a severely disabling mental illness owing to its intensity, the continuous and unchanging or deteriorative course of its symptoms and the disturbance in psychosocial functioning that they cause (Rasmussen and Tsuang, 1984; Koran et al., 1996; Antony et al., 1998; Skoog and Skoog, 1999).

Although the pathophysiology of OCD is still far from resolved, the existence of a biological basis for OCD is now clearly established and will be discussed from a phenomenological point of view, on the one hand, and in the light of our increasing knowledge of the physiology of prefrontal cortex-striatal-thalamic-cortical functional loops, on the other. The present chapter will then examine the therapeutic effects of various psychosurgical approaches used for the management of OCD forms, which were unresponsive to the prototypical treatments classically proposed in this psychiatric condition. All these procedures have consisted in performing lesions in order to produce an interruption of fibers connecting the thalamus to the prefrontal cortex through the anterior limb of the internal capsule. Although they have not been shown to generate serious complications and/or untoward effects in most cases, deep brain stimulation (DBS) has recently been considered as a potential alternative for treating resistant OCD.

1. Brief Overetview of the Pathophysiology of OCD

1.1 Phenomenological Aspects

The heart of the obsessional process is the subject's underlying impression that "something is wrong" (Schwartz, 1998, 1999). In other words, obsessions may be thought of as the permanent perception of a mistake and/or error in certain behavioral situations. Compulsions occur as behavioral responses aiming to relieve the tensions or anxiety generated by the situation. If obtained, this relief may be felt to be a form of reward. Nevertheless, it is only transient, thereby creating a feeling of considerable anxiety. This leads to immediately reproduce the behavior in a cyclic manner on the basis of an internal motivational state through an expectation of the reward. Although it is undoubtedly simplistic, this phenomenological view is of interest because it suggests that several malfunctioning processes are altered within the OCD: 1) error recognition; and, 2) emotion and motivation and their activational aspects, e.g. activations for initiation and sustaining behavioral reactions and tendency to work for reward. Therefore, it can be expected in OCD that there is a dysfunction of the brain regions that mediate the processes of error detection and/or management of the reward and emotional systems, including orbitofrontal and anterior cingulate cortices and ventral striatum, respectively (Devinsky et al., 1995; Le Moal, 1995; Piazza and Le Moal, 1996; Koob and Le Moal, 1997; Piazza and Le Moal, 1997; Schwartz, 1998, 1999; Bush et al., 2000; Paus, 2001; Bush et al., 2002).

1.2 Anatomo-functional Data

Several studies have found a dysregulation in the frontal-subcortical circuits originating in the orbitofrontal and anterior cingulate cortices, respectively, in the pathogenesis of OCD. These loops concern discrete regions of the striatum and the pallidum and receive clearly delimited inputs from the cortex, which are subsequently integrated as far as the thalamus. Although they are part of a parallel model of organization, these circuits are permanently interrelated (Cummings, 1993).

The orbitofrontal cortex (OFC) and ventromedial areas are involved in appraisal in determining the emotional and motivational values of environmental information, and in integrating the subject's prior experience, which is crucial in decision-making (Charney and Bremner, 1999; Tremblay and Schultz, 1999, 2000a, 2000b; Krawczyk, 2002; Ramnani and Owen, 2004). The OFC also contributes to the selection, comparison and judgment of stimuli and error detection process (Rosenkilde et al., 1981; Thorpe et al., 1983; Ramnani and Owen, 2004).

The anterior cingulate cortex (ACC) is comprised of 1) a ventral or affective region which is intimately connected to the orbitofrontal cortex, ventral striatum, amygdala, hippocampus and hypothalamus. This subdivision could keep attention on the internal emotional and motivational status and participates to the regulation of autonomic responses; and, 2) a dorsal or cognitive region which is interconnected to the dorsolateral prefrontal cortex, parietal cortex, and premotor and supplementary motor areas. This cortical area serves a wide range of cognitive functions including attention, working memory, error detection, conflict monitoring and response selection with decisional and planning aspects in situations with high likelihood of making an error, and anticipation of incoming information (Niki and Watanabe, 1979; Devinsky et al., 1995; Shima and Tanji, 1998; Schwartz, 1999; Bush et al., 2000; Akkal et al., 2002; Bush et al., 2002; Shidara and Richmond, 2002).

Ventral striatum that is received important inputs from the OFC and ACC, is primarily implicated in the preparation, initiation and execution of behavioral responses oriented toward reward delivery after cognitive and emotional integration of behaviorally relevant information at the cortical level (Hollerman et al., 1998; Tremblay et al., 1998; Hassani et al., 2001).

The medial dorsal nucleus (MD) is the principal thalamic nucleus related to the prefrontal cortex. It is composed of several subdivisions, the main portion being centrally located and represented by the parvicellular part (MDpc), and its most medial portion corresponding to the magnocellular part (MDmc; Goldman-Rakic and Porrino, 1985). The MDpc receives inputs from the substantia nigra, which has a major role in cognition, and projects preferentially to the ACC (Barbas, 2000; McFarland and Haber, 2002). On the other hand, the MDmc, which receives inputs from the limbic portions of the basal ganglia (ventral striatum) and from the amygdala, projects mainly to the OFC (Barbas, 2000; McFarland and Haber, 2002).

1.3 Functional Neuroimagery

Functional imaging research has shown that several brain structures in OCD patients have abnormal functional activity. Most teams have reported an increased functional activity in the OFC, ACC, head of the caudate nucleus and thalamus (Saxena et al., 1998; Baxter, 1999; Aouizerate et al., 2004a). These functional abnormalities have been found in basal conditions and during provocation tests. Moreover, the therapeutic efficacy of antidepressants and cognitive-behavioral therapies seems to be associated with a progressive reduction in activity of the OFC, ACC and the caudate nucleus, thereby strengthening other data suggesting a functional deterioration in the orbitofrontal and anterior cingulate cortex system in the pathogenesis of OCD (Saxena et al., 1998; Baxter, 1999).

In conclusion, it seems in OCD that there is a dysfunction of the brain regions that belong to the orbitofrontal and anterior cingulate loops in view of evidences obtained from separate and complementary approaches

2. Psychosurgical Treatments

Over the last 30 years, distinct therapeutic approaches have been developed ranging from psychotropic drugs to psychotherapies and are now considered as effective for the management of OCD. In this respect, an ample body of literature has emerged and proven the efficacy of antidepressant agents for treating OCD. They preponderantly block the serotonin transporter located in the outer membrane of presynaptic axonal terminals of the brainstem raphe neurons, and thereby inhibit neurotransmitter reuptake (Flament and Bisserbe, 1997; Piggot and Seay, 1998; Goodman, 1999; McDougle, 1999; Pigott and Seay, 1999). Psychological treatments primarily based on cognitive-behavioral therapy with the current procedure termed "exposure with self-imposed response prevention" also appear to be effective in the treatment of OCD, alone or in combination with pharmacotherapy (Greist, 1994; Foa et al., 1998; 2002). However, at least 20-30 % of patients with OCD fail to respond adequately, with minimal to no change during these conventional treatments (Pigott and Seay, 1998; Pallanti et al., 2002). Therefore, psychosurgical approaches have been considered for the management of these chronic, severely distressing forms of OCD resistant to all currently available traditional treatments. The most frequently described procedures, which are anterior capsulotomy, anterior cingulotomy, subcaudate tractotomy and limbic leucotomy, have shown to be of significant benefit in the treatment of refractory OCD.

2.1 Anterior Capsulotomy

Developed in Sweden, anterior capsulotomy targets the fiber bundles in the anterior limb of the internal capsule connecting the medial dorsal nucleus of the thalamus and the frontal lobes. Two surgical techniques have been used, the radiofrequency thermolesion, or thermocapsulotomy and the newer radiosurgical, or gamma knife capsulotomy techniques (Mindus and Jenike, 1992; Jenike, 1998; Binder and Iskandar, 2000; Greenberg et al., 2000; Greenberg et al., 2003). The first report by Herner (1961) showed that at follow-up ranging from 24 to 80 months there were either good or fair results in 78 % of the 18 patients with OCD who underwent this surgical procedure. Bingley et al. (1977) found that all 35 patients with OCD responded favorably to this type of operation. Sixteen (46 %) were free of symptoms, 9 (26 %) were much improved, and 10 (28 %) were slightly improved at the mean 35-month follow-up. There was an improvement in the degree of social rehabilitation and working capacity. In the study by Kullberg (1977), general improvement, reflecting symptom reduction and social capacity, was considered as "excellent" in 1 (12.5 %), "good" in 2 (25 %), "moderate" in 2 (25 %), "slight" in 1 and "none" in 2 (25 %) of the 8 patients treated with capsulotomy at the end of the follow-up period (1 to 9 years). Fodstad et al. (1982) reported that two patients with OCD were much improved during the 24-month period following capsulotomy. In the review by Mindus et al. (1994), it has been mentioned that 5 (23 %) of the 22 patients with OCD exhibited a clinical aggravation at the 8-year follow-up after capsulotomy while 2 (9 %) were improved by 1 % to 25 %, 5 (23 %) improved by 26 % to 50 %, 3 (13 %) improved by 51 % to 75 %, and 7 (32 %) improved by 75 % to 100 %. Adverse effects of anterior capsulotomy in the initial series of 116 patients observed by Herner (1961) may be summarized as follows: three patients died 11, 28 and 33 months, respectively after the intervention; two from suicide and the third from a cardiac infarction. Operative complications were considerably few: stenosis of the aqueduct of the mid-brain in one case and epilepsy in four (3.4 %). The side effects on the emotional, the volitional and the intellectual status, as found in 55.5 % of the 18 patients with OCD, were mild and transient. Other untoward effects were urinary (and fecal) incontinence and weight gain but were not serious. In the study by Bingley et al. (1977), transient hemiparesis due to small subcortical hemorrhage was described in 2 (6 %) of the 35 OCD cases treated with capsulotomy. EEG showed abnormalities localized mainly to the frontal regions in 28 of these patients at 10-day follow-up before normalization after a more prolonged post-operative period. Post-operative mental confusion also occurred in some cases and lasted less than 1-3 weeks after the operation. Other mental changes consisted of diminution of inhibition, elevation of mood, and loss of initiative, but were not disturbing in most cases (Bingley et al., 1977; Kullberg, 1977; Chiocca and Martuza, 1990). At the 1-year follow-up, capsulotomy contributed to reverse personality changes observed pre-operatively (Mindus et al., 1988; Mindus and Nyman, 1991; Mindus et al., 1999).

2.2 Anterior Cingulotomy

Developed in the United States and Canada, anterior cingulotomy was the most currently neurosurgical procedure applied to the treatment of anxiety disorders including refractory OCD. Bilateral thermolesions are created by the radiofrequency in the anterior cingulate cortex (Broadman areas 24 and 32; Mindus and Jenike, 1992; Jenike, 1998; Binder and Iskandar, 2000; Greenberg et al., 2000; Greenberg et al., 2003). Whitty et al. (1952) first reported the satisfactory results of this surgical procedure in two patients with OCD. The therapeutic effects were much less favorable in the study by Kullberg (1977) showing that cingulotomy produced a slight reduction in OCD symptoms severity only in 1 (33 %) of the three OCD cases at the end of the follow-up period (1-8 years). In a larger sample, Ballantine et al. (1987) found that 8 (25 %) of the 32 patients with OCD were slightly improved, 10 (31.3 %) were markedly improved, 4 (12.5 %) were functionally normal on medication and/or psychotherapy maintenance, and 4 (12.5 %) were essentially well without any treatment. The remaining 6 patients (18.7 %) showed unchanged or worsened OCD symptoms at the mean follow-up of 8.6 years. Jenike et al. (1991), using Y-BOCS for assessment of OCD symptom severity, described that 6 (43 %) of the 14 patients with OCD treated with cingulotomy showed no improvement, while the remaining 8 (57 %) exhibited moderate to marked improvement at the mean 13.1-year follow-up, defined by a 50 % or greater reduction in Y-BOCS scores. However, 2 of these 8 patients considered their improvement related to the current treatment with SRI (fluoxetine) and CBT rather than cingulotomy. In the most recent prospective study, Dougherty et al. (2002) reported favorable effects of this surgical procedure in 44 patients with intractable OCD. At a mean follow-up of 32 months, 14 (32 %) were considered as responders according to the conservative criteria for treatment response and 6 others (14 %) were partial responders after one or more cingulotomies. Serious operative complications were relatively few including hemiplegias (0.03 %) and controllable seizure disorders (1 %) in the series of 696 bilateral cingulotomies (Ballantine et al., 1987). Death by suicide was observed in 18 patients over the mean 8.6-year follow-up, but all 18 of these patients had preoperative suicidal ideation and 13 had made suicide attempts before the operation. Transient mental confusion was reported in 2 (15.4 %) of the 13 patients treated with cingulotomy during the first post-operative days (Kullberg, 1977). Memory deficits were described in two (5 %) of the 44 patients who underwent this type of surgical intervention, but had resolved within 6 to 12 months. Apathy with loss of energy was noted in one patient (2 %) following cingulotomy. Urinary disturbances were reported in three (7 %) patients, which resolved within the first days postoperatively (Dougherty et al., 2002).

2.3 Subcaudate Tractotomy

Developed in the United Kingdom, subcaudate tractotomy is characterized by bilateral lesions made by radioactive yttrium-90 seeds placed in the substantia innominata, which is located close to the ventral part of the anterior capsule beneath the head of the caudate nucleus. The goal is to interrupt connections from orbitofrontal cortex to subcortical regions such as ventral caudate, nucleus accumbens, which then send projections to the ventromedial pallidum and thalamus (Mindus and Jenike, 1992; Jenike, 1998; Binder and Iskandar, 2000; Greenberg et al., 2000; 2003). There were relatively few reports of the efficacy of this surgical procedure in the treatment of refractory OCD. In the series of Strom-Olsen and Carlisle (1971), it has been found that at the follow-up ranging from 16 months to 8 years, 7 (35 %) of the 20 patients with OCD had no symptoms, 3 (15 %) were improved but with slight residual symptoms for which no treatment was needed, 3 (15 %) were improved but with persistent symptoms requiring treatment. The remaining 7 (35 %) patients exhibited unchanged or worsened symptoms. In most cases, the reducing effects on OCD symptom severity were delayed within 4-5 months after the operation. Bridges et al. (1973) also reported favorable effects of subcaudate tractotomy in 24 patients intractable OCD. Sixteen (67 %) of these patients showed a good outcome, as defined by no symptoms or mild residual symptoms after three years of follow-up. The remaining eight (33 %) patients had poor outcome with persistence of significant symptoms responsible for functional impairment in the patient's life. These results were confirmed by Goktepe et al. (1975) showing that nine (50 %) of the 18 patients with OCD had satisfactory response after a 2.5-year period of follow-up. In the most recent report by Hodgkiss et al. (1995), good outcome was only observed in 5 (33.3 %) of the 15 patients with OCD within one year after surgery. There was no post-operative mortality in the series of Strom-Olsen and Carlisle (1971), conducted on 150 patients with psychiatric conditions operated. However, there were three deaths by suicide in the series of 208 cases of Goktepe et al. (1975). The incidence of post-operative epilepsy in this series was 2.2 % (Goktepe et al., 1975). Weight gain was observed (Strom-Olsen and Carlisle, 1971). Psychological and behavioral changes occurred (Strom-Olsen and Carlisle, 1971; Goktepe et al., 1975). The commonly reported symptoms were tiredness and lethargy lasting for up to three months or irritability, outspokenness and volubility, which most often failed to have repercussions on family and social relationships. Neuropsychological testing revealed frontal lobe dysfunction 6 months after the operation (Kartsounis et al., 1991).

2.4 Limbic Leucotomy

Introduced in the United Kingdom, limbic leucotomy is based on bilateral lesions of cingulotomy, in addition to those of the original subcaudate tractotomy (Mindus and Jenike, 1992; Jenike, 1998; Binder and Iskandar, 2000; Greenberg et al., 2000; Greenberg et al., 2003). In the early report of Kelly et al. (Kelly and Mitchell-Heggs, 1973; Kelly et al., 1973), 13 (76 %) of the 17 patients with OCD were clinically improved within six weeks after the intervention. Of these 13 patients, 1 (8 %) was rated as "symptom free", 6 (46 %) as "much improved" and 6 (46 %) as "improved". The favorable effects even persisted after a mean 16- or 17-month period of follow-up (Kelly and Mitchell-Heggs, 1973; Kelly et al., 1973; Mitchell-Heggs et al., 1976). These data confirmed the efficacy of this surgical procedure in the treatment of OCD, as reported in the early controlled retrospective study by Tan et al. (1971) showing a more profound reduction in OCD symptom severity in 24 patients with OCD operated compared with their 13 controls at three months after the operation, and at the end of the five years of follow-up. Post-operative complications were as follows: subarachnoid hemorrhage in one patient (4 %) and death in three patients (12.5 %; of whom one committed suicide; Tan et al., 1971). There also were transient confusion, headache, apathy, laziness, incontinence of urine, and rarely feces, which currently lasted from one to several days. Weight gain was observed. Poorer memory and concentration capacities, outspokenness or irritability were inconsistently reported (Tan et al., 1971; Kelly and Mitchell-Heggs, 1973; Kelly et al., 1973; Mitchell-Heggs et al., 1976).

Therefore, functional neurosurgical procedures, leading to an interruption of reciprocal connections between the frontal lobes and subcortical structures, have been demonstrated to be effective in the management of OCD unresponsive to both pharmacological and psychological strategies typically used in this condition.

2.5 Deep Brain Stimulation

Although the lesion techniques have been shown to cause relatively few serious undesirable effects, the reversible procedure deep brain stimulation (DBS) in the context of recent technological advances is becoming an important strategy in the treatment of severe forms of Parkinson's disease and other movement disorders (Malhi and Sachdev, 2002). This approach has recently been proposed as a potential therapeutic alternative in resistant OCD. When applied bilaterally in the anterior limb of internal capsule instead of bilateral anterior capsulotomy, DBS has been found to markedly improve OCD symptoms in three of the four OCD patients who underwent this procedure. The beneficial effects occurred almost immediately after the beginning of DBS (Nuttin et al., 1999). Headache was experienced during the first 10 seconds of stimulation and then disappeared. Long-term follow-up studies have confirmed the favorable effects of chronic anterior capsular stimulation. There was a sustained 35 % and greater reduction in Y-BOCS scores in two of the three cases of long-standing treatment-resistant OCD during the 33-month period of follow-up. At 1-year DBS, there was no deleterious effect or harmful consequence on neuropsychological functioning and personality traits (Gabriels et al., 2003). It has also been shown that a gradual decline in OCD symptom severity with recovery defined by scores in Y-BOCS below 8, which was obtained within the first 3 months of DBS application and remained stable over the seven following months. This was paralleled by a dramatic improvement in global psychosocial functioning (Anderson and Ahmed, 2003). Other brain regions have been proposed as target for DBS. In this context, a reduction in OCD manifestations by approximately 60 % was reported in two Parkinsonian patients with comorbid OCD after 6-month DBS of the subthalamic nucleus. However, symptomatic improvement was observed immediately after discharge from the neurosurgery unit (Mallet et al., 2002). The nucleus accumbens that represents the ventral and limbic part of the caudate nucleus has also been chosen as target for DBS. There was a clinical amelioration in three of the four patients with OCD and related anxiety disorders, which was achieved a few days to several weeks after beginning of DBS. No side effect was reported during the 24- to 30-month period of follow-up (Sturm et al., 2003). We also found favorable effects of DBS of the ventral caudate nucleus, including the nucleus accumbens and ventromedial head of the caudate nucleus in one patient suffering from resistant OCD with comorbid major depression (Aouizerate et al., 2004b). Reduction in depressive symptom severity occurred early during the first three months of DBS until remission obtained at 6 months while there was a delayed onset of the anti-obsessional effects, which was observed at 12-month DBS. This was parallel by a progressive improvement in global functioning. No adverse effect of any kind was noted. There was no deterioration of neuropsychological testing exploring specifically executive and mnemonic functions.

Conclusion

To summarize, a disturbance in frontal-subcortical loops originating in the OFC and ACC has extensively been documented to play a major role in the pathogenesis of OCD. Numerous neuroimaging studies have consistently shown abnormalities in functional activity in the OFC, ACC, ventral striatum and medial thalamus. These brain regions have been found implicated in cognitive and emotional processes that can be thought disrupted in OCD in the light of phenomenological considerations. Data collected from psychosurgery proposed in resistant OCD forms, which failed to successfully respond to both conventional pharmacological treatments and psychotherapies, confirm the involvement of such brain regions in the pathophysiology of OCD. The most widely used approaches (anterior capsulotomy, anterior cingulotomy, subcaudate tractotomy and limbic leucotomy) intended to perform lesions within the frontal-subcortical loops have been shown to produce an improvement in OCD symptoms in 40 to 60% of cases. They were relatively well-tolerated. However, chronic DBS has been proposed as reversible procedure for the management of refractory OCD. This surgical technique has benefited from methodological advances made in the field of Parkinson's disease and other movement disorders. Different target regions have been considered for DBS in OCD, such as the anterior limb of the internal capsule, the subthalamic nucleus or the nucleus accumbens. Although DBS seems to be the first-line choice since it is the least invasive, there are still many unknown factors. The most critical issue is to determine the optimal targets both in terms of their possible efficacy and their risks and benefits. In this perspective, further preclinical studies in laboratory animals would be helpful in order to provide more precise information about the anatomo-functional bases of OCD. The promising anti-obsessional effects and safety of DBS remain to be confirmed in larger populations of patients with intractable OCD.

References

Akkal D, Bioulac B, Audin J, Burbaud P (2002) Comparison of neuronal activity in the rostral supplementary and cingulate motor areas during a task with cognitive and motor demands. *Eur J Neurosci* **15**:887-904.

Anderson D, Ahmed A (2003) Treatment of patients with intractable obsessive-compulsive disorder with anterior capsular stimulation. Case report. *J Neurosurg* **98**:1104-1108.

Antony MM, Downie F, Swinson RP (1998) Diagnostic issues and epidemiology in obsessive-compulsive disorder. In: *Obsessive-compulsive disorder*. Theory, research, and treatment (Swinson RP, Antony MM, Rachman S, Richter MA, eds), pp 3-32. New-York: The Guilford Press.

Aouizerate B, Guehl D, Cuny E, Rougier A, Bioulac B, Tignol J, Burbaud P (2004a) Pathophysiology of obsessive-compulsive disorder: a necessary link between phenomenology, neuropsychology, imagery and physiology. *Prog Neurobiol* **72**:195-221.

Aouizerate B, Cuny E, Martin-Guehl C, Guehl D, Amieva H, Benazzouz A, Fabrigoule C, Allard M, Rougier A, Bioulac B, Tignol J, Burbaud P (2004b) Deep brain stimulation of the ventral caudate nucleus in the treatment of obsessive-compulsive disorder and major depression. Case report. *J Neurosurg* **101**:682-686.

Ballantine HT, Jr., Bouckoms AJ, Thomas EK, Giriunas IE (1987) Treatment of psychiatric illness by stereotactic cingulotomy. *Biol Psychiatry* **22**:807-819.

Barbas H (2000) Connections underlying the synthesis of cognition, memory, and emotion in primate prefrontal cortices. *Brain Res Bull* **52**:319-330.

Baxter LR (1999) Functional imaging of brain systems mediating obsessive-compulsive disorder: Clinical studies. In: *Neurobiology of mental illness* (Charney DS, Nestler EJ, Bunney BS, eds), pp 534-547. New York: Oxford University Press.

Binder DK, Iskandar BJ (2000) Modern neurosurgery for psychiatric disorders. *Neurosurgery* **47**:9-21; discussion 21-23.

Bingley T, Leksell L, Meyerson BA, Rylander G (1977) Long-term results of stereotactic anterior capsulotomy in chronic obsessive-compulsive neurosis. In: *Neurosurgical treatment in Psychiatry, Pain and Epilepsy* (Sweet WH, Obrador S, Martin-Rodriguez JG, eds), pp 287-299. Baltimore: University Park Press.

Bridges PK, Goktepe EO, Maratos J (1973) A comparative review of patients with obsessional neurosis and with depression treated by psychosurgery. *Br J Psychiatry* **123**:663-674.

Bush G, Luu P, Posner MI (2000) Cognitive and emotional influences in anterior cingulate cortex. *Trends Cogn Sci* **4**:215-222.

Bush G, Vogt BA, Holmes J, Dale AM, Greve D, Jenike MA, Rosen BR (2002) Dorsal anterior cingulate cortex: a role in reward-based decision making. *Proc Natl Acad Sci U S A* **99**:523-528.

Charney DS, Bremner JD (1999) The neurobiology of anxiety disorders: Clinical studies. In: *Neurobiology of mental illness* (Charney DS, Nestler EJ, Bunney BS, eds), pp 494-517. New York: Oxford University Press.

Chiocca EA, Martuza RL (1990) Neurosurgical therapy of obsessive-compulsive disorder. In: *Obsessive-compulsive disorders: Theory and management* (Jenike MA, Baer L, Minichiello WE, eds), pp 283-294. Chicago: Year Book Medical Publishers.

Cummings JL (1993) Frontal-subcortical circuits and human behavior. *Arch Neurol* **50**:873-880.

Devinsky O, Morrell MJ, Vogt BA (1995) Contributions of anterior cingulate cortex to behaviour. *Brain* **118** (Pt 1):279-306.

Dougherty DD, Baer L, Cosgrove GR, Cassem EH, Price BH, Nierenberg AA, Jenike MA, Rauch SL (2002) Prospective long-term follow-up of 44 patients who received cingulotomy for treatment-refractory obsessive-compulsive disorder. *Am J Psychiatry* **159**:269-275.

Flament MF, Bisserbe JC (1997) Pharmacologic treatment of obsessive-compulsive disorder: comparative studies. *J Clin Psychiatry* **58** Suppl 12:18-22.

Foa EB, Franklin ME, Kozac MJ (1998) Psychosocial treatments for obsessive-compulsive disorder. Literature review. In: *Obsessive-compulsive disorder. Theory, research, and treatment* (Swinson RP, Antony MM, Rachman S, Richter MA, eds), pp 258-276. New-York: The Guilford Press.

Foa EB, Franklin ME, Moser J (2002) Context in the clinic: how well do cognitive-behavioral therapies and medications work in combination? *Biol Psychiatry* **52**:987-997.

Fodstad H, Strandman E, Karlsson B, West KA (1982) Treatment of chronic obsessive compulsive states with stereotactic anterior capsulotomy or cingulotomy. *Acta Neurochir (Wien)* **62**:1-23.

Gabriels L, Cosyns P, Nuttin B, Demeulemeester H, Gybels J (2003) Deep brain stimulation for treatment-refractory obsessive-compulsive disorder: psychopathological and neuropsychological outcome in three cases. *Acta Psychiatr Scand* **107**:275-282.

Goktepe EO, Young LB, Bridges PK (1975) A further review of the results of sterotactic subcaudate tractotomy. *Br J Psychiatry* **126**:270-280.

Goldman-Rakic PS, Porrino LJ (1985) The primate mediodorsal (MD) nucleus and its projection to the frontal lobe. *J Comp Neurol* **242**:535-560.

Goodman WK (1999) Obsessive-compulsive disorder: diagnosis and treatment. *J Clin Psychiatry 60 Suppl* **18**:27-32.

Greenberg BD, Murphy DL, Rasmussen SA (2000) Neuroanatomically based approaches to obsessive-compulsive disorder. Neurosurgery and transcranial magnetic stimulation. *Psychiatr Clin North Am* **23**:671-686, xii.

Greenberg BD, Price LH, Rauch SL, Friehs G, Noren G, Malone D, Carpenter LL, Rezai AR, Rasmussen SA (2003) Neurosurgery for intractable obsessive-compulsive disorder and depression: critical issues. *Neurosurg Clin N Am* **14**:199-212.

Greist JH (1994) Behavior therapy for obsessive compulsive disorder. *J Clin Psychiatry* **55** Suppl:60-68.

Hassani OK, Cromwell HC, Schultz W (2001) Influence of expectation of different rewards on behavior-related neuronal activity in the striatum. *J Neurophysiol* **85**:2477-2489.

Herner T (1961) Treatment of mental disorders with frontal stereotactic thermo-lesions. A follow-up study of 116 cases. *Acta Psychiatr Scand Suppl*. **36**.

Hodgkiss AD, Malizia AL, Bartlett JR, Bridges PK (1995) Outcome after the psychosurgical operation of stereotactic subcaudate tractotomy, 1979-1991. *J Neuropsychiatry Clin Neurosci* **7**:230-234.

Hollerman JR, Tremblay L, Schultz W (1998) Influence of reward expectation on behavior-related neuronal activity in primate striatum. *J Neurophysiol* **80**:947-963.

Jenike MA (1998) Neurosurgical treatment of obsessive-compulsive disorder. Br J Psychiatry Suppl:79-90.

Jenike MA, Baer L, Ballantine T, Martuza RL, Tynes S, Giriunas I, Buttolph ML, Cassem NH (1991) Cingulotomy for refractory obsessive-compulsive disorder. A long-term follow-up of 33 patients. *Arch Gen Psychiatry* **48**:548-555.

Karno M, Golding JM, Sorenson SB, Burnam MA (1988) The epidemiology of obsessive-compulsive disorder in five US communities. *Arch Gen Psychiatry* **45**:1094-1099.

Kartsounis LD, Poynton A, Bridges PK, Bartlett JR (1991) Neuropsychological correlates of stereotactic subcaudate tractotomy. *A prospective study. Brain* **114** (Pt 6):2657-2673.

Kelly D, Mitchell-Heggs N (1973) Stereotactic limbic leucotomy--a follow-up study of thirty patients. *Postgrad Med J* **49**:865-882.

Kelly D, Richardson A, Mitchell-Heggs N, Greenup J, Chen C, Hafner RJ (1973) Stereotactic limbic leucotomy: a preliminary report on forty patients. *Br J Psychiatry* **123**:141-148.

Koob GF, Le Moal M (1997) Drug abuse: hedonic homeostatic dysregulation. *Science* **278**:52-58.

Koran LM, Thienemann ML, Davenport R (1996) Quality of life for patients with obsessive-compulsive disorder. *Am J Psychiatry* **153**:783-788.

Krawczyk DC (2002) Contributions of the prefrontal cortex to the neural basis of human decision making. *Neurosci Biobehav Rev* **26**:631-664.

Kullberg G (1977) Differences in effects of capsulotomy and cingulotomy. In: *Neurosurgical treatment in Psychiatry, Pain and Epilepsy* (Sweet WH, Obrador S, Martin-Rodriguez JG, eds), pp 301-308. Baltimore: University Park Press.

Le Moal M (1995) Mesocorticolimbic dopaminergic neurons. Functional and regulatory roles. In: *Psychopharmacology: The fourth generation of progress* (Bloom FE, Kupfer DJ, eds), pp 283-294. New York: Raven Press.

Malhi GS, Sachdev P (2002) Novel physical treatments for the management of neuropsychiatric disorders. *J Psychosom Res* **53**:709-719.

Mallet L, Mesnage V, Houeto JL, Pelissolo A, Yelnik J, Behar C, Gargiulo M, Welter ML, Bonnet AM, Pillon B, Cornu P, Dormont D, Pidoux B, Allilaire JF, Agid Y (2002) Compulsions, Parkinson's disease, and stimulation. *Lancet* **360**:1302-1304.

McDougle CJ (1999) The neurobiology and treatment of obsessive-compulsive disorder. In: *Neurobiology of mental illness* (Charney DS, Nestler EJ, Bunney BS, eds), pp 518-533. New York: Oxford University Press.

McFarland NR, Haber SN (2002) Thalamic relay nuclei of the basal ganglia form both reciprocal and nonreciprocal cortical connections, linking multiple frontal cortical areas. *J Neurosci* **22**:8117-8132.

Mindus P, Nyman H (1991) Normalization of personality characteristics in patients with incapacitating anxiety disorders after capsulotomy. Acta Psychiatr Scand 83:283-291.

Mindus P, Jenike MA (1992) Neurosurgical treatment of malignant obsessive compulsive disorder. *Psychiatr Clin North Am* **15**:921-938.

Mindus P, Rasmussen SA, Lindquist C (1994) Neurosurgical treatment for refractory obsessive-compulsive disorder: implications for understanding frontal lobe function. J Neuropsychiatry *Clin Neurosci* **6**:467-477.

Mindus P, Edman G, Andreewitch S (1999) A prospective, long-term study of personality traits in patients with intractable obsessional illness treated by capsulotomy. *Acta Psychiatr Scand* **99**:40-50.

Mindus P, Nyman H, Rosenquist A, Rydin E, Meyerson BA (1988) Aspects of personality in patients with anxiety disorders undergoing capsulotomy. *Acta Neurochir Suppl (Wien)* **44**:138-144.

Mitchell-Heggs N, Kelly D, Richardson A (1976) Stereotactic limbic leucotomy--a follow-up at 16 months. *Br J Psychiatry* **128**:226-240.

Niki H, Watanabe M (1979) Prefrontal and cingulate unit activity during timing behavior in the monkey. *Brain Res* **171**:213-224.

Nuttin B, Cosyns P, Demeulemeester H, Gybels J, Meyerson B (1999) Electrical stimulation in anterior limbs of internal capsules in patients with obsessive-compulsive disorder. *Lancet* **354**:1526.

Pallanti S, Quercioli L, Koran LM (2002) Citalopram intravenous infusion in resistant obsessive-compulsive disorder: an open trial. *J Clin Psychiatry* **63**:796-801.

Paus T (2001) Primate anterior cingulate cortex: where motor control, drive and cognition interface. *Nat Rev Neurosci* **2**:417-424.

Piazza PV, Le Moal ML (1996) Pathophysiological basis of vulnerability to drug abuse: role of an interaction between stress, glucocorticoids, and dopaminergic neurons. *Annu Rev Pharmacol Toxicol* **36**:359-378.

Piazza PV, Le Moal M (1997) Glucocorticoids as a biological substrate of reward: physiological and pathophysiological implications. *Brain Res Brain Res Rev* **25**:359-372.

Piggot TA, Seay SM (1998) Biological treatments for obsessive-compulsive disorder. Literature review. In: *Obsessive-compulsive disorder. Theory, research, and treatment* (Eds R. P. Swinson MMA, S. Rachman, M. A. Richter., ed), pp pp. 298-326.: The Guilford Press: New-York.

Pigott TA, Seay SM (1999) A review of the efficacy of selective serotonin reuptake inhibitors in obsessive-compulsive disorder. *J Clin Psychiatry* **60**:101-106.

Ramnani N, Owen AM (2004) Anterior prefrontal cortex: insights into function from anatomy and neuroimaging. *Nat Rev Neurosci* **5**:184-194.

Rasmussen SA, Tsuang MT (1984) The epidemiology of obsessive compulsive disorder. *J Clin Psychiatry* **45**:450-457.

Robins LN, Helzer JE, Weissman MM, Orvaschel H, Gruenberg E, Burke JD, Jr., Regier DA (1984) Lifetime prevalence of specific psychiatric disorders in three sites. *Arch Gen Psychiatry* **41**:949-958.

Rosenkilde CE, Bauer RH, Fuster JM (1981) Single cell activity in ventral prefrontal cortex of behaving monkeys. *Brain Res* **209**:375-394.

Saxena S, Brody AL, Schwartz JM, Baxter LR (1998) Neuroimaging and frontal-subcortical circuitry in obsessive-compulsive disorder. *Br J Psychiatry Suppl*:**26**-37.

Schwartz JM (1998) Neuroanatomical aspects of cognitive-behavioural therapy response in obsessive-compulsive disorder. An evolving perspective on brain and behaviour. *Br J Psychiatry Suppl*:**38**-44.

Schwartz JM (1999) A role of volition and attention in the generation of new brain circuitry. Toward a neurobiology of mental force. *J Consciousness studies* **6**:115-142.

Shidara M, Richmond BJ (2002) Anterior cingulate: single neuronal signals related to degree of reward expectancy. *Science* **296**:1709-1711.

Shima K, Tanji J (1998) Role for cingulate motor area cells in voluntary movement selection based on reward. *Science* **282**:1335-1338.

Skoog G, Skoog I (1999) A 40-year follow-up of patients with obsessive-compulsive disorder [see commetns]. *Arch Gen Psychiatry* **56**:121-127.

Strom-Olsen R, Carlisle S (1971) Bi-frontal stereotactic tractotomy. A follow-up study of its effects on 210 patients. *Br J Psychiatry* **118**:141-154.

Sturm V, Lenartz D, Koulousakis A, Treuer H, Herholz K, Klein JC, Klosterkotter J (2003) The nucleus accumbens: a target for deep brain stimulation in obsessive-compulsive- and anxiety-disorders. *J Chem Neuroanat* **26**:293-299.

Tan E, Marks IM, Marset P (1971) Bimedial leucotomy in obsessive-compulsive neurosis: a controlled serial enquiry. *Br J Psychiatry* **118**:155-164.

Thorpe SJ, Rolls ET, Maddison S (1983) The orbitofrontal cortex: neuronal activity in the behaving monkey. *Exp Brain Res* **49**:93-115.

Tremblay L, Schultz W (1999) Relative reward preference in primate orbitofrontal cortex. *Nature* **398**:704-708.

Tremblay L, Schultz W (2000a) Modifications of reward expectation-related neuronal activity during learning in primate orbitofrontal cortex. *J Neurophysiol* **83**:1877-1885.

Tremblay L, Schultz W (2000b) Reward-related neuronal activity during go-nogo task performance in primate orbitofrontal cortex. *J Neurophysiol* **83**:1864-1876.

Tremblay L, Hollerman JR, Schultz W (1998) Modifications of reward expectation-related neuronal activity during learning in primate striatum. *J Neurophysiol* **80**:964-977.

Whitty CW, Duffield JE, Tov PM, Cairns H (1952) Anterior cingulectomy in the treatment of mental disease. *Lancet* **1**:475-481.

In: Deep Brain Stimulation
Editors: Mark H. Rogers and Paul B. Anderson

ISBN 978-1-60692-895-0

Chapter VII

Deep Brain Stimulation in Adult and Pediatric Dystonia*

Laura Cif, Simone Hemm, Nathalie Vayssiere and Philippe Coubes†
Research Group on Movement Disorders, Department of Neurosurgery
(Professor Philippe Coubes, Montpellier University Hospital,
34295 Montpellier, Cedex 5, France

Abstract

In numerous medical conditions, abnormal movements (dystonia, dyskinesia, myoclonus and tremor) are present, isolated or associated to other neurological deficits. Deep brain stimulation has been validated as a safe and efficient neurosurgical procedure in treating Parkinson's disease and essential tremor. Following the experience with ablative surgery for dystonia and high frequency stimulation for Parkinson's disease, chronic electrical stimulation of the internal globus pallidus (GPi) has been proposed to treat dystonic syndromes. Based on etiology and spread of symptoms, 82 patients were divided in subgroups separating, for each of them, children and adults: primary DYT1 dystonia, primary dystonia without DYT1 mutation, primary segmental dystonia, post anoxic cerebral palsy, pantothenate kinase associated neurodegeneration (PKAN) and mitochondrial diseases. Assessment was performed pre- and postoperatively by the Burke-Fahn's Marsden Dystonia Rating Scale, motor and disability sections. Bilateral electrode implantation was performed under general anaesthesia. High frequency (130 Hz), 450 microseconds pulse width and monopolar stimulation were used. Clinical improvement at three years was comparable for the groups of primary dystonia (82% for the motor scores) and for secondary dystonia and degenerative diseases, improvement was less important but still interesting (40%). The originality of the method consisted in the use of stereotactic MR imaging for the target selection without microelectrode recordings. This reduced the duration of the procedure and the risk of haemorrhage.

---

* A version of this chapter was also published in *Recent Reakthroughs in Basal ganglia Research* , edited by Erwan Bezard published by Nova Science Publishers, Inc. It was submitted for appropriate modification in an effort to encourage wider dissemination of research

† Correspondence should be addressed to Philippe Coubes: Tel/Fax: +33 (0) 4.67.33.74.64. E-mail address: p-coubes@chu-montpellier.fr or urmae@chu-montpellier.fr

Chronic high frequency stimulation of the GPi can be considered as an efficient and lasting treatment in primary dystonia and proposed in selected cases of secondary dystonia and degenerative disease.

Background and Purpose

In a wide range of medical conditions, a movement disorder can be the only symptom or associated with other neurological deficits. Most of them are of unknown origin. Dystonia, dyskinesia, myoclonus, tremor, atethosis are abnormal movements susceptible to be influenced by high frequency modulation of the basal ganglia. Nevertheless, the control of these symptoms is highly depending on the etiology. Movement disorders (primary dystonia, myoclonus dystonia, tardive dyskinesia), which are not associated to other neurologic deficits are more likely to be controlled by high frequency stimulation.

The first validated medical condition successfully treated by DBS was Parkinson's disease (Benabid et al., 1987). Gradually, the indications of this therapy were enlarged to include other diseases associating movement disorders as dystonia and dyskinesia of various etiologies. Based on the experience of our group (Gros et al., 1976) with brain lesioning surgery (pallidotomy) in a young patient with idiopathic generalized dystonia (Iacono et al., 1996) and deep brain stimulation in Parkinson's disease dyskinesias (Benabid et al., 1987; 1993), we reported, in 1996 the efficacy of DBS in a young lady presenting with severe life threatening primary generalized dystonia after chronic bilateral stimulation of the GPi (Coubes et al., 1999). Since then, 105 dystonic patients have been treated for bilateral stimulation of the Internal Globus Pallidus (GPi) in the department of Neurosurgery in Montpellier.

The originality of our method consists in the use of stereotactic MR imaging for the target determination, without microelectrode recordings. This considerably reduces the procedure's duration, which is important especially in children, as well as for the risk of hemorrhage (0 cases). Furthermore, the surgery, performed under general anesthesia is more adapted in patients with permanent involuntary movements.

We will present the population, the surgical procedure, the clinical management of the patients and the results obtained by DBS. In order to discuss the criteria for selecting the patients with dystonia-dyskinesia, we will briefly remember this medical condition. Whatever, others movement disorders being influenced by the DBS are sometimes associated to dystonia in patients to be operated.

Dystonia has been defined as a neurological syndrome characterized by involuntary, sustained muscle contractions, causing twisting and repetitive movements or abnormal postures (Fahn, 1988).

Its classification is a difficult task and can be done in several ways: according to the spread of the symptoms to different body parts, to the age of onset or to etiology.

According to distribution, dystonia is classified into one of the following categories: focal, segmental, multifocal, hemidystonia and generalized dystonia.

The age of onset is another important criterion for characterizing a patient. In case of early onset, the disease is more likely to generalize and severely worsen than for adult-onset dystonias.

Dystonia can also be classified by etiology. In primary dystonia, dystonia is the only symptom and can be sporadic or inherited (DYT1 dystonia; Ozelius et al., 1997). Dystonia-plus is a group of syndromes where dystonia is usually associated to another neurological condition such as parkinsonism or myoclonus (Dopa responsive dystonia, myoclonus-dystonia syndrome). The group of heredodegenerative dystonia includes numerous diseases and in this group, dystonia is typically not pure. Amino acid disorders, lipid disorders, Lesch-Nyhan disease, pantothenate kinase-associated neurodegeneration (PKAN), mitochondrial diseases, Wilson's disease, Huntington's disease, Juvenile parkinsonism-dystonia (Dwork et al., 1993; Ishikawa and Takahashi, 1998) and many others are heredodegenerative dystonias. Secondary dystonias are generated by insults such as drugs, strokes, tumors, infections (Fahn, 1988) and this subgroup includes also dystonia-dyskinesia secondary to cerebral palsy (CP).

In 40 % of the patients with early-onset dystonia a specific cause can be found. The etiologic diagnosis is established by clinical evaluation, neuroimaging and molecular analysis in primary dystonias. When the history of the disease, the clinical examination and the brain MRI suggest a heredogenerative dystonia, further investigations are performed such as blood work-up, urine sample analysis, CSF testing, electrophysiologic studies, muscle, skin, liver biopsies, PET, eye slit-lamp examination.

The identification of the etiology is very important for the prognosis of the disease and because of the existence of very few medical conditions having a specific treatment such as Dopa-Responsive dystonia, creatine deficiency or Wilson's disease.

Several drugs are available to treat dystonic symptoms but their efficacy is often limited, transient and difficult to assess (often because of the fluctuation of the symptoms). The most important drugs to be used are Levodopa (also as a diagnosis trial in Dopa responsive dystonia), anticholinergics, benzodiazepines, baclofen (Ford et al., 1998) and Botulinum toxin injections especially for the treatment of focal dystonias (Tsui et al., 1987)

Because of the poor efficacy of the pharmaceutical treatment in front of the very severe forms of movement disorders (especially generalized dystonias with onset in childhood) we were led to propose deep brain stimulation as another therapeutic strategy in order to control the symptoms generating life-threatening complications.

Patients (Population)

In the following report, we will present the results of 82 patients presenting with segmentary or generalized dystonia treated by bilateral chronic electrical stimulation of the GPi. The population was divided in subgroups separating, for each of them, children from adults. Group 1 included patients with primary generalized DYT1 dystonia, group 2 primary generalized dystonia without DYT1 mutation, group 3 primary segmentary dystonia (cervico-axial dystonia), group 4 generalized dystonia-dyskinesia due to postanoxic cerebral palsy, group 5 generalized dystonia secondary to PKAN and group 6 one generalized dystonia secondary to mitochondrial disease. For the reported patients, the follow-up was at least of 6 months.

Clinical Evaluation

Dystonic movements and abnormal postures were evaluated using the Burke-Fahn-Marsden-Dystonia-Rating scale (BFMDRS, motor and disability part; Burke et al., 1985) before the surgical procedure, several times during the post-operative hospital stay, every month during the first year and every three months afterwards.

Surgical Procedure

Bilateral electrode implantation was performed in a single surgical session under general anesthesia (Vayssiere et al., 2000; Coubes et al., 2002a; Vayssiere et al., 2002). The MR-compatible Leksell stereotactic frame was applied and a 3D-SPGR (spoiled gradient recall) acquisition was performed. The postero-ventral part of the GPi was located through axial, sagittal and coronal MRI studies (Figure 1A). The target coordinates (x, y, z) and the trajectory angles (α,β) were calculated using a dedicated software.

Two four contact electrodes (DBS 3389, Medtronic, Minneapolis) were implanted under strict profile radioscopic control. Immediate postoperative control MRI (Figure 1B) was obtained with the stereotactic frame on. Electrodes were connected to a pulse generator five days later (Itrel II or III, Kinetra and Soletra Medtronic, Minneapolis, USA), which was subcutaneously introduced in the abdominal area. In each patient final placement of the implanted devices and their connections were checked by a radiographic control during the postoperative hospital stay (Figure 2).

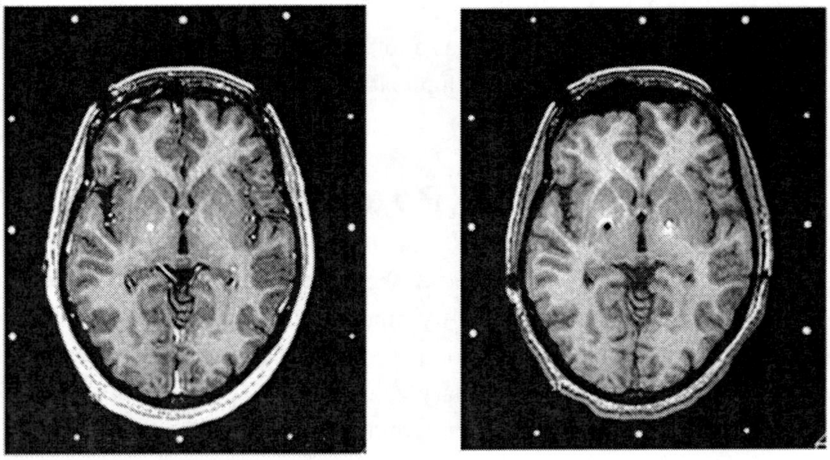

Figure 1. Stereotactic MRI. A. Pre-operative planning. B. Post-operative MRI to control the final electrode position (black points = electrode artefacts).

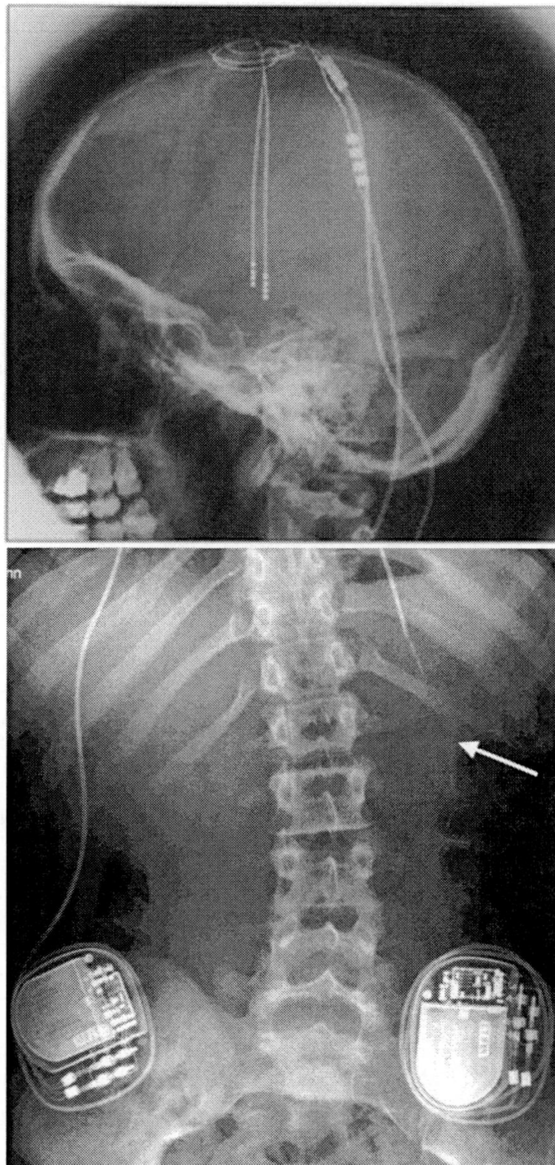

A B

Figure 2. Radiographic control of the implanted devices. A. Electrodes connected to the extensions. B. Neurostimulators with extension length reserve. Arrow indicates an extension fracture during sports.

Electric Parameter Settings

After implantation, stimulators were switched on. Electrical variables were set at high frequency (130 Hz), 450 μsec for the pulse width with one contact negatively activated. Intensity was progressively increased according to the needs of each patient (Hemm et al., 2004) and the clinical evolution. Usually the first levels for the voltage were between 0.5 V-

0.8 V. Over the time, we modified the electric parameters in several patients, by increasing the voltage or activating a second contact when requested. The mean steady state value of the voltage was 1.6 ± 0.3 V (Hemm et al., 2002).

Clinical Results

Motor and disability scores' evolution (BMFDRS) for primary and secondary dystonia is presented in tables I and II. Within each group, the improvement was progressive over time. With more than 3 years of follow-up, the clinical improvement was comparable for the two groups of primary dystonia (82% of improvement on the motor scale). The results obtained in the group of secondary dystonia and heredodegenerative diseases are less important but yet around 40 % with 3 years of follow-up. After three years, the disability score improvement was superior in the group of primary DYT1 dystonia (80 %) compared to non-DYT1 primary dystonia (56 %) and to secondary dystonia (19 %). The group of secondary dystonia and heredodegenerative diseases is a very heterogeneous group. This is why results for all etiologies should be presented separately.

Discussion

We report here our experience with bilateral chronic electrical stimulation of the GPi in the treatment of primary DYT1 positive and DYT1 negative generalized dystonia (Coubes et al., 1999; 2000; 2002b; Cif et al., 2004; Coubes et al., 2004), generalized dystonia–dyskinesia secondary to post-anoxic cerebral palsy, generalized dystonia secondary to PKAN syndrome and to mitochondrial diseases. We also report the results obtained by DBS in primary segmentary dystonia. Since the first child has been operated, 126 other patients underwent surgery for DBS in our department (Dystonia + Parkinson).

While at the beginning DBS was proposed in children with primary generalized dystonia (with or without DYT1 mutation), selection criteria were revisited and enlarged for including now other types of dystonia in children and adults. Several patients with generalized dystonia associating myoclonus underwent surgery for chronic electrical stimulation of the GPi and we could see an early and complete control of myoclonus. These findings led us to propose this treatment in a child with genetically proven myoclonus-dystonia syndrome (Cif et al., 2004) MDS, DYT11, mutation in the epsilon-amino sarcoglycan gene, (Gasser, 1998; Zimprich et al., 2001) and we obtained a very satisfactory improvement of his symptoms. We confirmed in a second patient with MDS the efficiency of GPi stimulation.

Being confronted with very severe clinical conditions in patients with secondary dystonia and heredodegenerative diseases, in which the efficacy of the medical treatment was poor and in which dystonic movements and postures were comparable with those met in primary dystonia, we proposed DBS in several selected patients of these groups.

The criteria for patient selection in this group were clinical, electrophysiological and based on brain imaging as well as on etiology.

Table I. Motor scores (BMFDRS) of dystonic children treated by DBS. Mean values ±SD. The values in brackets represent the mean improvement in percent. A reduction in the score indicates an improvement in function. BMFDRS denotes Burke-Marsden Fahn's Dystonia Rating Scale.

Motor score		6 months after surgery/120 (%)[1]	1 year after surgery/120 (%)[1]	2 years after surgery/120 (%)[1]	>3 years after surgery/120 (%)[1]
PGD[2] DYT1+[3]	Children	80±20 n[5]=14	77±28 n[5]=13	76±25 n[5]=12	82±18 n[5]=10
	Adults	75±17 n[5]=10	75±21 n[5]=8	70±16 n[5]=5	73±13 n[5]=2
PGD[2] DYT1-	Children	72±15 n[5]=12	74±15 n[5]=12	66±26 n[5]=11	72±21 n[5]=9
	Adults	53±31 n[5]=19	64±33 n[5]=19	73±26 n[5]=16	71±26 n[5]=7
Cervico-axial dystonia	Children	77±0 n[5]=1	93±0 n[5]=1	93±12 n[5]=1	100±10 n[5]=1
	Adults	70±34 n[5]=7	88±20 n[5]=7	85±21 n[5]=7	84±12 n[5]=4
Post-anoxic cerebral palsy	Children	31±8 n[5]=5	37±6 n[5]=2	45±0 n[5]=1	51±0 n[5]=1
	Adults	41±25 n[5]=5	38±10 n[5]=5	45±15 n[5]=3	62±0 n[5]=1
PKAN[4]	Children	51±29 n[5]=4	59±25 n[5]=4	22±5 n[5]=2	33±13 n[5]=2
	Adults	71±12 n[5]=2	73±10 n[5]=2	74±1 n[5]=2	88±0 n[5]=1
Mitochondrial disease	Children	27±17 n[5]=3	46±30 n[5]=2	25±10 n[5]=2	42±6 n[5]=2

[1]The improvement in percent is calculated based on the maximal possible gain ($Score_{preop}$-$Score_{postop}$)/($Score_{preop}$).
[2]Primary generalized dystonia
[3]DYT1 mutation
[4]Pantothenate kinase-associated neurodegeneration
[5]Number of patients

Table II. Disability scores (BMFDRS) of dystonic children treated by DBS. Mean values ±SD. The values in brackets represent the mean improvement in percent. A reduction in the score indicates an improvement in function. BMFDRS denotes Burke-Marsden Fahn's Dystonia Rating Scale.

Disability score		6 months after surgery/120 (%)[1]	1 year after surgery/120 (%)[1]	2 years after surgery/120 (%)[1]	>3 years after surgery/120 (%)[1]
PGD[2] DYT1+[3]	Children	58±39 n[5]=14	62±39 n[5]=13	63±27 n[5]=12	80±14 n[5]=10
	Adults	61±25 n[5]=10	64±29 n[5]=8	74±14 n[5]=52	58±3 n[5]=2
PGD[2] DYT1-	Children	42±23 n[5]=12	52±21 n[5]=12	54±24 n[5]=11	49±29 n[5]=9
	Adults	35±34 n[5]=19	52±31 n[5]=19	67±30 n[5]=16	58±36 n[5]=7
Cervico-axial dystonia	Children	100±0 n[5]=1	92±0 n[5]=1	92±0 n[5]=1	100±0 n[5]=1
	Adults	55±36 n[5]=7	74±22 n[5]=7	86±18 n[5]=7	74±12 n[5]=4
Cerebral palsy	Children	4±3 n[5]=5	11±4 n[5]=2	19±0 n[5]=1	19±0 n[5]=1
	Adults	21±22 n[5]=5	28±21 n[5]=5	17±12 n[5]=3	27±0 n[5]=1
PKAN[4]	Children	35±32 n[5]=4	28±28 n[5]=4	2±2 n[5]=2	7±14 n[5]=2
	Adults	31±20 n[5]=2	43±10 n[5]=2	62±7 n[5]=2	65±0 n[5]=1
Mitochondrial disease	Children	8±5 n[5]=3	10±3 n[5]=2	11±3 n[5]=2	8±1 n[5]=2

[1]The improvement in percent is calculated based on the maximal possible gain ($Score_{preop}$-$Score_{postop}$)/($Score_{preop}$).
[2]Primary generalized dystonia
[3]DYT1 mutation
[4]Pantothenate kinase-associated neurodegeneration
[5]Number of patients

We performed surgery for DBS in patients in whom dystonia and dyskinesia were prominent compared to other neurological deficits (especially motor deficit and spasticity), the motor pattern was preserved and in patients presenting with severe or life threatening symptoms due to dystonia-dyskinesia (swallowing difficulties, permanent opisthotonos, painful muscle spasms).

Electroencephalogram, electroretinogram, visual and brainstem, somatosensory evoked responses were obtained. Motor evoked potentials were performed in elder children to identify pyramidal tract impairment. In order to exclude brain abnormalities contraindicating surgery (major cortical atrophy, severe periventicular leucomalacia especially met in cerebral palsy, basal ganglia and thalamic lesions), brain MR under general anesthesia was performed in all patients.

As shown in tables I and II, best results were obtained within the group of patients with DYT1 mutation (Coubes et al., 1999; 2000; Roubertie et al., 2000; Coubes et al., 2004). The surgery of abnormal movements should intervene before the occurrence of skeletal deformities, which always diminish the outcome. Within the population of non-DYT1 dystonia and especially in secondary and heredodegenerative dystonias, results are not so predictable. The improvement of dysarthria is variable and often very few influenced by DBS.

Stimulation's switch-off systematically causes the recurrence of symptoms within some hours or days. Whatever, in several patients we could see a long lasting preservation of the clinical improvement for several weeks without stimulation.

In the secondary dystonia group, the efficacy of stimulation is far more limited. We were led to propose it for very handicapped patients for whom other therapeutic strategies failed to improve dystonia, as already mentioned. The clinical and etiological heterogeneity among this group almost prevents any global interpretation of these results. In this group, a frequently associated hypertonia of pyramidal origin influences the dystonic component.

An important negative prognostic factor under stimulation is the existence of a permanent hypertonia at rest, whatever may be its origin. Although we are not yet able to predict the long-term prognosis, we observed an interesting improvement with dyskinesia-dystonia secondary to a perinatal anoxia (dyskinetic forms of cerebral palsy accounting for less than 10 % of all forms CP; Lin, 2003), PKAN and mitochondrial diseases treated by GPi stimulation. A constant control of pain associated with muscle spasms was obtained in patients suffering from secondary dystonia.

The progression of the causal disease is of critical importance for patient's prognosis.

Using this surgical method based on MRI alone (Vayssiere et al., 2000; Coubes et al., 2002a; Vayssiere et al., 2002), the associated morbidity is low. We didn't observe hemorrhage due to the intracerebral tracts as reported before in other series (our experience reaches 236 electrodes; Starr et al., 1999). Secondary infection of the stimulation system remains the major complication of this technique and was observed in 4 patients. We summarize the complications observed in our population in table III.

Table III. Complications

Complications	Number
Hemorrage	0
Infection	4
Lead fracture	3
Extension fracture	3

The remarkable tolerance of the internal pulse generator must be also emphasized in children. We never observed any complication due to displacement with growth (loss of efficacy linked to the displacement of the electrode). As shown in figure 2 and 3, a residual length was enrolled around the battery and the electrode in order to compensate for growth in children and to provide some flexibility with movements in the system (Figure 2). Furthermore, it appears that growth does not interfere with stimulation, and the implantation of a single 90 cm extension compensates adequately for the growth of the child. We observed in two patients (1 child, 1 adult) an extension fracture due to adherences fixing the extension and limiting its mobility and flexibility.

The children's physical development (height, body weight) was followed as well as hormonal levels (Insuline-like Growth Factor-IGF1, Insuline–like Growth Factor Binding Protein 3-IGF-BP3, Estradiol, Testosterone, Folliculine Stimulating Hormone-FSH and Luteinizing Hormone-LH) in order to check puberty development.

Conclusion

Despite cost and complexity of the follow-up, bilateral chronic electrical stimulation can be proposed as first line treatment for early onset primary generalized dystonia when pharmacologically intractable and also early considered in segmentary dystonia in adults and in well-selected cases of secondary dystonia. It is conservative, adaptable, reversible and well tolerated by the whole population. It must be applied soon, especially in primary dystonia before neuro-ortopaedic sequels occur. The complication rate remains low.

For secondary dystonia, pallidal stimulation can partially improve dystonic syndromes with important control of pain and swallowing difficulties.

References

Benabid AL, Pollak P, Louveau A, Henry S, de Rougemont J (1987) Combined (thalamotomy and stimulation) stereotactic surgery of the VIM thalamic nucleus for bilateral Parkinson disease. *Appl Neurophysiol* **50**:344-346.

Benabid AL, Pollak P, Seigneuret E, Hoffmann D, Gay E, Perret J (1993) Chronic VIM thalamic stimulation in Parkinson's disease, essential tremor and extra-pyramidal dyskinesias. *Acta Neurochir Suppl (Wien)* **58**:39-44.

Burke RE, Fahn S, Marsden CD, Bressman SB, Moskowitz C, Friedman J (1985) Validity and reliability of a rating scale for the primary torsion dystonias. *Neurology* **35**:73-77.

Cif L, Valente EM, Hemm S, Coubes C, Vayssiere N, Serrat S, Di Giorgio A, Coubes P (2004) Deep brain stimulation in myoclonus-dystonia syndrome. *Mov Disord* **19**:724-727.

Coubes P, Roubertie A, Vayssiere N, Hemm S, Echenne B (2000) Treatment of DYT1-generalised dystonia by stimulation of the internal globus pallidus. *Lancet* **355**: 2220-2221.

Coubes P, Vayssiere N, El Fertit H, Hemm S, Cif L, Kienlen J, Bonafe A, Frerebeau P (2002a) Deep brain stimulation for dystonia. Surgical technique. *Stereotact Funct Neurosurg* **78**:183-191.

Coubes P, Echenne B, Roubertie A, Vayssiere N, Tuffery S, Humbertclaude V, Cambonie G, Claustres M, Frerebeau P (1999) [Treatment of early-onset generalized dystonia by chronic bilateral stimulation of the internal globus pallidus. Apropos of a case]. *Neurochirurgie* **45**:139-144.

Coubes P, Cif L, El Fertit H, Hemm S, Vayssiere N, Serrat S, Picot MC, Tuffery S, Claustres M, Echenne B, Frerebeau P (2004) Electrical stimulation of the globus pallidus internus in patients with primary generalized dystonia: long-term results. *J Neurosurg* **101**:189-194.

Coubes P, Cif L, Azais M, Roubertie A, Hemm S, Diakonoya N, Vayssiere N, Monnier C, Hardouin E, Ganau A, Tuffery S, Claustre M, Echenne B (2002b) [Treatment of dystonia syndrome by chronic electric stimulation of the internal globus pallidus]. *Arch Pediatr* **9** *Suppl* **2**:84s-86s.

Dwork AJ, Balmaceda C, Fazzini EA, MacCollin M, Cote L, Fahn S (1993) Dominantly inherited, early-onset parkinsonism: neuropathology of a new form. Neurology 43:69-74.

Fahn S (1988) Concept and classification of dystonia. *Adv Neurol* **50**:1-8.

Ford B, Greene PE, Louis ED, Bressman SB, Goodman RR, Brin MF, Sadiq S, Fahn S (1998) Intrathecal baclofen in the treatment of dystonia. *Adv Neurol* **78**:199-210.

Gasser T (1998) Inherited myoclonus-dystonia syndrome. Adv Neurol 78:325-334.

Gros C, Frerebeau P, Perez-Dominguez E, Bazin M, M PJ (1976) Long term results of stereotaxic surgery for infantile dystonia and dyskinesia. *Neurochirurgia (Stuttg)* **19**: 171-178.

Hemm S, N D, G M, N V, L C, P C (2002) Stimulated volume and energy consumption in improved dystonic patients treated by high frequency GPi stimulation. *Movement Disorders* **17**:S302.

Hemm S, Vayssiere N, Mennessier G, Cif L, Zanca M, Ravel P, Frerebeau P, P C (2004) Evolution of brain impedance in dystonic patients treated by GPi electrical stimulation. *Neuromodulation* **7**:67-75.

Iacono RP, Kuniyoshi SM, Lonser RR, Maeda G, Inae AM, Ashwal S (1996) Simultaneous bilateral pallidoansotomy for idiopathic dystonia musculorum deformans. *Pediatr Neurol* **14**:145-148.

Ishikawa A, Takahashi H (1998) Clinical and neuropathological aspects of autosomal recessive juvenile parkinsonism. *J Neurol* 245:P4-9.

Lin JP (2003) The cerebral palsies: a physiological approach. *J Neurol Neurosurg Psychiatry* **74** Suppl 1:i23-29.

Ozelius LJ, Hewett JW, Page CE, Bressman SB, Kramer PL, Shalish C, de Leon D, Brin MF, Raymond D, Corey DP, Fahn S, Risch NJ, Buckler AJ, Gusella JF, Breakefield XO (1997) The early-onset torsion dystonia gene (DYT1) encodes an ATP-binding protein. *Nat Genet* **17**:40-48.

Roubertie A, Echenne B, Cif L, Vayssiere N, Hemm S, Coubes P (2000) Treatment of early-onset dystonia: update and a new perspective. *Childs Nerv Syst* **16**:334-340.

Starr PA, Vitek JL, DeLong M, Bakay RA (1999) Magnetic resonance imaging-based stereotactic localization of the globus pallidus and subthalamic nucleus. *Neurosurgery* **44**:303-313; discussion 313-304.

Tsui JK, Fross RD, Calne S, Calne DB (1987) Local treatment of spasmodic torticollis with botulinum toxin. *Can J Neurol Sci* **14**:533-535.

Vayssiere N, Hemm S, Zanca M, Picot MC, Bonafe A, Cif L, Frerebeau P, Coubes P (2000) Magnetic resonance imaging stereotactic target localization for deep brain stimulation in dystonic children. *J Neurosurg* **93**:784-790.

Vayssiere N, Hemm S, Cif L, Picot MC, Diakonova N, El Fertit H, Frerebeau P, Coubes P (2002) Comparison of atlas- and magnetic resonance imaging-based stereotactic targeting of the globus pallidus internus in the performance of deep brain stimulation for treatment of dystonia. *J Neurosurg* **96**:673-679.

Zimprich A, Grabowski M, Asmus F, Naumann M, Berg D, Bertram M, Scheidtmann K, Kern P, Winkelmann J, Muller-Myhsok B, Riedel L, Bauer M, Muller T, Castro M, Meitinger T, Strom TM, Gasser T (2001) Mutations in the gene encoding epsilon-sarcoglycan cause myoclonus-dystonia syndrome. *Nat Genet* **29**:66-69.

In: Deep Brain Stimulation
Editors: Mark H. Rogers and Paul B. Anderson

ISBN 978-1-60692-895-0

Chapter VIII

Deep Brain Stimulation of the Subthalamus: Neuropsychological Effects*

Rita Moretti, Paola Torre, Rodolfo M. Antonello and Antonio Bava[1]

[1] Dip. Fisiologia e Patologia, Università di Trieste, Italy

The basal ganglia were considered as a site for integrating diverse inputs from the entire cerebral cortex and funneling these influences via the ventrolateral thalamus to the motor cortex (Alexander, 1994). The subthalamic nucleus (STN) has generally been considered as a rely station within frontal-subcortical motor control circuitry. The function of the STN in the current model of the basal ganglia organization was developed from animal model and neurodegenerative diseases with hypo- and hyperkinetic movement disorders (Alexander et al, 1986): in this model, the STN represents a relay in the so-called "indirect" pathway of the parallel basal ganglia-thalamocortical circuits. STN excitatory efferents reinforce the inhibition of basal ganglia output nuclei, the internal globus pallidus (GPi) and the reticular substantia nigra (SNr) on thalamo-frontal neurons. A "direct" striato-pallidal pathway opposes the STN by normally inhibiting basal ganglia outflow, facilitating thalamo-frontal drive (Schroeder et al., 2002).

Clinicians maintain firm conviction on the fundamental role of the basal ganglia, and of STN, in motor syndromes such as Parkinson Disease. Lesions at the level of STN lead to hemiballism and involuntary movements of the contralateral extremities (Guridi and Obeso, 2001).

The limits of drug therapy in severe forms of Parkinson's Disease have led to a renewed interest in functional surgery of the basal ganglia and the thalamus. Deep brain stimulation of

* A version of this chapter was also published in *Basal Ganglia and Thalamus: Their Role in Congition and Behavior*, edited by Rita Moretti published by Nova Science Publishers, Inc. It was submitted for appropriate modification in an effort to encourage wider dissemination of research.

these structures was developed with the aim of reducing the morbidity of surgery and of offering an adaptive treatment. This type of stimulation was first applied to the thalamus in patients with severe tremor and has recently been applied to the subthalamic nucleus and the internal pallidum. The physiological expectation for this approach is based on the nigro-striatal dopaminergic defect common of Parkinson Disease: i.e., that it induces over-activity of the excitatory glutaminergic subthalamic nucleus-globus pallidus pathway and thus, when the activity is decreased by stimulation, it should lead to an improvement of levodopa-responsive symptoms (akinesia, rigidity, rest tremor, and gait impairment) (Pollak, 2001).

Deep Brain Stimulation (DBS) has become widely used to treat medically refractory tremor, Parkinson's Disease (PD) and primary dystonia. DBS of the thalamus for tremor and of the subthalamic nucleus (STN) and the internal segment of the Globus Pallidus (GPi) for PD is now FDA approved. As the number of DBS procedures for movement disorders, epilepsy and pain increase, more neurologists will need to acquire the knowledge of DBS programming.

DBS comprises chronic high frequency electrical stimulation of the target nucleus, a brain pacemaker, which might work by entraining neuronal firing patterns and pathological synchronization of neuronal activity. The DBS electrode has 4 contacts, which can be used singly in a monopolar mode of stimulation or in combinations of contacts in a bipolar mode. The adjustable parameters of stimulation are the rate or frequency of stimulation, the pulse width, and the voltage. Thus the number of stimulation parameters possible for programming are huge and DBS programming can be a time consuming and daunting task unless a clear protocol is followed. An advantage of DBS compared to ablative procedures is that the stimulation parameters can be adjusted over time, to optimize the clinical benefit while minimizing side effects (Bronte-Stewart, 2003).

As general accordance, the bilateral stimulation of subthalamic nucleus has as a direct consequence a significant bilateral reduction in Parkinson' disability (Kumar et al., 2000). High frequency deep brain stimulation of the STN improves motor function in Parkinson's Disease patients and has therefore become a strategy to treat medically intractable PD patients (Deep Brain Stimulation for Parkinson's Disease Study Group, 2001). Nevertheless, the physiologic mechanism underlying the beneficial effect of deep brain stimulation is not completely understood, but one can argue that it has reversible suppressive effects on the nuclei, and it leads to the hypothesis that high frequency electrical stimulation is neuro-inhibitive, due to the stimulation of GABAergic fibers. In particular, focusing our interest on subthalamic stimulation, there is evidence that, in epileptic animals, modifications in subthalamic nucleus activity can block the ectopical discharges of epileptic foci (Vercueil et al., 1998).

Using functional imaging, it has previously been shown that STN stimulation enhances movement associated activation of supplementary motor area (SMA) (Ceballos-Baumann et al., 1999). Overactivation of the lateral premotor cortex has been shown in an event-related fMRI study investigating joystick movements as well as in block design fMRI studies on complex finger movements (Haslinger et al., 2001; Sabatini et al., 2000). However, facilitation of movement related frontal activity is not necessarily coupled with improvement in frontal executive function as suggested by neuropsychological studies in Parkinson's disease with DBS. Still controversial and debated are the possible consequences on cognition due to DBS-STN, considering that STN role in cognition has not yet been investigated in detail. Clinical studies suggest that the STN participates in non-motor functions which can now be probed in Parkinson's disease patients with deep brain stimulation of the STN, allowing selective and reversible modulation of this nucleus. Bilateral DBS-STN for PD can cause subtle impairments in various aspects of frontal executive functioning, particularly in older patients (Saint Cyr et al., 2000; Jahanshahi et al.; 2000 Pillon, 2002), but results are quite controversial.

In these aspects the striatum may play a more central role, providing important information for subsequent cortical processing.

Though, linguistic aspects have never been strenuously investigated in the subjects with subthalamic nucleus stimulation. There have been attempts to follow some patients with subthalamic nucleus deep brain stimulation (Zanini, et al., 2000; Moretti et al., 2001; Moretti et al., 2002), during which different patients underwent linguistic assessment, before and after surgery. These Authors have found a small, but significant amelioration in linguistic performance during electrical stimulation.

In order to better define the eventual modification of the cognitive profile of patients who underwent to subthalamic nucleus-deep brain stimulation, we have followed nine Parkinson disease patients before and after surgery.

Our study (Moretti et al., 2003- A) included 9 patients (6 men and 3 women) with idiopathic Parkinson's disease (UK Parkinson's Disease Society Brain Bank Clinical diagnostic criteria) (Hughes et al., 1992). All the patients could be fully studied (mean age 68.7 ± 7.89 years, range= 60-76 years; average age at onset= 48.34 ± 7.89 years, range= 41-56 years). All the patients suffered for 8.91 ± 2.34 years from Parkinson disease and had been treated for several years with levodopa preparations, then developed motor fluctuations and dyskinesias difficult to control by adapting their drug regimen. They were selected as candidates for deep brain stimulation of the subthalamic nucleus because of severe motor fluctuations. In the off medication state, the mean Hohen and Yahr (Hohen and Yahr, 1967) score was 4.01 and the mean Unified Parkinson's Disease Rating Scale (UPDRS II) (Fahn, Elton, and the members of the UPDRS Development Committee, 1987) score was 32.1(activity of daily living) and UPDRS III score was 61.72 (motor examination). The mean preoperative levodopa equivalent dosage was 1432 mg/day. Before surgery, three and eight months later they underwent a neuropsychological evaluation.

All the subjects were right-handed following the criteria of Briggs and Nebes (+ 22.34 ± 1.32, for the Briggs and Nebes test, 1975). Their average educational levels, represented by school years, is of 11.34 ± 5.67 years.

The stereotaxic implant was carried out bilaterally in the subthalamic nucleus, with platinum-iridium electrodes, model Medtronic ® 3389, connected to a subcutaneous impulse generator. Stimuli were provided continuously at 140-180 Hz (square waves of 0.2 ms, voltage less than 3.6 V, intensity 40 μA). Patients responded to neurosurgery, in particular decreasing motor fluctuations and increasing daily living independency.

The stereotaxic implant was carried out bilaterally in the subthalamic nucleus, with platinum-iridium electrodes, Model Medtronic® 3389. The target visualization was determined using a preoperative stereotactic T1 and T2 weighted MRI. The STN was best identified on the coronal T2 weighted sequences.

The AC-PC line and the midline of the third ventricle were used to define the target coordinates corresponding to the STN in a brain atlas (3 mm posterior to the midpoint of the biscommissural line, 4 mm inferior to AC-PC, 12.5 mm lateral to midline). The electrodes were implanted stereotactically in a single session in accordance (left: x=-13.80; y=8.01; z= 1.75; right: x= 9.87; y=7.71; z= 1.75) with preoperative MRI and intraoperative microrecordings and connected to a subcutaneous impulse generator stimulation. The implanted quadripolar electrodes were positioned as closely as possible to the location where motor benefit was induced by the lowest electrical intensity and adverse effects by the highest electrical intensity using monopolar stimulation. Electrical parameters (pulse width, frequency, and voltage) were progressively adjusted by telemetry, using a console programmer, until an optimal effect was reached, in both the "on" and "off" drug conditions. The stimulation was unipolar, using one contact of the quadripolar electrode. At the time of the study, the mean voltage of stimulation was 2.3 ± 1.02 V; the mean pulse width was of 68 ± 11.34 μs; the mean frequency was 130 ± 23.45 Hz. MRI of the brain was performed the day after electrode implantation to verify the final electrode placement and the lack of significant bleeding. No haemorrhage, infection or ischaemic stroke directly related to the surgery was noted (Moretti et al., 2003- A).

Patients were examined before surgery, after three, six and twelve months after surgery (Moretti et al., 2003-A).

The patients underwent to a Zung self-evaluation for depression (Zung, 1965).

The general cognitive profile was tested by a battery of tests, which comprises: Stroop Test (Stroop, 1935; Perret, 1974), Raven Standard Progressive Matrices (Raven, 1960), digit span backwards and forwards (Wechsler, 1981), retrieval of a story (Wechsler 1945), Syntactic comprehension test and Morphological test (from the Bilingual aphasia test, part B –italian language- Paradis and Canzanella, 1990), alternating verbal semantic fluency (Wechsler, 1981), alternating verbal phonological fluency (Wechsler, 1981), Benton Line Orientation Test (Benton et al, 1983). Moreover, the patients underwent to an alternating syllabic-phonological test, which we have prepared.

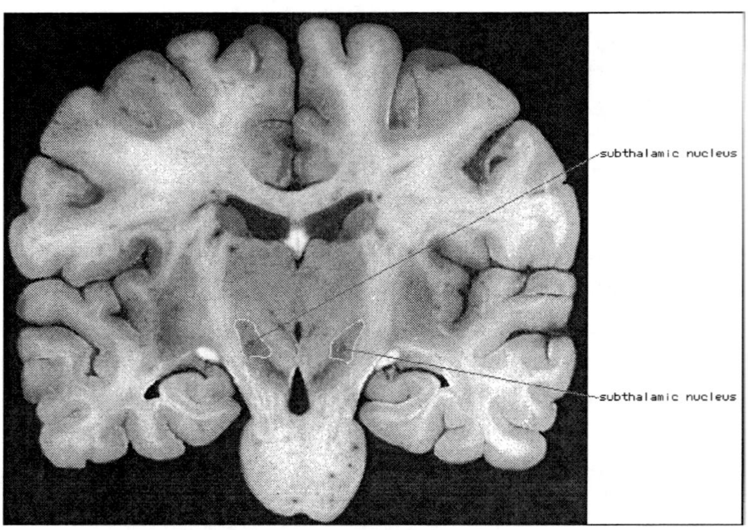

Figure 1. A schematic vision of the subthalamic nucleus.

Subjects were strained to produce in 1 minute time the highest number of words beginning with a given syllable ("per", "tra", and "di"): we test the total number of words produced and the number of intrusion mistakes (e.g.: if syllabic given target is "tra", we count the number of different nouns beginning with "ter", or "ta", or "tr") eventually produced (Moretti et al., 2002). The order of test' presentation was constant in all the sessions.

The scores obtained by the patients were compared with those obtained by a group of 9 patients (6 men and 3 women) with idiopathic Parkinson' s disease (UK Parkinson's Disease Society Brain Bank Clinical diagnostic criteria) (Hughes et al., 1992) not submitted to DBS, matched for age, educational level, handedness, and disease degree, who previously agreed to participate and gave their informed consent for testing. All the patients could be fully studied (mean age 69.45 ± 7.12 years, range= 60-76 years; average age at onset= 47.64 ± 7.12 years, range= 41-56 years). All the patients suffered for 8.71 ± 1.46 years from Parkinson disease and had been treated for several years with levodopa preparations.

Statistical analyses were performed using the Statistical Package for the Social Sciences (SPSS, version 10.0). Changes from baseline between Groups with DBS and control group were compared using the two-sample Wilcoxon test. This was done for each efficacy variable. Results are presented as means with standard deviations and *p*-values are presented where appropriate (Table 1).

Table 1. Statistical differences obtained on the three trials: a comparison has been made with the results obtained before surgery during the 2nd and 3rd session. Differences from the control population have been made during the 1st session.

Tests	1st session	2nd session	3rd session	controls
Stroop	67.45 seconds ($p<0.05$; χ^2 test); 1 mistakes	71.24 sec. 1 mistakes (n.s)	78 sec. 2 mistakes (n.s)	58.2 seconds; 1 mistake
Raven Standard Progressive Matrices (correct)	36/60 (ns)	36/60 (n.s)	36/60 (n.s)	39/60
Digit span forward (WAIS-R)	4 ($p<0.05$; χ^2 test)	6 ($p<0.05$)	6 ($p<0.05$)	7.5
Digit span backwards (Wais-r)	4 (ns)	3 (n.s)	3 (n.s)	4.3
Retrieval of a story (Wais-memory)	13/22 (ns)	14/22 (n.s)	14/22 (n.s)	17.8/22
Synctactic comprehension (Bilingual aphasia test-b: errors)	17 ($p<0.05$; χ^2 test)	14 (n.s)	14 (n.s)	11
Morphological tasks (Bilingual aphasia test-b: errors)	8 (ns)	8 (n.s)	8 (n.s)	8

Table 1. (Continued)

Tests	1st session	2nd session	3rd session	controls
Alternating verbal semantic fluency (WAIS-R)	46	38 (p<0.05)	37 (p<0.05)	49.32
Alternating verbal phonological fluency	38	26 (ns)	24 (p<0.05)	42.34
Alternating syllabic verbal fluency	26 (3 interference mistakes) (p<0.01 χ2 test)	21 (3 inter-ference mistakes) (p<0.05)	23 (0 inter-ference mistakes) (p<0.01)	36.9
Benton line orientation test (errors)	1 (ns)	1 (n.s)	1 (n.s)	0.2

Testing before surgery was conducted when the patients were on medication. At baseline, there were no statistical differences between the two groups on any of the scales, a part from an evident increase in time of Stroop execution (72.34 ± 1.42 seconds) in DBS group, when compared to control group (p<0.05, paired samples, t-test). No other differences were evident, indicating that the two groups were matched for cognitive performances.

At one-month, patients submitted to DBS showed significant increase in the total time to execute Stroop test, of 5.55 points over baseline (p<0.01) and -10.89 over control Group (p<0.001), and in number of mistakes in Stroop test, of 3.44 over baseline (p<0.01) and –3.34 over control Group (p<0.01); there was a significant decrease of correct recall, of –2.3 over baseline (p0.05), of total words produced in semantic fluency tasks, of –7.19 over baseline (p<0.001), and of –5.89 over control (p<0.001), in phonological fluency tasks, of –3.9 over baseline (p<0.01), and of –3.27 over control (p<0.01), in syllabic fluency, of –8.3 over baseline (p<0.001), and of –9.6 over control (p<0.001); on the contrary, there was a significant increase in number of intrusion mistakes, of 5.78 over baseline (p<0.001), and of -5.89 over control group (p<0.001).

At six-month, patients with DBS showed significant increase in the total time to execute Stroop test, of 12.1 points over baseline (p<0.001) and -16.11 over control Group (p<0.001), and in number of mistakes in Stroop test, of 2.33 over baseline (p<0.01) and –2 over control Group (p<0.01); there was a significant decrease of correct recall, of –1.6 over baseline (p<0.05), of total words produced in semantic fluency tasks, of –10.97 over baseline (p<0.001), and of –9.23 over control (p<0.001), in phonological fluency tasks, of –6.2 over baseline (p<0.01), and of –6.67 over control (p<0.01), in syllabic fluency, of –10.52 over baseline (p<0.001), and of –9 over control (p<0.001); on the contrary, there was a significant increase in number of intrusion mistakes, of 4.34 over baseline (p<0.001), and of –4.56 over control group (p<0.001).

At twelve-month, patients with DBS showed significant increase in the total time to execute Stroop test, of 16.33 points over baseline (p<0.001) and -20.11 over control Group (p<0.001), and in number of mistakes in Stroop test, of 1.88 over baseline (p<0.01) and –1.44 over control Group (p<0.01); there was a significant decrease of total mistakes in syntactic comprehension tasks, of –3.12 over baseline (p<0.01), and of -3.11 over control (p<0.01), of total words produced in semantic fluency tasks, of –10.63 over baseline ($p<0.001$), and of –9 over control ($p<0.001$), in phonological fluency tasks, of –5.87 over baseline ($p<0.01$), and of –6.34 over control ($p<0.01$), in syllabic fluency, of –10.41 over baseline ($p<0.001$), and of –8.89 over control ($p<0.001$); on the contrary, there was a significant increase in number of intrusion mistakes, of 1.34 over baseline ($p<0.01$), and of –1.56 over control group ($p<0.05$).

Subthalamic stimulation has been shown to present an advantage as it induces a higher antiakinetic effect and has positive effects on all parkinsonian symptoms (Dujardin et al., 2001; Iansek et al., 2002).

The subthalamus has generally been considered as a rely station within frontal-subcortical motor control circuitry. It has connections to the substantia nigra, pars reticulata, output pathways from the basal ganglia (Jahanshahi, et al., 2000): the dorsolateral prefrontal cortex is the final target of the thalamic projection from the substantia nigra pars reticulata. A PET study (Limousin et al. 1997) showed that there was a greater activation of dorsolateral prefrontal cortex during effective stimulation of the subthalamus nucleus. Direct cortico-STN projections and indirect connections, via the nucleus accumbens and ventral pallidum from prelimbic and medial orbital cortex, have an excitatory influence on the STN (Maurice et al., 1998).

On the other hand, subthalamic nucleus may be connected with the frontal-caudate-pulvinar circuits, and therefore be involved in verifying the semantic acceptability of the linguistic production and in the so-called language planning-loop (Wallesch and Papagno, 1988; Cummings, 1995; Fabbro et al., 1997). Information processing in the circuits is not strictly sequential, and it seems to control the preparatory linguistic activity (Cummings, 1995).

Having accepted that bilateral stimulation of the subthalamic nucleus has as a direct consequence a significant bilateral reduction in Parkinson's disability, the most interesting aspect of deep brain stimulation of the subthalamic nucleus is the possible consequence on cognitive process, extending basal ganglia's role from motor to cognitive control. Different authors sustained that there was no significant change in memory or executive functions in a sample of 62 patients treated by bilateral subthalamic nucleus or globus pallidus stimulation (Ardouin et al., 1999) when compared to results obtained before surgery, however other authors obtained previously opposite results (Troster et al., 1997) on the same points. Two recent studies have attempted to study cognition in deep brain stimulation. The first (Pillon, 2002) showed that in "on" phases, deep brain stimulation of the subthalamic nucleus patients had no cognitive deficit at 12 months, except for a decrease in lexical fluency (not explicated by the authors), and no differential effect associated with subthalamic nucleus or globus pallidus stimulation. The second study (Jahanshahi et al., 2000) assessed the effects of bilateral deep brain stimulation on subthalamic nucleus and globus pallidus on executive function, assessed with Reitan Trail Making test or on Wisconsin Card Sorting Test (data and literature in: Jahanshahi, et al., 2000; Schubert et al, 2002). The results showed a significant better performances obtained in subthalamic nucleus stimulation, when compared to globus pallidus stimulation, in particular of executive function. The conditional associative learning, and in general change in performance became more erroneous too. Thus, the significant deterioration in learning of arbitrary conditional associations lends some support to the proposal of Marsden and Obeso (Marsden and Obeso, 1994) that following subcortical surgery, patients with Parkinson's disease should exhibit some deficits in situations that require changing behaviour in novel context. In these aspects the striatum may play a more central role, providing important information for subsequent cortical processing.

As demonstrated by Schroeder et al. (2002), DBS in the STN decreased cerebral blood flow responses in the anterior cingulate cortex during the Stroop task, while impairing task performance at the same time. Decreased activation was also located in the ventral striatum, the structure receiving input from the anterior cingulate cortex in the current model of basal ganglia organization. The angular gyrus is associated with encoding of words (Menard et al., 1996; Peterson et al., 1999). The increased activation during stimulation therefore most likely corresponds to difficulties in suppressing the habitual response, i.e. word processing, when patients had actually to name the font colour of the colour word. Alternatively, during off stimulation, anterior cingulate cortex might effectively modulate language processing in the angular gyrus, resulting in decreased activation compared with the on state. This is in good correspondence to a factorial analysis of cognitive processes in the Stroop task, revealing suppression of language processing to facilitate colour naming (Peterson et al., 1999; Schroeder et al, 2002). Schroeder et al. (2002) results are consistent with the emerging identification of the role of the STN as an important basal ganglia input and output structure not only in the motor, but also in the cognitive/limbic domain.

According to a classical model, STN stimulation should result in facilitation of projections to cortical areas, on the contrary, Schroeder et al. (2002) found the reverse effect, namely impaired cognitive performance coupled to reduced activation in the anterior cingulate cortex circuit. The Stroop task requires a high level of conflict monitoring and response inhibition. The differential impact of STN stimulation on cognitive and motor circuitry supports the two opposite predictions of the so-called paradox of stereotactic surgery in Parkinson's disease (Marsden and Obeso, 1994). The motor system devoid of the important basal ganglia input structure STN could continue to function in routine, predictable and automatic movement. "Releasing the brake" on frontal function with STN stimulation improves aspects of motor functions (Limousin et al., 1995). However, in new and unexpected situations, requiring non-automated behaviour, disruption of basal ganglia input at the level of the TN may lead to inflexibility of mental and motor responses, as shown in the Stroop task.

Thus, we decided to study these aspects of cognitive process, in particular relating them with linguistic process. Therefore, our patients underwent to three different alternating test of verbal fluency, which could give us information on our patients capabilities to adapt themselves in linguistic situations that require changing behaviour and to implement effective strategies to select and produce different words with a given root (in our case a syllable). Attention, working memory, and speediness are indispensable to a good performance on this test. In addition to these aspects, some of the other processes that are necessary for performance of this task are: intrinsic generation of responses partly through suppression of habitual responses, monitoring of one's output and switching attention between different stimulus in a set. These are all processes that are strongly dependent on the integrity of the dorsolateral prefrontal cortex.

Our previous work (Moretti, et al., 2001; Moretti et al., 2002) confirmed a general stability of cognitive performances, with a decrease in fluency tasks (confirming the findings of other studies, such those of Troster, et al., 1997 and those of Ardouin, et al., 1999, in the traditional semantic or phonological tasks) associated with a significant reduction of interference errors in syllabic task. This data seem in accordance to what has been found in literature: in addition to being a potential site of storage of learned habits or procedures (Packard and Knowlton, 2002), the basal ganglia also appears to be able to switch between various tasks depending on the demands present. This process is also known as the ability to shift cognitive set in response to the environment. Patients with damage to basal ganglia circuitry exhibit performance costs that are greater than controls when switching from one task to another (Lawrence et al., 2000). In addition, neuroimaging evidence suggests that frontal corticostriatal loops are activated when subjects must select between many possible responses (Desmond et al., 1998). Observations of these stimulated patients supports the prior research; verbal production is decreased in semantic and syllabic tasks, along with an increase in time required to execute the Stroop test, but the quality of production is better preserved, as showed by a significant reduction of interference mistakes in syllabic tasks, and a concomitant reduction of errors in Stroop execution. Mutatis mutandis, syllabic tasks might be considered as a suppression language process task, tightly bound to attention, selection and verbal production. Defects in focal attention has been described as a consequence of the disruption of the fronto-striatal circuit, which can cause a significant impairment in visual search (Chari, et al., 1996). Therefore, better execution on an attention task (Stroop) may be in part dependent on the "releasing the brake", as Jahanshahi said, over frontal cortical function during subthalamus stimulation (Jahanshahi et al., 2000). This situation may be caused by a possible disinhibition of thalamic nuclei, or may simply be related to a facilitation of prefrontal cortical activation. Thus, it appears there is a reduced linguistic output corresponding to a more selective and precise performance.

Chronic stimulation may help restore of the control property on language exerted by deep brain circuits or may implement prefrontal cortex. The result may be consistent with a slowness of cognitive activity, with a reduction of quantitative production, but with an increase of control on the production, which may be more precise and definite. Long term effects on cognition and on language, in particular, need to be studied, and possible different sequel could emerge. This is an issue that requires longitudinal follow up of patients with chronic deep brain stimulation, in order to assess and verify the previous hypothesis.

Few patients were involved in the study, and considering the variability among Parkinson patients, the potential for generalization is seriously limited: though, the results obtained confirm the follow-up previously published (Moretti et al., 2002).

Many different reports seem to evidence the potential side-effect of DBS-STN on cognition, behaviour and social conduct of patients who undergo to this surgery.

It has been accepted that deep brain stimulation (DBS) may help cases of PD where pharmacological therapy could not manage the symptoms any more. Cognitive decline may follow deep brain stimulation (DBS) of the subthalamic nucleus (STN)Changes in cognition between stimulation on and off have also been described(Saint-Cyr et al.,2000; Dujardin et al., 2001; Witt et al., 2004) .

We have described a 68-year-old right-handed man, with a 14 – year history of PD, who had severe rigidity, severe akinesia, freezing of gait, and moderate tremor while resting, despite 1000 mg of L-dopa, and 2.1 mg of pramipexole daily, and disabling dyskinesias, underwent DBS-STN (Moretti et al., 2003-B).

His UPDRS III (Fahn et al., 1987) in off was 49, and in on is 25. Brain MRI was normal. The stereotaxic implant was carried out bilaterally in the STN, with platinum-iridium electrodes (Medtronic ® 3389). The electrodes were implanted stereotactically in a single session in accordance with preoperative MRI and intraoperative microrecordings. The stimulation was unipolar, using one contact of the quadripolar electrode (2.0 V, 90 μs, 130 Hz). MRI of the brain was performed the day after electrode implantation to verify the final electrode placement and the lack of significant bleeding.

After surgery the patient interrupted all the oral therapy: his UPDRS-III in off (DBS –) was 35; in off, (DBS +) was 14. Stimulation status was significantly associated with a better motor score in tremor, rigidity, bradykinesia, gait and postural stability. The general cognitive profile was tested by a battery of tests, as seen in table 1. One month and after five months, we resubmitted the patient to further evaluation. The scores obtained were compared with those of a group of 15 volunteers (data have been presented before). In this period, language was fluid, without semantically deviant sentences. Auditory and reading comprehension was maintained, and repetition skills were preserved. One month after surgery, a CT of the head was normal. The patient reported a difficulty of initiate his speech. Initial stuttering is very limiting for the patient, who, began a target word three or four time, repeating the first phoneme, or the initial syllable, but not being keen of proceeding. The hesitation was not correlated with "freezing of speech". He knew what he had to say (since he could point to, or indicate in a multiple choice, either visually either verbally presented, the defined word and his verbal working memory was well preserved). Automatic speech was conserved (both when the patient cursed to his misfortune, or when he pronounced automatic expression). Spared were his writing and reading capabilities. The situation remains stable five months later (Table 2). A single study reported one case of worsening of dysartria and gait freezing which had existed before the implantation (Thobois et al., 2002). To our knowledge, speech start-hesitation has not been previously described as a consequence of DBS-STN (Moretti et al., 2003-B).

Trying to make some speculation, start-hesitation (by definition that of gait) is a typical initial symptom of the freezing phenomenon (Fahn and Quinn, 2000). Our patient, who had freezing of gait before surgery, manifested speech start hesitation, without other motor symptoms, after DBS-STN. One might say that the mechanism of action of DBS remains to be defined (Ashby, 2000). By whatever mechanism, stimulation mirrors the effects of a destructive lesion.

Subthalamus may be related to speech control by its connections to the substantia nigra, pars reticulata, output pathways from the basal ganglia (Ojemann, 1982): the dorsolateral prefrontal cortex is the final target of the thalamic projection from the substantia nigra pars reticulata. A PET study (Ojemann, 1982) showed that there was a greater activation of dorsolateral prefrontal cortex during effective stimulation of the subthalamus nucleus. With the cortico-striato-thalamo-cortical loop the cortical structures of all cerebral lobes can control the cognitive – motor activity of the frontal lobe structures. The latter are involved in the generation and coordination of voluntary movements (Ojemann, 1982), and maybe in language control. Echolalia, i.e., additional characteristic disorders presented in left basal ganglia lesions, results from the inability of the speaker to inhibit the motor internalisation of verbal expressions produced by the patient (Ojemann, 1982). Chronic stimulation may help to restore the control property on language exerted by deep brain circuits or may implement prefrontal cortex. The result may be consistent with a slowness of cognitive activity, with a reduction of quantitative production . May we say that speech start-hesitation is an excess of control? If so, why has this control been exercised in speech output and not in motor act? (Moretti et al. 2003)

Table 2. Neurolinguistic evaluation of 5 minutes spontaneous speech. A comparison with healthy control.

	1st session	2nd session	3rd session	Control
Number of utterances	29	28	26	32
Total word's number	345	231	267	478
Words/minute	78	56	61	92
Types	123	109	76	137
Neologism	0	0	0	0
Semantic paraphasia	0	0	0	0
Verbal paraphasia	0	0	0	0
Substitution of free grammatical mormorphemes	0	0	0	1
Omission of Free grammatical morphemes	0	0	0	0
Circumlocutions	2	4	5	1
Perseverations of words	1	9	11	0
Semantically deviant sentences	0	5	2	0

Smeding et al (2007) describe a patient with severe decline after STN DBS and postoperative electrode displacement. The patient is a 43-year-old woman diagnosed with Parkinson disease 8 years prior to DBS STN for severe response fluctuations and dyskinesias. Neuropsychological evaluation was normal. She used levodopa/carbidopa slow release 400/100 mg daily. Surgery was performed using MRI, four-tract microrecordings, and macrostimulation for target localization (12 mm lateral, 2 mm posterior, and 4 mm inferior to the midcommissural point [MCP]). The left electrode (model 3389; Medtronic) was implanted in the central trajectory, with the deepest contact 7 mm below MCP. There was considerable CSF leakage from the burr holes. On the right side, no typical STN activity could be recorded. Because test stimulation along the medial trajectory induced a large reduction in rigidity and bradykinesia, the DBS electrode was implanted with the deepest contact 4 mm below MCP (Smeding et al., 2007). Postoperatively, a stereotactic CT scan showed intracranial air bifrontally with posterior and caudal brain shift. The electrode contacts were at the intended position. Confusion resolved within 1 day. At discharge, the stimulation settings were monopolar, contact 0, pulse width 60 microseconds, frequency 130 Hz, and on the right side amplitude 1.8 V and left side 1.3 V. The levodopa/carbidopa slow-release dosage was reduced to 200/50 mg; 2 mg of pergolide was added. Six months after surgery, motor functioning was satisfactory. Neuropsychological testing showed decline of verbal memory, selective and divided attention, and verbal fluency Her relatives confirmed increased forgetfulness, word-finding difficulties, slowed comprehension, and increased irritability. One year postoperatively, she had progressive memory decline. Neurologic examination showed no changes in motor functioning. Compared with 6 months after surgery, there was a progressive decline in verbal fluency but not in memory. Subsequently, both neurostimulators were turned off. Neuropsychological examination 1 week later showed complete recovery of her cognitive functioning (Smeding et al., 2007). The neurostimulator settings were changed to monopolar at contact 2. One month later, she had no cognitive complaints and motor functioning was satisfactory. Formal testing demonstrated a decline in verbal fluency, but other scores were comparable with the preoperative state. A new stereotactic CT scan was made and co-registered with the preoperative MRI. On the left side, contact 0 was located 12.5 mm lateral, 2 mm anterior, and 3 mm inferior to MCP, in the internal capsule lateral to the anterodorsal STN. Contact 2 was located at the border of the internal capsule and the zona incerta adjacent to the globus pallidus internus (13 mm lateral, 4 mm anterior, 0.5 mm superior relative to MCP). On the right side, contact 0 was in the dorsomedial globus pallidus externus (17 mm lateral, 8.5 mm anterior, 3.5 mm superior to MCP). Contact 2 was in the dorsolateral globus pallidus externus close to the putamen (17 mm lateral, 10.5 mm anterior, 7.5 mm superior to MCP). Cognitive decline resolved after switching off DBS. Adjustment of stimulation settings to the dorsal contacts led only to a minor setback in cognition (Smeding et al., 2007). The electrodes were probably displaced as a result of brain shift caused by CSF leakage during surgery and subsequent unfolding of the brain in the postoperative period. Since this incident, we close the burr holes during surgery with Tissuecol to reduce CSF leakage. Cognitive decline was worst with the ventral contacts activated, which were located outside the STN, on the left side in the internal capsule close to the anterodorsal lateral STN, and on the right side in the dorsomedial globus pallidus externus. Adjustment of stimulation settings did not lead to an improvement in off-phase parkinsonism measured with the Unified Parkinson's Disease Rating Scale, though there was an evident decrease of dyskinesias and less on–off fluctuations possibly related to stimulation of the globus pallidus (Smeding et al., 2007).

Concerns have been raised about the possibility that subthalamic deep brain stimulation (STN-DBS) could also produce cognitive changes and mood and behavioural alterations. Valldeoriola et al. (2006)report the clinical and neuropathological features of a patient with advanced PD who developed behavioural changes and dementia while on STN-DBS. A 74 year old man suffering from PD for 11 years presented troublesome dyskinesias and unpredictable motor fluctuations that did not respond to multiple changes in medication. The Hoehn and Yahr stage was IV while "off" and III while "on" medication. The Schwab and England scale score was 40% in the "off" and 80% in the "on" condition. The UPDRS-III score was 56 while "off" and 21 while "on". No clinically evident signs of cognitive impairment were present. The Mini-Mental State Examination (MMSE) score was 28/30.

Neuropsychological assessment was considered to be normal except for the presence of mild cognitive processing slowness and free recall impairment.

Dyskinesias and motor fluctuations had disappeared 3 months after STN-DBS. The Hoehn and Yahr stage was III and the Schwab and England score was 70%. Dopaminergic medication was initially reduced to 20% but the patient later developed restless legs syndrome (attributed to the reduction in dopaminergic medication) and levodopa was reintroduced (400 mg/day). Motor performance remained stable during the following months. There were no significant changes in neuropsychological performance 6 months after STN-DBS. However, shortly afterwards the patient developed mood changes consisting of apathy, anhedonia without sadness, and diurnal hypersomnolence. Levodopa was then increased and antidepressants were started. Changing stimulation electrical parameters and stimulation poles did not change the patient's mood. The patient developed fluctuating confusion, visual hallucinations, and paranoid ideations 1.5 years after surgery. The MMSE score was 22/30. He became violent with his relatives. Clozapine (100 mg/day) reduced aggression but confusion persisted. The possible role of STN-DBS on these cognitive and behavioural changes was assessed by switching off the stimulators for 1 week. Mental status remained unchanged but parkinsonism worsened until the stimulators were again switched on. Later in the course of the disease, the patient received galantamine which improved psychiatric symptoms and temporal-spatial orientation. The patient died from bronchopneumonia 3.5 years after surgery (Valldeoriola et al., 2006). Macroscopic examination of the brain disclosed important loss of pigmentation in the substantia nigra pars compacta and locus coeruleus. The electrode tips were placed within the boundaries of the subthalamus on both sides. On microscopic examination moderate inflammatory infiltrates of T lymphocytes and mild astrocytic gliosis were observed surrounding the leads. Lewy bodies (LB) and Lewy neurites were found in the substantia nigra pars compacta, locus coeruleus, raphe nuclei, the dorsal nucleus of the vagus, and the hypoglossal nerve. Dystrophic neurites and cytoplasmatic inclusions were found in the nucleus of Meynert and the subthalamus (Valldeoriola et al., 2006). Cortical type LB were observed in the gyrus cinguli, transentorhinal cortex, the amygdala, and the parietal and temporal cortex. The density of LB was maximal in the sub-cortical nuclei and the limbic areas. A few neurons showing neurofibrilar degeneration were found in the transentorhinal and entorhinal cortex, amygdalar complex, locus coeruleus, and raphe nuclei. Neocortical senile plaques were scarce and signs of amyloid angiopathy were absent. The pathological diagnosis was diffuse Lewy body disease, transitional type (Valldeoriola et al., 2006). This report (Valldeoriola et al., 2006) is the second clinicopathological description of a patient with PD, dementia, and STN-DBS. The first report by Jarraya et al (2003) described a parkinsonian patient who had some cognitive impairment before STN-DBS and whose mental condition worsened after surgery. Post-mortem examination confirmed the diagnosis of PD. The authors concluded that the bad outcome after surgery was due to the inadequate selection of a candidate who had cognitive deterioration before surgery, but the cause of the worsening mental status after STN-DBS remained unclear. In the case reported here, post-mortem examination disclosed changes typical of diffuse Lewy body disease. In addition, the cognitive and behavioural alterations were not thought to be related to STN-DBS since mental problems appeared late after STN-DBS and changes in stimulation parameters or even disconnection did not result in any mental or behavioural change. The clinical manifestations, the course of the disease, the presence of hallucinations, and the good response to cholinesterase inhibitors were also typical of so called Parkinson's disease-dementia in which the main pathological substrate is the presence of LB in limbic and neo-cortical areas (Cummings, 2005). The case report (Valldeoriola et al., 2006) supports the view that mental problems observed after STN-DBS in some patients are not related to STN-DBS and suggests alternative explanations. A better understanding of the predictive factors for the development of dementia in PD will help to improve candidate selection for STN-DBS (Valldeoriola et al., 2006).

References

Alexander G. A. Basal ganglia thalamocortical circuits: their role in control of movement. *Journal of Clinical Neurophysiolgy* 1994; 11: 420-431.

Alexander G.E., DeLong M.R, Strick P.L Parallel organization of functionally segregated circuits linking basal ganglia and cortex. *Annu. Rev. Neurosci.*1986; 9, 357-381.

Ardouin C., Pillon B., Peiffer E., Bejjani P., Limousin P., Damier P., Arnulf I., Benabid, A.L., Agid Y., Pollak P. Bilateral subthalamic or pallidal stimulation for Parkinson's Disease affects neither memory nor executive functions: a consecutive series of 62 patients. *Annals of Neurology* 1999; 46(2): 217-223.

Ashby P. What does stimulation in the brain actually do? *Prog. Neurol. Surg.,* 2000, 15, 236-245.

Benton AL., Hamshe K., Varney N., Spreen O. Contributions to neuropsychological assessment. New York: Oxford University Press, 1983.

Briggs G., Nebes R. Patterns of hand preference in a student population. *Cortex* 1975; 11: 230-238.

Bronte-Stewart H Deep brain stimulation for movement disorders- general principles. American Academy of Neurology, Minneapolis, 2003. (Ac.003 pdf. 1-23.

Ceballos-Baumann AO, Boecker H, Bartenstein P, von Falkenhayn I, Riescher H, Conrad B et al. A positron emission tomographic study of subthalamic nucleus stimulation in parkinson disease: enhanced movement-related activity of motor association cortex and decreased motor cortex resting activity. *Arch. Neurol.* 1999; 56: 997-1003.

Chari G., Shaw PJ., Sahgal A. Non-verbal visual attention but not recognition memory of learning processes are impaired in motor neuron disease. *Neuropsychologia* 1996; 34(5): 377-385.

Cummings J.L. Anatomic and behavioural aspects of frontal-subcortical circuits. In: Grafman J., Holyoak KJ, Boller F (Eds) Structure and function of the human prefrontal cortex. *Ann. NY Acad. Sci.* 1995; 769: 1-14.

Cummings JL. Cholinesterase inhibitors for treatment of dementia associated with Parkinson's disease. *J. Neurol. Neurosurg. Psychiatry* 2005; 76: 903–4.

DEEP BRAIN STIMULATION FOR PARKINSON'S DISEASE STUDY GROUP. Deep Brain Stimulation of the Subthalamic nucleus or the pars interna of the globus pallidus in Parkinson's Disease. *New Engl. J. Med.* 2001; 345: 956-963.

Desmond JE, Gabrieli JDE, Glover GH. Dissociation of frontal and cerebellar activity in a cognitive task: evidence for a distinction between selection and search. *Neuroimage* 1998; 7: 368-378.

Dujardin K., Defebvre L., Krystkowiak P., Blond S., Destée, A. Influence of chronic bilateral stimulation of the subthalamic nucleus on cognitive function in Parkinson's disease. *Journal of Neurology* 2001; 248: 603-611.

Fabbro F. Subcortical aphasia. *Journal of Neurolinguistics*, 1997; 10: 251-367.

Fahn S, Quinn N. Unusual movement disorders. American Academy of Neurology, San Diego, 2000; 3AG.003-1-24.

Fahn S., Elton R.L., the members of the UPDRS Development Committee The Unified Parkinson's disease rating scale. In: S. Fahn, C. D. Marsden, D. B. Calne, M. Goldstein (Eds) Recent developments in Parkinson's disease. Florham Park, NJ: *Macmillan Healthcare*. 1987. Vol. 2. Pp. 153-163.

Guridi J, Obeso JA. The subthalamic nucleus, hemiballismus and Parkinson's disease: reappraisal of a neurosurgical dogma. *Brain* 2001; 124: 5-19.

Haslinger B, Erhard P., Kampfe N, Boecker H, Rummeny E, Schwaiger M, et al. Event-related functional magnetic resonance imaging in Parkinson's Disease before and after levo-dopa. *Brain* 2001; 124: 558-570.

Hohen, M.M, Yahr MD. Parkinsonism: onset, progression and mortality. *Neurology*. 1967; 17: 427-442.

Hughes AJ, Daniel SE, Kilford L, Lees AJ. Accuracy of clinical diagnosis of idiopathic Parkinson's disease: a clinico-pathological study of 100 cases. *J. Neurol. Neurosurg. Psychiatry* 1992; 55: 181-184.

Iansek R, Rosenfeld JV, Huxham FE. Deep brain stimulation of the subthalamic nucleus in Parkinson's disease. *MJA,* 20002: 177 (3): 142-146

Jahanshahi M, Ardouin CMA., Brown RG., Rothwell JC., Obeso J., Albanese A., Rodriguez-Oroz .MC., Moro E, Benabid AL., Pollak P, Limousin-Dowsey P. The impact of deep brain stimulation on executive function in parkinson's disease. *Brain* 2000; 123, 1142-1154.

Jarraya B, Bonnet A-M, Duyckaerts C, et al. Parkinson's disease, subthalamic stimulation and selection of candidates: a pathologic study. *Mov. Disord.* 2003; 18: 1517–20.

Kumar R., Lozano A. M., Montgomery E., Lang A. E. Pallidotomy and deep brain stimulation of the pallidum and subthalamic nucleus in advanced Parkinson's disease. *Movement Disorders*, 1998; 13(S1): 73-82.

Lawrence AD, Watkins LHA, Sahakian BJ Hodges JR, Robbins TW. Visual object and visuospatial cognition in Huntington's disease: implications for information processing in corticostriatal circuits. *Brain* 2000 ; 123: 1349-1364

Limousin P, Pollack P, Benazzouz A, Hoffmann D, Le Bas JF, Brousolle E et al. Effect of parkinsonian signs and symptoms of bilateral subthalamic nucleus stimulation. *Lancet* 1995; 345: 91-95

Limousin P., Greene J., Pollak P., Rothwell J., Benabid A.L., Frackowiak R. Changes in cerebral activity pattern due to subthalamic nucleus or internal pallidum stimulation in Parkinson's disease. *Annals of Neurology*, 1997, 42, 283-291.

Marsden C.D., Obeso J.A. The functions of the basal ganglia and the parodox of stereotaxic surgery in Parkinson's disease. *Brain* 1994; 117: 877-897.

Maurice N, Deniau JM, Glowinski J, Thierry AM Relationships between the prefrontal cortex and the basal ganglia in the rat: physiology of the corticosubthalamic circuits. *J. Neurosci.* 1998; 18: 9539-9546.

Menard MT, Kosslyn SM, Thompson WL, Alert NM, Rauch SL. Encoding words and pictures: a positron emission tomography study. *Neuropsychologia* 1996; 34: 185-194.

Moretti R, Torre P, Antonello R M.,Capus L, Gioulis M, Zambito Marsala S,Cazzato G, Bava A. "Speech start-hesitation" following subthalamic nucleus stimulation in Parkinson Disease. *European Neurology*, 2003; 49: 251-253.- B

Moretti R, Torre P., Antonello RM, Capus L, Zambito Marsala S, Cattaruzza T, Cazzato G., Bava A. Neuropsychological changes after subthalamic nucleus stimulation: a 12-month follow-up in nine patients with Parkinson Disease. *Parkinsonism and Related disorders*, 2003; 10: 73-79. A

Moretti R, Torre P., Antonello RM, Cazzato G., Bava A. Subcortical-cortical lesions and two-step aplasia in a bilingual patient. In: S.P.Shohov (Ed). *Advances in psychology research.* Vol. 23. Novascience Publisher, New York, 2003. Pp. 33-44. C

Moretti R, Torre P., Antonello RM., Capus L, Gioulis M, Zambito Marsala S., Cazzato G, Bava A. Cognitive changes following subthalamic nucleus stimulation in two patients with parkinson disease. *Perceptual and motor skills*, 2002, 95: 477-486.

Moretti R., Torre P., Antonello R.M., Capus L., Gioulis M., Zambito Marsala, S., Cazzato G, Bava A. Effects on cognitive abilities following subthalamic nucleus stimulation in Parkinson Disease. *European Journal of Neurology* 2001; 8: 726-727.

Ojemann G.A. Models of the brain organization for higher integrative functions derived by electrical stimulation techniques. *Human Neurobiology*, 1982; 1,:243-249.

Packard MG, Knowlton BJ. Learning and memory functions of the basal ganglia. *Ann. Rev. Neurosci.* 2002; 25: 563-593.

Paradis M., Canzanella M. Test per l'afasia in un bilingue. Versione italiana. Hillsdale, N.J:. 1990. Erlbaum.

Peterson BS, Skudlarski P, Gatenby JC, Zhang H, Anderson AW, Gore JC. An fMRI study of Stroop word-color interference: evidence for cingulated subregions subserving multiple distributed attentional systems. *Biol. Psychiatry* 1999; 45: 1237-1258

Pillon B, Boller F, Levy R, Dubois B Cognitive deficits in Parkinson's disease. In: Boller F, Grafman J (Eds) Handbook of neuropsychology Amsterdam: *Elsevier*. 2002.

Pollak, P. Deep brain stimulation. American Academy of Neurology (AAN), Philadelphia, 2001: 3PC. 005-16-52.

Raven J. Guide to the Standard Progressive Matrices. London: H. K. Lewis 1960.

Sabatini U, Boulanouar K, Fabre N, Martin F, Carel C, Colonnese C et al.. Cortical motor reorganization in akinetic patients with Parkinson's Disease: a functional MRI study. *Brain* 2000; 123: 394-403.

Saint-Cyr JA, Trepanier LL, Kumar R, Lozano AM, Lang AE. Neuropsychological consequences of chronic bilateral stimulation of the subthalamic nucleus in Parkinson's Disease. *Brain* 2000; 123: 2091-2108.

Schroeder U, Kuehler A, Haslinger B, Erhard P, Fogel W, Tronnier VM, Lange KW, Boecker H, Ceballos-Baumann AO. Subthalamic nucleus stimulation affects striato-anterior cingulated cortex circuit in a response conflict task: a PET study. *Brain* 2002; 125 (9): 1995-2004.

Schubert T, Volkmann J, Muller U, Sturm V, Voges J, Freund HJ, von Cramon DY (2002). Effects of pallidal deep brain stimulation and levodopa treatment on reaction-time performance in Parkinson's disease. *Exp. Brain Res*. 144: 8-16.

Smeding H.M.M., van den Munckhof P., Esselink R. A.J., Schmand B., Schuurman P. R., Speelman J. D. Reversible cognitive decline after DBS STN in PD and displacement of electrodes. *Neurology* 2007; 68 (15): 1235-1236.

Stroop JR. Studies of interference in serial verbal reactions. *Journal of Experimental Psychology* 1935; 18: 643-662.

Thobois S, Mertens P, Guenot M, Hermier M, Mollion H, Bouvard M, Chazot G, Broussolle E, Sindou M. Subthalamic nucleus stimulation in parkinson's disease. Clinical evaluation of 18 patients. *Journal of Neurology*, 2002; 249, 529-534.

Troster AI, Fields JA, Wilkinson SB, Pahwa R., Miyawaki E., Lyons K.E., Koller WC. Unilateral pallidal stimulation for Parkinson's disease: neurobehavioural functioning before and 3 months after electrode implanatation. *Neurology* 1997; 49: 1078-1083.

Valldeoriola F, Tolosa E, Alegret M, Rey MJ, Morsi O, Pilleri M, Rumià J. Cognitive changes in Parkinson's disease during subthalamic stimulation: a clinicopathologic study Journal of Neurology, *Neurosurgery, and Psychiatry* 2006;77:565-566

Vercueil L., Benazzouz A., Deransart C., Bressand K., Marescaux C., Depaulis A., Benabid A. L. (1998) High frequency stimulation of the subthalamic nucleus suppresses absence seizures in the rat: comparison with neurotoxic lesions. *Epilepsy Research* 1998; 31(1): 39-46.

Wallesch C. W., Papagno C. Subcortical aphasia. In F. Clifford Rose, R. Whurr and M. Wukye (Eds.), Aphasia. London: Whurr. 1988. Pp. 256-287.

Wechsler D. WAIS- Revised manual. New York: The Psychological Corp 1981.

Wechsler D. A standardized memory scale for clinical use. *Journal of Psychology* 1945; 19: 87-97.

Witt K, Pulkowski U, Herzog J, et al. Deep brain stimulation of the subthalamic nucleus improves cognitive flexibility but impairs response inhibition in Parkinson disease. *Arch. Neurol.* 2004;61:697–700.

Zanini S., Melatini A, Vassallo A., Moretti R., Bava A. Speech and language improvement in Parkinson disease after electrical stimulation of the subthalamic nucleus: a case study. *European Journal of Physiology*, 2000; 440: R35-63.

Zung WWK. A self-rating depression scale. *Archives of General Psychiatry* 1965; 12: 63-70.

In: Deep Brain Stimulation
Editors: Mark H. Rogers and Paul B. Anderson

ISBN 978-1-60692-895-0

Chapter IX

Subthalamic High-Frequency Deep Brain Stimulation Evaluated by Positron Emission Tomography in a Porcine Parkinson Model

Mette S. Nielsen*[*1], Flemming Andersen[2], Paul Cumming[2], Arne Møller[2], Albert Gjedde[2], Jens. C. Sørensen[3] and Carsten R. Bjarkam[1]

[1]Department of Neurobiology, Institute of Anatomy, University of Aarhus, Denmark

[2]PET Center, University Hospital of Aarhus, Denmark

[3]Department of Neurosurgery, University Hospital of Aarhus, Denmark

Abstract

Background: Subthalamic high-frequency deep brain stimulation (STN DBS) has during the last decade been widely used in the treatment of Parkinson's disease (PD) complicated by motor fluctuations and medicine-induced adverse effects. The exact mechanism of STN DBS is, however, still unelucidated. Objective: To evaluate whether STN DBS changes regional cerebral blood flow (rCBF) and oxygen consumption, by positron emission tomography (PET) in a non-primate large animal PD model of STN DBS. Methods: Three MPTP (1-methyl-4-phenyl-1,2,3,6-tetrahydropyridine) intoxicated female Göttingen minipigs (age 8-12 months, weight 16-20 kg) were stereotaxically implanted unilaterally with a DBS electrode (Medtronic, model 3387) connected to a pulse generator (Medtronic, model 7424) placed subcutaneously in the neck region. Four to six weeks later the animals were anesthetized and placed in a PET scanner. Three water ($H_2{}^{15}O$) and three oxygen ($^{15}O_2$) scans were performed, before stimulation with

* Correspondence to: Mette Slot Nielsen. Department of Neurobiology, Institute of Anatomy, University of Aarhus, DK-8000 Aarhus C, Denmark. Phone: (+45) 8942 3027. Fax: (+45) 8942 3060. E-mail: ml@neuro.au.dk

clinical parametres (continuous unipolar stimulation (electrode negative, case positive), amplitude 3V, frequency 160 Hz, and pulse-width 60 μs) was initiated and followed by 5 water and oxygen scans 5, 30, 60, 120 and 240 min thereafter. The obtained data (the three baseline scans versus the five poststimulation scans) were analysed by parametric DOT-analysis after semiautomatic coregistration to an average MRI pig brain. Results: rCBF was significantly increased (t-value = 5.47, p-value < 0.05) at the electrode tip after initiation of stimulation, and non-significant increases of oxygen consumption occurred in the ipsilateral- (t-value = 3.67, p-value < 0.1), and contralateral cortex (t-value = 3.34, p-value < 0.1). Conclusion: Our results indicate that STN DBS increases local midbrain rCBF and oxygen consumption in centrally placed cortical areas. The minipig may thus be a well-suited animal model for further studies of the mechanism of STN DBS in PD.

Keywords: animal model, basal ganglia, cerebral oxygen consumption, Göttingen minipig, MPTP, regional cerebral blood flow (rCBF)

Introduction

Subthalamic high-frequency deep brain stimulation (STN DBS) has during the last 15 years proven its value in the treatment of Parkinson's disease (PD) complicated by motor fluctuations and levodopa-induced dyskinesias [14,18,35-37,40,49,53,55]. However, many aspects of subthalamic DBS such as the mechanism of action, potential long-term adverse or neuroprotective effect still remain unelucidated [6,10,26,34,42,45,46,48,54].

Clinical studies may resolve some of these unanswered questions, but are often hampered by the inclusion of a limited number of patients exhibiting a diverse disease and medication pattern. Many experimental procedures are likewise impossible to perform in humans due to ethical concerns. Reliable animal models are therefore necessary for further elucidation of the role of STN DBS in the treatment of PD. Few studies of STN DBS have been conducted in animals and only two animal models of STN DBS in PD have been described. One model is based on primates [7,9,28,31] whereas the other is based on rats [8,10,20,23,28,43,50,57].

The use of rats is economically advantageous compared to use of larger laboratory animals. Stereotaxic targeting of the STN is furthermore eased by the availability of a superb rat brain atlas of stereotaxic coordinates related to external skull structures [44]. However, the small size of the rat brain naturally excludes the use of DBS devices intended for human use, and functional neuroimaging with PET or MRI for such small brains require special equipment. Due to the small size of the rat STN, one would also expect considerable spillover of the stimulation effect to adjacent brain structures.

The use of primates as an experimental model for STN DBS is on the other hand hampered by the high cost of these animals, ethical considerations and the danger of transfer of simian viruses [29]. Thus, many studies using primate models include no more than three to four animals [7,9,28,31]. To address these concerns we have recently developed a new large non-primate animal model for STN DBS in PD employing 1-methyl-4-phenyl-1,2,3,6-tetrahydropyridine (MPTP) intoxicated Göttingen minipigs implantated with clinical DBS devices [17]. The present chapter will accordingly describe the first positron emission tomography (PET) results from this animal model and relate these findings to existing PET results on DBS in humans.

Materials and Methods

Animals: Three female young adult Göttingen minipigs (age 8-12 months, weight 16-20 kg) were used in the study, in accordance with a protocol approved by the Danish Council on Animal Research Ethics (DANCARE). All animals were kept separately in a large stable on a 12-hour light/dark cycle at constant temperature and humidity, with free access to food and water.

MPTP-intoxication: The three animals were initially intoxicated with MPTP injected subcutaneously at a dose of 1 mg/kg bodyweight every other day over a period of 17 days, receiving a total dose of 8 mg/kg bodyweight [24]. All intoxicated animals displayed behavioral signs of parkinsonism by the end of the treatment period, evaluated by scores for motility, rigidity and coordination [41].

Stereotaxic DBS electrode implantation: Six months after MPTP-intoxication the animals were anesthetized with ketamine and midazolam, intubated and artificially ventilated with 60/40% N_2O/O_2 and 1.5% isoflurane. The animals were then stereotaxically implanted unilaterally with a DBS electrode (Medtronic, model 3387) that was connected to a pulse generator (Medtronic, model 7424) placed subcutaneously in the neck region [17]. The electrode was fixated to the skull with dental cement. The position of the electrode was verified by postoperative MRI before the animals were extubated and awakened.

PET: Four to six weeks later the animals were anesthetized as described above. The animals were placed prone in a PET scanner (Siemens ECAT HR+ tomograph). Three water ($H_2{}^{15}O$) and three oxygen ($^{15}O_2$) scans were then performed before DBS stimulation with clinical parametres (continuous unipolar stimulation (electrode negative, case positive), amplitude 3V, frequency 160 Hz, and pulse-width 60 μs) was initiated by telemetry and followed by 5 water and oxygen scans at 5, 30, 60, 120 and 240 min (Fig. 1). The duration of each scan was 3 min and consisted of a 3 min long dynamic positron emission sequence in 3D acquisition mode preceeded by an intravenous injection of min 300 MBq $H_2{}^{15}O$ or inhalation by single-breath of $^{15}O_2$ followed by 10 s breath holding [47]. Arterial blood samples were collected from the femoral artery every 5 s for the first min, every 10 s for the next min, and every 20 s for the last min during the scan sequence for measurement of the respective plasma input function for $H_2{}^{15}O$ or $^{15}O_2$. Attenuation correction was applied on the basis of an initially performed 15 min transmission scan (Fig. 1).

The obtained data (the three baseline scans versus the five poststimulation scans) were analysed by parametric DOT-analysis after semiautomatic coregistration to an average MRI pig brain [4,5,56] (Fig. 2).

Perfusion and postmortem analysis: The animals were euthanized with pentobarbital 6-12 months after the described PET-procedure, followed by a transcardial perfusion with 5 l of phosphate buffered 4% paraformaldehyde (pH 7.4). The brain was removed from the skull and the electrode was retracted. The brain was then embedded and oriented in HistOmer (HistOtech ApS, Denmark) according to an MRI-atlas of the Göttingen minipig [56] followed by sectioning into 6-9 mm thick coronal tissue slabs [15,52] enabling identification of the exact electrode position and related changes in the brain tissue.

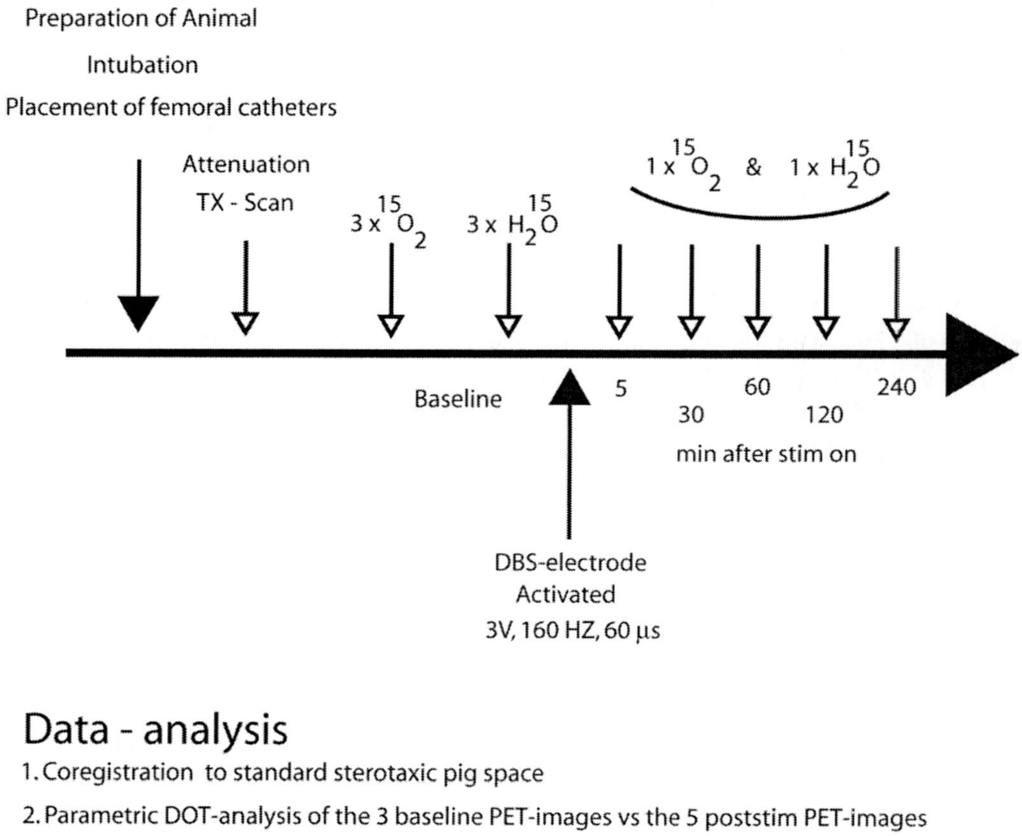

Figure 1. Flow-chart illustrating the time course and interventions of the PET-study. The total procedure would last approximately 6-7 hrs. During this period the animal would be intubated and anesthetized with its ECG, blood pressure and temperature closely monitored. Approximately 1 L of isotonic saline was administered during the procedure, and the body temperature was maintained at 37-38°C with an electrical heating blanket.

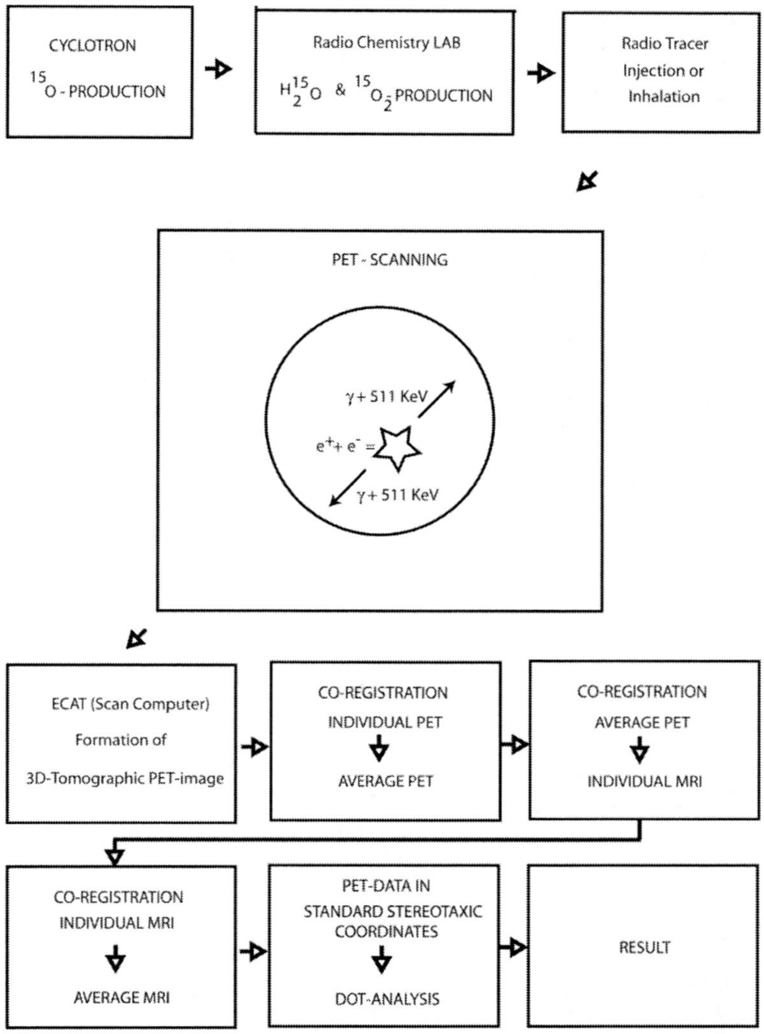

Figure 2. Schematic drawing illustrating the PET procedure from production of ^{15}O in the cyclotron to the formation of the individual 3D-tomographic PET-image and the elaborate process of co-registration [4,5,56] necessary for the DOT-analysis.

Results

Surgical procedure: The three animals survived for more than 6 months with active DBS electrodes. Postoperative infections were not encountered. Unilateral stimulation caused initial rotational behavior in all animals, which dissapeared after a few days. The implanted electrodes were generally tolerated well by the minipigs, and all animals were able to resume normal daily activities shortly after the surgical procedure without any change in consciousness or other non-motor functions.

Postoperative MRI (Fig. 3): In all three animals, the electrode was located ventrally in the caudal diencephalon (MPTP 2 and 9) or the rostral mesencephalon (MPTP 4) within 5 mm of the subthalamic area depicted with arrow on MPTP 2 and 9.

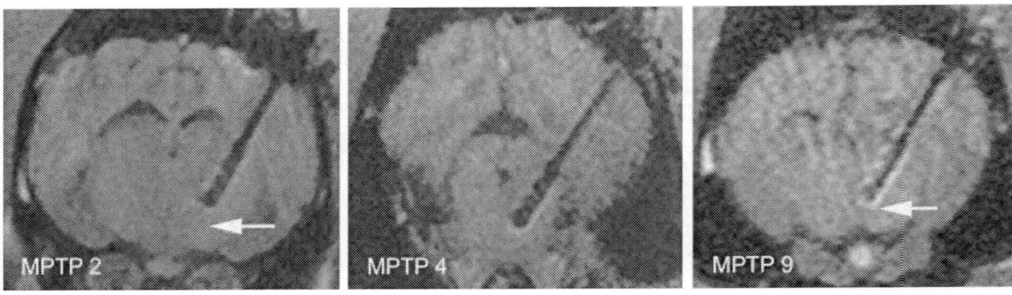

Figure 3. Postoperative MR images illustrating the electrode placement in the three animals MPTP 2, 4 and 9, respectively. The electrode was in all three cases located ventrally in the caudal diencephalon (MPTP 2 and 9) or the rostral mesencephalon (MPTP 4) within 5 mm of the subthalamic area (depicted with arrow on MPTP 2 and 9).

Postmortem examination (Fig. 4). After brain removal 6-12 months postoperatively, it was noticed that the electrodes in MPTP 2 and MPTP 9 had migrated due to insufficient fixation of the electrodes, while the electrode of MPTP 4 had kept its position in the mesencephalon. The meninges and the brain surface around the electrodes were, however, devoid of any apparent signs of inflammation or bleeding.

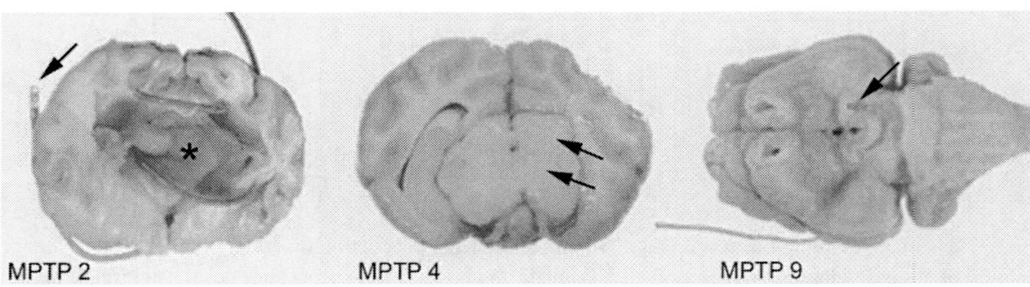

Figure 4. Photographic montage of brain images from MPTP 2, 4 and 9 after postmortem removal. Severe electrode migration was noted in MPTP 2, resulting in the formation of a large cavity in the forebrain (*). Arrow points to electrode tip. Electrode migration was also seen but to a lesser extent in MPTP 9 where the electrode penetrated out through the ventral brain surface at the mesencephalic/diencephalic transition (arrow). It was accordingly only possible to verify the postoperative MRI-visualized electrode placement in MPTP 4 at the postmortem examination (arrows: electrode tract).

PET results (Figs. 5 and 6). Regional cerebral blood flow (rCBF) was significantly increased (t-value = 5.47, p-value between 0.05 and 0.02) after stimulation onset at the mesencephalic/diencephalic transition zone (Fig. 5) corresponding to the MRI-verified postoperative placement of the electrode tip (Fig. 3). No significant increase in rCBF was noted elsewhere in the minipig brain after stimulation onset (Fig. 5).

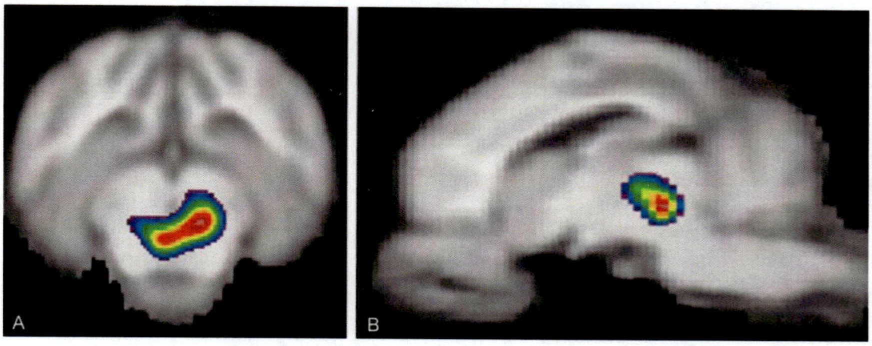

Figure 5. t-statistical coronal (A) and sagittal (B) maps showing change in rCBF after stimulation onset. Note that rCBF is significantly increased (t-value = 5.47, coresponding to a p-value between 0.05 and 0.02) at the mesencephalic/diencephalic transition zone corresponding to the MRI-visualized postoperative placement of the electrode tip.

A non-significant increase in cerebral oxygen consumption after stimulation onset was noted in the ipsilateral centrally placed dorsolateral neocortex (t-value = 3.67, p-value < 0.1) (Fig. 6B, C and D), and in the contralateral dorsomedial neocortex situated close to the central (Fig. 6A, B and D) and posterior part (Fig. 6A and B) of the cingulate sulcus (t-value = 3.34, p-value < 0.1).

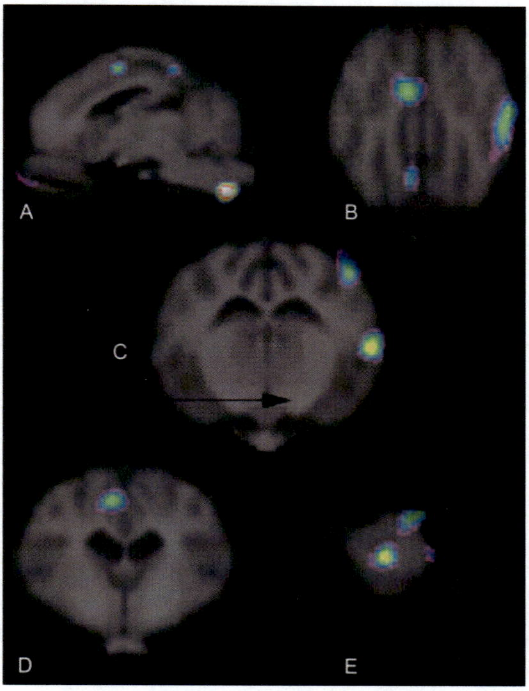

Figure 6. t-statistical mid-sagittal (A), dorsal (B), mid-coronal (C), anterior-coronal (D) and lateral-sagittal (E) maps showing change in cerebral oxygen consumption after stimulation onset. An non-significant increase in cerebral oxygen consumption is seen in the ipsilateral dorsolateral neocortex (t-value = 3.67, corresponding to a p-value between 0.1 and 0.05), and contralateral dorsomedial cortex (t-value = 3.34, corresponding to a p-value between 0.1 and 0.05). The increase noted in the brain stem at the ventral ponto-medular junction is a commonly occurring artifact caused by the anatomy of minipig vascular system. Arrow on (C) indicates the position of the subthalamic nucleus [38].

Discussion

This chapter describes for the first time that immediate initiation of subthalamic DBS may lead to a local increase in rCBF around the electrode tip and increased cerebral oxygen consumption in the centrally placed ipsi- and contralateral neocortex. It is tempting to interpret the results on cerebral oxygen consumption after stimulation onset as support to the hypotheses claiming that the activity of the somatomotor neocortex is suppressed in PD due to decreased thalamocortical activity caused by an increased inhibitory output from the basal ganglia globus palidus pars interna (GPi) originating partly from excessive activity of the subthalamic nucleus in Parkinson disease [1-3,12-14,18,21,25]. Presuming that subthalamic DBS results in decreased subthalamic activity leading to reduced inhibitory output from GPi, causing a release of thalamocortical motor activity, increased neocortical motor activity would be expected after STN DBS, leading to increased neocortical oxygen consumption. The rCBF which normally is closely linked to cerebral oxygen consumption is, however, not increased in the neocortex in this study but only around the electrode tip, which could reflect that the immediate initiation of DBS with full clinical stimulation parameters could cause local vasodilatation on a direct electrical or inflammatory basis, or in fact increases neuronal firing (see below). Caution should be made, however, when interpreting these data due to several factors. Firstly, placement of clinical DBS electrodes is difficult in the relative small subthalamic nucleus of the minipig [17,38]. None of our electrodes were directly situated within the STN but all within 5 mm of the target. The electrodes should, accordingly, be close enough to the STN to influence it, but influence on neighboring structures such as the thalamus and medial lemniscus, which may also lead to increased neocortical oxygen consumption, cannot be excluded. Secondly, two of the electrodes migrated (Fig. 4) during the 6-12 months postoperative follow-up period. The migration occurred between the day of the postoperative MRI visualization of the electrode placement (Fig. 3) and the day of sacrifice, which furthermore makes interpretation of the PET results difficult, if this migration occurred before the PET study was performed. We cannot prove that the electrode migration took place after the PET study was carried out, but the clear increase in rCBF (Fig. 5) at the level corresponding so well with the electrode tip visualized on the postoperative MRI (Fig. 3) gives us some support that the electrode migration had not occurred at the time of the PET study. Thirdly, although the use of MPTP-intoxicated minipigs as an experimental model for PD has been well characterized behaviorally [41], biochemically [5,24,41] and histologically [41], precise mapping of the minipig neocortex has yet to be performed. We are therefore unable to precisely identify the functional importance of the neocortical areas that display a tendency towards increased oxygen consumption after stimulation onset. It is tempting to identify the ipsilateral dorsolateral neocortex as being sensory-motor, but in reality such as statement would require histological staining and neural tracing studies that are ongoing, but have not yet been completed.

Previous PET-studies examining rCBF changes in PD patients undergoing effective STN DBS find, in accordance with our results from the minipig, an increase in rCBF directly in or in close proximity to the stimulated STN, globus pallidus or ventral thalamus [22,32,33]. A SPECT-study by Sestini et al. [51] showed increased rCBF in several cortical areas such as the rostral supplementary motor area (SMA), the anterior cingulate cortex and dorsolateral prefrontal cortex (DLPFC), which is in accordance with the hypotheses on basal ganglia circuitry and mechanism of effect of STN DBS described above. However, several other PET studies of cortical rCBF in PD patients at rest undergoing clinically effective STN DBS describe a decreased rCBF in the SMA, sensorimotor cortex (pre- and postcentral gyrus), and lateral premotor cortex and to a varying extent prefrontal cortex [22,30,32,33,39]. When studying rCBF in STN-stimulated PD patients performing motor tasks, there is general agreement of increased rCBF in the SMA [22,30,39], and some authors additionally find increased rCBF in the DLPFC and cingulated cortex [39], premotor cortex [22] and superior parietal cortex and cerebellum [30]. This suggests a normalization of cortical activity in STN DBS-treated PD patients when performing motor tasks. The decrease in cortical rCBF seen at rest is consistent with the opposite proposal of mechanism of effect of STN DBS described above, suggesting that DBS in fact increases activation of STN output neurons, leading to increased inhibitory pallidal output and a following decrease in cortical activity [33]. Increased activation of STN output neurons may thus serve to normalize pathological neuronal networks as reflected by decreased cortical rCBF [30]. Thus, relief of tremor, rigidity and dystonia in PD in addition to bradykinesia may restore an otherwise attenuated motor cortical activity, resulting in an overall decreased rCBF despite a clearly improved motor performance [39]. In addition it has been suggested that direct cortico-subthalamic projections could very well play an important role in the modulation of subcortical-cortical pathways [32].

The result on rCBF in the minipig corresponds well with the human findings of increased activity in the stimulated midbrain area. Significant results from cortical areas could perhaps have been obtained if it had been possible to include more animals. The observed trend towards increased oxygen consumption in central cortical areas does not correspond with the substantial evidence of reduced rCBF at rest in STN DBS-treated patients, but perhaps the cortical response is different immediately following activation of electrical stimulation rather than in the chronic state examined in patients. In addition, a larger number of animals would be preferred just as caution should be made when comparing anesthetized animals directly with awake though resting patients. Naturally with the minipig we do not have the opportunity to study response to motor tasks with PET, but this animal model still may prove helpful in future studies of STN DBS in PD as the animals can be studied in a variety of different parkinsonian stages without results being hampered by previous medical treatments as seen in patients.

Conclusion

Initiation of STN DBS in a porcine model of PD leads to a local increase in rCBF around the electrode tip and trend towards increased cerebral oxygen consumption in centrally placed neocortical areas. Our study illustrates that MPTP-intoxicated minipigs are suitable for long-term implantation of DBS electrodes and related devices intended for human use, if these are properly placed and fixated [16,19]. The Göttingen minipig may under such circumstances serve as a useful experimental model for further elucidation of the mechanisms underlying the benefits of acute and chronic DBS in PD.

Acknowledgments

The authors acknowledge with gratitude the skillful assistance of Ms. D. Jensen, Mr. A. Meier, and the staff at the Påskehøjgård Animal Care Facility, Clinical Institute, University of Aarhus. This study was supported by the Lundbeck Foundation, the Aarhus University Research Foundation, the Alice Brenaa Foundation, the Danish Medical Research Council, the Danish Parkinson Association, the Foundation for the Advancement of Medical Science, the Lily Benthine Lund Foundation, the Medical Society of Aarhus County, the Novo Nordisk Foundation, the Aase and Ejnar Danielsen Foundation, the Foundation of 2/7 1984 against Parkinson's Disease, the Foundation of Ib Henriksen and the Foundation of King Christian the 10th.

References

[1] Albin, RL; Young, AB; Penney, B. (1989). The functional anatomy of basal ganglia disorders. *Trends Neurosci 12*, 366-375

[2] Alexander, GE; Crutcher, MD. (1990). Functional architecture of basal ganglia circuits: neural substrates of parallel processing. *Trends Neurosci 13*, 266-271.

[3] Alexander, GE. (1994). Basal ganglia-thalamocortical circuits: Their role in control of movements. *J Clin Neurophysiol 11*, 420-431

[4] Andersen, F. (2001). Automation methods for analysis of the porcine brain: A study on the Göttingen minipig brain. Ph.D. Thesis, Faculty of Health Sciences, University of Aarhus, Denmark.

[5] Andersen, F; Watanabe, H; Bjarkam, CR; Danielsen, EH; Cumming, P; The DaNeX Study Group. (2005). Pig brain stereotaxic standard space: Mapping of cerebral blood flow normative values and effect of MPTP-lesioning. *Brain Res Bull 66(1)*, 17-29.

[6] Benabid, AL; Benazzouz, A; Pollak, P. (2002). Mechanisms of deep brain stimulation. *Mov Disorders 17/Suppl. 3*, S73-S74.

[7] Benazzouz, A; Gross, C; Fegér, J; Boraud, T; Bioulac, B. (1993). Reversal of rigidity and improvement in motor performance by subthalamic high-frequency stimulation in MPTP-treated monkeys. *Eur J Neurosci 5*, 382-389.

[8] Benazzouz, A; Piallat, B; Pollak, P; Benabid, AL. (1995). Responses of substantia nigra pars reticulata and globus pallidus complex to high frequency stimulation of the subthalamic nucleus in rats: electrophysiological data. *Neurosci Lett 189*, 77-80.

[9] Benazzouz, A; Boraud, T; Fegér, J; Burbaud, P; Biolac, B; Gross, C. (1996). Alleviation of experimental hemiparkinsonism by high-frequency stimulation of the subthalamic nucleus in primates: A comparison with L-dopa treatment. *Mov Disord 11/6*, 627-632.

[10] Benazzouz A, Gao DM, Ni ZG; Piallat, B; Bouali-Benazzouz, R; Benabid AL. (2000). Effect of high-frequency stimulation of the subthalamic nucleus on the neuronal activities of the substantia nigra pars reticulata and ventrolateral nucleus of the thalamus in the rat. *Neurosci 99/2*, 289-295.

[11] Benazzouz, A; Hallett, M. (2000). Mechanism of action of deep brain stimulation. *Neurology 55(Suppl 6)*, S13-S16.

[12] Bergman, H; Wichmann, T; DeLong, MR. (1990). Reversal of experimental parkinsonism by lesions of the subthalamic nucleus. *Science 249*, 1436-1438.

[13] Bergman, H; Wichmann, T; Karmon, B; DeLong, MR. (1994). The primate subthalamic nucleus. II. Neuronal Activity in the MPTP model of Parkinsonism. *J Neurophysiol 72/2*, 507-520.

[14] Bjarkam, CR; Sørensen, JC; Sunde, NÅ; Geneser, FA; Østergaard, K. (2001). New strategies for the treatment of Parkinson's disease hold considerable promise for the future management of neurodegenerative disorders. *Biogerontology 2*, 193-207.

[15] Bjarkam, CR; Pedersen, M; Sørensen, JC. (2001). New strategies for embedding, orientation and sectioning of small brain specimens enable direct correlation to MR-images, brain atlases, or use of unbiased stereology. *J Neurosci Methods 108*, 153-159.

[16] Bjarkam, CR; Cancian, G; Larsen, M; Rosendal, F; Ettrup, KS; Zeidler, D; Blankholm, AD; Østergaard, L; Sunde, N; Sørensen JC. (2004). A MRI-compatible stereotaxic localizer box enables high-precision stereotaxic procedures in pigs. *J Neurosci Methods 139(2)*, 293-298.

[17] Bjarkam, CR; Larsen, M; Watanabe, H; Röhl, L; Simonsen, CZ; Pedersen, M; Ringgaard, S; Andersen, F; Cumming, P; Dalmose, AL; Møller, A; Jensen, LW; Danielsen, EH; Dalmau, I; Finsen, B; Öttingen, Gv; Gjedde, A; Sørensen, JC. Title: A porcine model of subthalamic high-frequency deep brain stimulation in Parkinson's disease. Willow MJ, editor. *Title: Parkinson's Disease: New Research.* New York, USA: Nova Science Publishers; 2005; Chapter 5. ISBN-1-59454-352-6.

[18] Bjarkam, CR; Sørensen, JC. Title: Progress and development in Parkinson disease therapy. Rattan S, Kassem M editors. *Title: Prevention and Treatment of Age-related Diseases*. Dordrecht, The Netherlands: Springer Publishers; 2006; Chapter 3; 31-48. ISBN 1-4020-4884-X.

[19] Bjarkam, CR; Jørgensen, RL; Jensen, KN; Sunde, NAa; Sørensen, JC. (2008). Deep brain stimulation electrode anchoring using BioGlue®, a protective electrode covering, and a titanium microplate. *J Neurosci Methods 168*, 151-155.

[20] Bruet, N; Windels, F; Bertrand, A; Feuerstein, C; Poupard, A; Savasta, A. (2001). High frequency stimulation of the subthalamic nucleus increase the extracellular contents of striatal dopamine in normal and partially dopaminergic denervated rats. *J Neuropathol Exp Neurol 60(1)*, 15-24.

[21] Ceballos-Baumann, AO; Obeso, JA; Vitek, JL; DeLong, MR; Bakay, R; Linazasoro, G; Brooks, DJ. (1994). Restoration of thalamocortical activity after posteroventral pallidotomy in Parkinson's disease. *Lancet 344,* 814.

[22] Ceballos-Baumann, AO; Boecker, H; Bartenstein, P; Falkenhayn, Iv; Riescher, H; Conrad, B; Moringlane, JR; Alesch, F. (1999). A positron emission tomographic study of subthalamic nucleus stimulation in Parkinson disease. *Arch Neurol 56*, 997-1003.

[23] Chang, J-Y; Shi, L-H; Luo, F; Woodward, DJ. (2003). High frequency stimulation of the subthalamic nucleus improves treadmill locomotion in unilateral 6-hydroxydopamine lesioned rats. *Brain Res 983*, 174-184.

[24] Danielsen, EH; Cumming, P; Andersen, F; Bender, D; Brevig, T; Falborg, L; Gee, A; Gillings, NM; Hansen, SB; Hermansen, F; Johansen, J; Johansen, TE; Dahl-Jørgensen, A; Jørgensen, HA; Meyer, M; Munk, O; Pedersen, EB; Poulsen, PH; Rodell, AB; Sakoh, M; Simonsen, CZ; Smith, DF; Sørensen, JC; Østergaard, L; Zimmer, J; Gjedde, A; Møller, A. (2000). The DaNeX study of embryonic mesencephalic, dopaminergic tissue grafted to a minipig model of Parkinson's disease: preliminary findings of effect of MPTP poisoning on striatal dopaminergic markers. *Cell Transplant 9*, 247-259.

[25] DeLong, MR. (1990). Primate models of movement disorders of basal ganglia origin. *Trends Neurosci 13*, 281-285.

[26] Dostrovsky, JO; Lozano, AM. (2002). Mechanisms of Deep Brain Stimulation. *Mov Disorders 17/Suppl.3*, S63-S68.

[27] Gao, D; Benazzouz, A; Bressard, K; Piallat, B; Benabid, AL. (1997). Roles of GABA, glutamate, acetylcholine and STN stimulation on thalamic VM in rats. *Neuroreport 8*, 2601-2605.

[28] Gao, D; Benazzouz, A; Piallat, B; Bressard, K; Ilinsky, IA; Kultas-Ilinsky, K; Benabid AL. (1999). High-frequency stimulation of the subthalamic nucleus suppresses experimental resting tremor in the monkey. *Neurosci 88/1*, 201-212.

[29] Goodman, S; Check, E. (2002). The great primate debate. *Nature 417*, 684-687.

[30] Grafton, ST; Turner, RS; Desmurget, M; Bakay, R; Delong, M; Vitek, J; Crutcher, M. (2006). Normalizing motor-related brain activity. *Neurology 66*, 1192-1199.

[31] Hashimoto, T; Elder, CM; Okun, MS; Patrick, SK; Vitek, JL. (2003). Stimulation of the subthalamic nucleus changes the firring pattern of pallidal neurons. *J Neurosci 23(5)*, 1916-1923.

[32] Haslinger, B; Kalteis, K; Boecker, H; Alesch, F; Ceballos-Baumann, AO. (2005). Frequency-correlated decreases of motor cortex activity associated with subthalamic nucleus stimulation in Parkinson's disease. *Neuroimage 28*, 598-606.

[33] Hershey, T; Revilla, FJ; Wernle, AR; McGee-Minnich, L; Antenor, JV; Videen, TO; Dowling, JL; Mink, JW; Perlmutter JS. (2003). Cortical and subcortical blood flow effects of subthalamic nucleus stimulation in PD. *Neurology 61*, 816-821.

[34] Krack, P; Pollak, P; Limousin, P; Hoffmann, D; Benazzouz, A; Le Bas, JF; Koudsie, A; Benabid, AL. (1998). Opposite motor effect of pallidal stimulation in Parkinson's disease. *Ann Neurol 43*, 180-192.

[35] Krack, P; Pollak, P; Limousin, P; Hoffmann, D; Xie, J; Benazzouz, A; Benabid AL. (1998). Subthalamic nucleus or internal pallidal stimulation in young onset Parkinson's disease. *Brain 121*, 451-457.

[36] Krack, P; Poepping, M; Weinert, D; Schrader, B; Deutschel, G. (2000). Thalamic, pallidal, or subthalamic surgery for Parkinson's disease? *J Neurol 247(Suppl 2)*, II/122-II/134.

[37] Kumar, R; Lozano, AM; Kim, YJ; Hutchison, WD; Sime, E; Halket, E; Lang, AE. (1998) Double-blind evaluation of subthalamic nucleus deep brain stimulation in advanced Parkinson's disease. *Neurology 51*, 850-855.

[38] Larsen, M; Bjarkam, CR; Østergaard, K; West, MJ; Sørensen, JC. (2004). The anatomy of the porcine subthalamic nucleus evaluated with immunohistochemistry and design based stereology. *Anat Embryol 208(3)*, 239-47.

[39] Limousin, P; Greene, J; Pollak, P; Rothwell, J; Benabid, AL; Frackowiak, R. (1997). Change in cerebral activity pattern due to subthalamic or internal pallidum stimulation in Parkinson's disease. *Ann Neurol 42*, 283-291.

[40] Limousin, P; Krack, P; Pollak, P; Benazzouz, A; Ardouin, C; Hoffman, D; Benabid, AL. (1998). Electrical stimulation of subthalamic nucleus deep brain stimulation in advanced Parkinson's disease. *N Engl J Med 339*, 1105-1111.

[41] Mikkelsen, M; Møller, A; Jensen, LH; Pedersen, A; Harajehi, JB; Pakkenberg, H. (1999). MPTP-induced Parkinsonism in minipigs: A behavioral, biochemical, and histological study. *Neurotoxicol Teratol 21*, 169-175.

[42] Montgomery Jr, EB; Baker, KB. (2000). Mechanisms of deep brain stimulation and future technical developments. *Neurol Res 22/3*, 259-266.

[43] Paul, G; Reum, T; Meissner, W; Marburger, A; Sohr, R; Morgenstern, R; Kupsch, A. (2000). High frequency stimulation of the subthalamic nucleus influences striatal dopaminergic metabolism in the naive rat. *Neuroreport 11(3)*, 441-444.

[44] Paxinos, G; Watson, C. The rat brain in stereotaxic coordinates, 4th edition. New York, USA: Academic Press. 1998

[45] Piallat, B; Benazzouz, A; Benabid, AL. (1996). Subthalamic nucleus lesion in rats prevents dopaminergic nigra neuron degeneration after striatal 6-OHDA injection: Behavioral and immunohistochemical studies. *Eur J Neurosci 8*, 1408-1414.

[46] Piallat, B; Benazzouz, A; Benabid, AL. (1999). Neuroprotective effect of chronic inactivation of the subthalamic nucleus in a rat model of Parkinson's disease. *J Neural Transm 55*, 71-77.

[47] Poulsen, PH; Smith, DF; Østergaard, L; Danielsen, EH; Gee, A; Hansen, SB; Astrup, J; Gjedde, A. (1997). In vivo estimation of cerebral blood flow, oxygen consumption and glucose metabolism in the pig by [^{15}O]water injection [^{15}O]oxygen inhalation and dual injections of [^{18}F]fluorodeoxyglucose. *J Neurosci Methods 77*, 199-209.

[48] Rodriguez, MC; Obeso, JA; Olanow, CW. (1998). Subthalamic nucleus-mediated excitotoxicity in Parkinson's disease: A target for neuroprotection. *Ann Neurol 44(3 Suppl 1)*, S175-S188.

[49] Rodriguez-Oroz, MC; Gorospe, A; Guridi, J; Ramos, E; Linazasoro, G; Rodriguez-Palmero, M; Obeso, JA. (2000). Bilateral deep brain stimulation of the subthalamic nucleus in Parkinson's disease. *Neurology 55(Suppl 6)*, S45-S51.

[50] Salin, P; Manrique, C; Forni, C; Kerkerian_Le Goff, L. (2002). High-frequency stimulation of the subthalamic nucleus selectively reverses dopamine denervation-induced cellular defects in the output structures of the basal ganglia in the rat. *J Neurosci 22(12)*, 5137-5148.

[51] Sestini, S; Luzio, ASd; Ammannati, F; Cristofaro, MTRD; Passeri, A; Martini, S; Pupi, A. (2002). Changes in regional cerebral blood flow caused by deep-brain stimulation of the subthalamic nucleus in Parkinson's disease. *J Nucl Med 43*, 725-732.

[52] Sørensen, JC; Bjarkam, CR; Danielsen, EH; Simonsen, CZ; Geneser, FA. (2000). Oriented sectioning of irregular tissue blocks in relation to computerized scanning modalities. Results from the domestic pig brain. *J Neurosci Methods 104*, 93-98.

[53] Tronnier, VM; Krause, M; Heck, A; Kronenbürger, M; Bonsanto, MM; Tronnier, J; Vogel, W. (1999). Deep brain stimulation for the treatment of movement disorders. *Neurol Psychiatr Brain Res 6*, 199-212.

[54] Vitek, JL. (2002). Mechanisms of Deep Brain Stimulation: Excitation or inhibition. *Mov Disord 17/Suppl.3*, S69-S72.

[55] Volkmann, J; Allert, N; Voges, J; Weiss, PH; Freund, HJ; Sturm, V. (2001). Safety and efficacy of pallidal or subthalamic nucleus stimulation in advanced PD. *Neurology 355*, 548-551.

[56] Watanabe, H; Andersen, F; Simonsen, CZ; Evans, SM; Gjedde, A; Cumming, P; The DaNeX Study Group. (2001). MR-based statistical atlas of the Göttingen minipig brain. *Neuroimage 14*, 1089-1096.

[57] Windels, F; Bruet, N; Poupard, A; Urbain, N; Chouvet, G; Feuerstein, C; Savasta, N. (2000). Effects of high frequency stimulation of subthalamic nucleus extracellular glutamate and GABA in substantia nigra and globus pallidus in the normal rat. *Eur J Neurosci 12(11)*, 4141-4146.

In: Deep Brain Stimulation
Editors: Mark H. Rogers and Paul B. Anderson

ISBN 978-1-60692-895-0

Chapter X

Current and Future Perspectives on Vagus Nerve Stimulation in Treatment-Resistant Depression

Bernardo Dell'Osso*, Giulia Camuri, Lucio Oldani and A. Carlo Altamura

Department of Psychiatry, University of Milan, Milano, Italy

Abstract

Treatment-resistant depression (TRD) is a leading cause of disability and therapeutic strategies used for this prevalent and impairing condition include pharmacological augmentation strategies and brain stimulation techniques. Vagus nerve stimulation (VNS) is a brain stimulation intervention that has shown to decrease seizure frequency in partial-onset seizure patients. Subsequent trials performed on treatment-resistant patients with major depression indicated that VNS may be an effective and safe treatment. VNS involves minor surgery in which an electrode pair is wrapped around the left vagus nerve in the neck and connected to a generator implanted in the chest wall subcutaneously. Several methodological approaches have been employed in order to better understand the mechanism of action of VNS and its effects on neurobiological circuits involved in mood regulation. Despite its invasive nature, the tolerability profile of VNS seems to be favourable given that, differently from other brain stimulation interventions (i.e., ECT, rTMS, tDCS), VNS is a continuous and chronic stimulation. Even though previous positive results from clinical trials have led VNS to be approved by the FDA and the EMEA for the use in TRD, researchers are now focusing their efforts in the identification of possible predictors of response to VNS. Further investigation of the effects of VNS in the long-term treatment (>2 years) of TRD is also required.

---

* Dr Bernardo Dell'Osso, Department of Psychiatry, University of Milan, Fondazione IRCCS , Ospedale Maggiore Policlinico, Mangiagalli e Regina Elena, Via Francesco Sforza 35, 20122 Milano, Italy. Phone.: 02-55035994. Fax:02-50320310.email:bernardo.dellosso@policlinico.mi.it.

Keywords: vagus nerve stimulation (VNS), treatment resistant depression (TRD), brain stimulation

Introduction

Partial response, lack of response and residual symptoms following antidepressant treatment are common in patients with Major Depression. In fact, it has been estimated that 30 to 45% of depressed patients show either partial response or no response to standard antidepressant treatments [1, 2]. In addition, depressed patients may develop treatment resistant depression (TRD) [3], defined as the lack of response to two antidepressant trials, given in succession, at adequate doses and for an adequate time, in compliant subjects [4]. In patients with TRD, different strategies of intervention have been proposed including pharmacological and psychotherapic augmentation as well as brain stimulation techniques [5, 6].

Brain stimulation interventions include different techniques which share the common feature to provide a selective electric stimulation of specific brain areas. These include electroconvulsive therapy (ECT), deep brain stimulation (DBS), repetitive transcranial magnetic stimulation (rTMS), transcranial direct current stimulation (tDCS), and vagus nerve stimulation (VNS) which, by means of direct or indirect (magnetic) electric stimulation, can alter neurocircuits in the brain. Among these techniques, only ECT and VNS have FDA-approved indications for Major Depression. VNS, in particular, has been approved as adjunctive treatment in patients with TRD, given that clinical studies with VNS were performed in combination with other pharmacological agents. Differently from other brain stimulation techniques, VNS requires an extracranial surgical implant to provide a continuous electric stimulation that can be maintained for many years. VNS is also a reversible and adjustable procedure.

Historically, VNS has been firstly tested in the late 80's in patients who had treatment-resistant epilepsy and were not candidates to surgical interventions [7]. Subsequent multicenter randomized clinical trials allowed the FDA to approve VNS as adjunctive treatment for adults and adolescents with treatment-resistant partial onset seizures in 1997 [8-10].

First anecdotal indications of the potential efficacy of VNS in depressed patients came from direct clinical observation and subsequent clinical evaluations through standard rating scales of improved mood and cognition in patients with epilepsy treated with VNS [11].

The aim of the present review is to provide a comprehensive and updated overview of the more recent neurobiological and clinical findings about VNS therapy with a detailed description of the procedure and a specific emphasis on tolerability issues. Potential new fields of research with VNS in psychiatry are discussed as well.

The Vagus Nerve Anatomy and Its Implications in Major Depression

It is not surprising that an anticonvulsant treatment, such as VNS, may have antidepressant effect: several anticonvulsant medications (Valproate, Carbamazepine, Lamotrigine, etc), in fact, have shown antidepressant properties as well as the capacity to prevent depressive recurrences in euthymic patients [12]. These indirect observations, have been subsequently supported by neurobiological studies which provided the rationale for the potential efficacy of VNS in Major Depression. The vagus nerve (VN), the longest cranial nerve, is a mixed nerve composed by 80% afferent and 20% efferent fibres and regulates several automatic functions of the body, many of which are important in a variety of emotional tasks [13]. The majority of the fibres in the vagus nerve are C-fibres. VN regulates a lot of functions such as heart rate, blood pressure and peristalsis. The sensory afferent cell bodies are placed in the nodose and the jugular ganglia and project to the nucleus of the solitary tract (NTS). Projections from NTS to the brain areas are widespread and many of these reach brain areas such as the Locus Coeruleus, the Amygdala, the Dorsal Raphe, the Hyppocampus etc, which are in turn connected to the Orbitofrontal Cortex, the Insula and the Anterior Cingulate Gyrus [14, 15]. Many of these regions are supposed to be involved in the pathophysiology of Major Depression [16, 17]. In this perspective, VNS is able to provide a widespread intermittent continuous stimulation of these areas by means of a stimulating electrode which is attached to the left VN.

The Surgical Procedure and the Implanted Device

VNS requires a relatively minor surgical intervention that can be completed in about one hour under local or general anaesthesia. A first small incision is made below the collarbone in the left upper chest area in order to place the VNS pulse generator which is controlled and programmed by physicians through a labtop. A second incision is made in the left side of the neck and a small helicoidal electrode, connected to the pulse generator through a wire placed subcutaneously, is wrapped around the VN. The implanted device delivers chronic, intermittent electrical impulses to the left VN. Once the device is turned on, patients can decide to stop the stimulation through a magnet when needed, by placing it in front of the pulse generator. The left VN is chosen in light of fewer potential heart interactions. Different effects between left and right VN, in fact, are due to their connections to the heart: the right vagus innervates the sinoatrial node whereas the left vagus innervates the atrioventricular node [18].

Once VNS is started, classical stimulation parameters include 30 seconds of stimulation followed by 5 minutes of pause with an initial current of 0.25 mA which is progressively increased by 0.25 mA up to 1.50 mA that is considered the optimal stimulation voltage.

Neurobiology and Neuroimaging Data on VNS Therapy

Several studies have been conducted to assess the effects of VNS therapy on major neurotransmitter systems [19]. The most studied neurotransmitters are Dopamine, Serotonin (5-HT) and Norepinephrine (NE).

With respect to a potential influence of VNS on the dopaminergic system, Carpenter and co-workers found a significantly elevated level of homovanillic acid in cerebrospinal fluid (CSF) samples obtained from 21 patients with TRD after 24 weeks of VNS therapy. The CSF was also analyzed in order to assess eventual changes in the concentration of other substrates (5-hydroxyindoleacetic acid, GABA, etc.), but no relevant changes were observed [20].

Recently, Dorr and Debonnel investigated 5-HT and NE neuronal firing rates in the brainstem nuclei—dorsal raphe nucleus (DRN) and locus coeruleus (LC)—after VNS therapy in rats. After short-term VNS treatment, firing rates were significantly higher for LC, whereas basal firing rates in the DRN and LC were significantly increased after long-term treatments. The authors suggested that VNS may have a novel mechanism of action, enabling its effectiveness in TRD [21].

Imaging studies with SPECT, PET, and functional magnetic resonance (fMRI) have been used to determine which areas of the brain are specifically affected by VNS therapy.

Previous SPECT studies have shown regional cerebral blood flow (rCBF) abnormalities in limbic and cortical structures (such as insula and temporal cortex) of depressed people [22]. In this perspective, a recent SPECT study exploring rCBF changes induced by VNS found decreased rCBF in the amygdala, left hippocampus, left subgenual cingulate cortex, left and right ventral anterior cingulum, right thalamus and brain stem. These effects are consistent with those reported after the administration of SSRIs [23].

PET studies assessing VNS effects have shown mixed results. On one hand, a previous study indicated a decreased metabolism compared to baseline in the substantia nigra, ventral tegmentum, hypothalamus, insula/claustrum and superior temporal gyrus after a 1-year course of VNS therapy [24]. On the other hand, Conway and colleagues recently reported that VNS therapy caused an increased metabolic activity in the orbitofrontal cortex, bilateral anterior cingulate cortex and right superior and medial frontal cortex, and a decreased rCBF in the bilateral temporal cortex and right parietal area [25].

As such, definitive conclusions from neuroimaging studies on VNS effects on specific brain areas cannot be drawn due to the small size of the samples studied and further investigation is required.

Clinical Efficacy Studies

With respect to short-term clinical trials conducted on TRD patients with VNS, a first 10-week open label trial was performed on 30 adult outpatients with nonpsychotic, treatment-resistant major depression who had failed at least two medication trials in the current episode (MDE) while on stable pharmacological regimens. Results showed that 40% of the sample achieved response, while 17% remission on the basis of HDRS total scores. In a further analysis, the authors found that more than half of the total reduction in depressive symptoms occurred after the first 6 weeks of VNS [26].

A subsequent open study conducted with a similar design by Sackeim and colleagues showed that 30.5% of the sample met the criteria for response and 15.3% the criteria for remission after 10 weeks of VNS. The authors concluded that VNS appears to be more effective in patients with low to moderate, but not extreme, antidepressant resistance [27].

A subsequent open study conducted on a very small group ($N = 7$) showed that VNS significantly improved depressive symptoms after 10 weeks of treatment with 4 out of 7 patients classified as HDRS responders and 2 of these remitters (HDRS$\leq$ 10) [28].

In the acute, sham-controlled, double-blind randomized trial published by Rush and co-workers and conducted on 235 patients treated with VNS, the authors reported mixed results. In fact, after 10 weeks of VNS, the mean HDRS response rates of both active VNS and sham groups did not show significant difference [29].

In a more recent study, a british group evaluated 11 patients with TRD who were treated with VNS therapy for 12 weeks [30]. Even though the clinical measures of depression decreased significantly, only one patient was classified as responder. Finally, Neuhaus and colleagues, in an exploratory study investigating the effects of VNS on auditory event-related potentials, reported that almost 40% of patients became responders after 10 weeks of treatment [31].

With respect to long-term effects of VNS, a follow-up study by Marangell and colleagues evaluated the efficacy of the stimulation at one year in the same sample previously treated in the short-term by Rush et al. [26]. The authors found a sustained response rate of 40% to 46% after 9 months. After one year of VNS, the remission rate significantly increased from 17% to 29%. Of note, the 91% of the responders at 3 months maintained their response at 12 months and among the non-responders at 3 months, 18% were considered responders at 12 months [32].

In a subsequent naturalistic follow-up study [33], including 205 patients, a significant improvement of depressive symptoms in the first 4 months of VNS therapy was reported. However, during the 12-month study, 30 patients were hospitalized due to a depressive relapse.

The only 2-year VNS follow-up study performed with a significant sample ($n = 59$) showed positive results [34] reporting the majority of antidepressant effects in the first 3 months of stimulation, even though additional improvements were shown at 12 months and maintained at 24 months.

The efficacy of adjunctive VNS to treatment as usual (VNS+TAU) has been compared to TAU in a 12-month, naturalistic, prospective study conducted on 229 treatment-resistant depressed patients [35]. Both groups, however, were different in terms of number of lifetime MDEs (higher in the TAU group), prior or past ECT exposure (greater in the VNS + TAU group), and pharmacological treatment (the VNS + TAU group showed a greater use of tricyclics, stimulants and neuroleptics in the current MDE). Analysis on the HDRS scores showed that 27% of the VNS + TAU group were responders at 12 months, compared to only 13% of the TAU group. In addition, a higher number of remitters, although not statistically significant, was found in the VNS + TAU group.

A recent open European multicenter study investigated the efficacy of adjunctive VNS therapy in 74 patients with TRD [36]. Treatment remained unchanged for the first 3 months whereas in the subsequent 9 months, medications and VNS parameters were altered as clinically indicated. After 3 months of VNS, response and remission rates reached respectively 37% and 17% of the sample on the basis of HDRS-28 scores. Response rates increased to 53% after 12 months of VNS, and remission rates reached 33% of the sample. Of clinical interest, median time to response was found to be of 9 months.

Side-Effects, Compliance and Tolerability of VNS

VNS related side-effects may rarely occur as a consequence of the neurosurgical intervention. Most frequent side-effects associated with VNS, in fact, are those involving the electrical stimulation of the left VN [37, 38]. When the device is implanted and the stimulation is started, rarely the device can cause cardiac rhythm disturbances. If this happens, the surgeon can readjust the electrodes to prevent this. During the initial phase of stimulation – when the current is increased – if patients experience disturbing side-effects (e.g., cough, voice alteration), the voltage can be readjusted to the previous level of good tolerability for additional time before a new attempt to increase it. Of clinical interest, VNS has not been reported to determine any systemic effect such as weight gain, sexual dysfunction, sedation, and other common side-effects associated with pharmacologic treatments.

During the active stimulation, the most common complications include voice alteration such as hoarseness and related symptoms which may occur in approximately the 50% of patients. In published clinical trials, these symptoms, however, were not serious enough to cause significant dropouts.

In the sham controlled trial, shortness of breath, neck pain, dysphasia, and paresthesias occurred in >10% of patients, and 25% to 35% experienced cough [26, 27]. Most of these symptoms gradually subsided, and the percentage of patients who experienced cough dropped to <10% at 2 years. Of clinical interest, in the acute pivotal trial [26], both sham control and active VNS patients reported similar rates of mild, moderate, or severe adverse effects. These results are consistent with subsequent studies showing a progressive reduction (within one year from the implant) of side-effects in terms of frequency and severity [32]. Taken as a whole, these studies indicate VNS as a safe and well-tolerated treatment.

With respect to the potential risk of a manic switch with VNS, published studies included both unipolar and bipolar patients, and it was reported that only a few patients became manic. On one hand, it is difficult to evaluate if patients spontaneously had a manic episode or if VNS induced it. On the other hand, it is well established that most effective antidepressant treatments have a propensity to increase the switch rate from depression to mania and, therefore, one might expect the same event to occur with VNS as well [39].

Finally, it needs to be taken into account that the device battery has a limited duration and that, as some VNS studies with follow-up at 45 months have shown [40, 41, 42], depressive symptoms may reappear with the end of the battery. Even though batteries with a longer duration are being developed, clinicians should expect that, after some years of stimulation, patients might need a new surgical intervention – which does not involve the electrode wrapped to the VN but only the pulse generator placed in the anterior chest – in order to replace battery and maintain the stimulation in the long-term.

Current and Future Perspectives with VNS

VNS may have some advantages over standard treatments of depression. One of these is represented by the compliance that is insured by a continuous stimulation and does not depend on patient. In addition, VNS has no influence on pregnancy because like other non-pharmacological treatments it does not pass through the placenta [43].

There are other clinical issues that should be further investigated with VNS and that might be of great clinical interest. A recent pivotal trial showed promising results in a small sample of patients with treatment-resistant rapid-cycling bipolar disorder. Over the 12-month study period, VNS was associated with a 38.1% mean improvement in the overall illness as compared to baseline, as well as with significant reductions in symptoms as measured by outcome rating scales [44]. In this perspective, it is noteworthy to highlight that VNS may exert a positive effect not only over depressive symptoms but, also, on the cyclicity that characterizes many forms of mood disorders. This putative effect may also be a *trait d'union* between the anticonvulsant effect of VNS and the clinical use of anticonvulsants as mood stabilizers in affective disorders.

Another clinical field of psychiatric interest for the use of VNS therapy is the one related to eating disorders, obesity in particular. In fact, it is well established that mood affects food craving, in particular the amount and kind of food consumed. On the basis of a relationship between the VN in hunger and satiety and the short-term regulation of food intake [45], Bodenlos and colleagues investigated whether acute VNS could temporarily alter food craving in people with TRD [46]. Thirty-three participants were recruited and divided in three groups: depressed patients treated with VNS, depressed patients who did not receive VNS, and healthy controls. At the endpoint, the authors found that VNS was associated with important changes in food cravings.

Recently, Pardo and colleagues, in a study with 14 depressed patients who received VNS and were followed up for 2 years, observed a significant and progressive weight loss, proportional to the initial BMI, hypothesizing for VNS a potential role in the treatment of obesity [47]. These preliminary positive results should encourage further studies specifically assessing the relationship between VNS and food intake and the potential role of this technique in the treatment of some eating disorders.

Finally, given that published trials investigated the efficacy of VNS in a follow-up period not longer than two years, it is important to evaluate the efficacy of the technique in the long-term. Another important issue is that VNS has been so far mostly investigated as augmentative treatment in TRD, and it would be interesting to assess its effect as monotherapy. In addition, it remains to be elucidated the optimal number of clinical trials failed before considering a patient potentially candidate to VNS. In fact, according to the results of the Sequenced Treatment Alternatives to Relieve Depression (STAR*D) study, chances of achieving remission dramatically drop after two failed adequate antidepressant trials [48, 49], indicating that this level of treatment-resistance has limited options. In this perspective, it should be further evaluated the possibility to administer VNS after a lower number of failed clinical trials.

Conclusions

VNS represents an approved adjunctive brain stimulation intervention for patients with TRD. Potential candidates should be patients with a history of chronic, recurrent depression who failed to respond to multiple adequate antidepressant trials during the index episode. Based on published clinical trials, clinicians may expect significant improvement of depressive symptoms in the first two years of VNS. Nevertheless, treatment studies with VNS have demonstrated different degrees of efficacy which varies depending on the study design (i.e., duration of stimulation, degree of treatment resistance, concomitant pharmacological treatment, etc.) which presented methodological limitations in some cases, making it difficult to compare study results.

On one hand, the high cost of the device, the invasive nature of the intervention and the need to perform further controlled trials to assess the efficacy of the technique in the very long-term and in specific subgroups of patients (i.e., unipolar vs bipolar patients, presence of rapid cycling patients) require some important precautions before prescribing such a treatment. On the other hand, the favourable tolerability profile and the lack of systemic side-effects combined to an optimal compliance encourage clinicians to consider VNS a novel and effective intervention for patients with TRD. Finally, it is mandatory to specify that VNS is not aimed to replace other brain stimulation interventions such as Electroconvulsive Therapy (ECT) which has a very different mechanism of action and has been also combined to VNS in a recent case series [50].

References

[1] Nierenberg Aa, Dececco Lm. Definitions Of Antidepressant Treatment Response, Remission, Nonresponse, Partial Response, And Other Relevant Outcomes: A Focus On Treatment-Resistant Depression. *J Clin Psychiatry.* 2001;62(16):5-9.

[2] Gayetot D, Ansseau M, Triffaux Jm. When Depression Does Not End. Resistant Depression: *Recent Clinical and Therapeutic Aspects. Rev Med Liege.* 2007;62:103-11.

[3] Fava M, Davidson Kg. Definition And Epidemiology Of Treatment-Resistant Depression. *Psychiatr Clin North Am.* 1996;19:179-200.

[4] Sackeim Ha. The Definition And Meaning Of Treatment-Resistant Depression. *J Clin Psychiatry.* 2001;62(S16):10-7.

[5] Preskorn Sh, Burke M. Somatic Therapy For Major Depressive Disorder: Selection Of An Antidepressant. *J Clin Psychiatry.* 1992;53(S):5-18.

[6] American Psychiatric Association. Practice Guidelines For The Treatment Of Patients With Major Depressive Disorder. *Am J Psychiatry.* 2000;157:1-45.

[7] Penry Jk, Dean Jc. Prevention Of Intractable Partial Seizures By Intermittent Vagal Stimulation In Humans: Preliminary Results. *Epilepsia.* 1990;31:(2)40-43.

[8] Rutecki P. Anatomical, Physiological, And Theoretical Basis For The Antiepileptic Effect Of Vagus Nerve Stimulation. *Epilepsia.* 1990;31 (S2):1-6.

[9] Ben-Menachem E, Mañon-Espaillat R, Ristanovic R, Wilder Bj, Stefan H, Mirza W Et Al. Vagus Nerve Stimulation For Treatment Of Partial Seizures. A Controlled Study Of Effect On Seizures. First International Vagus Nerve Stimulation Study Group. *Epilepsia.* 1994;35:616-626.

[10] The Vagus Nerve Stimulation Study Group. A Randomized Controlled Trial Of Chronic Vagus Nerve Stimulation For Treatment Of Medically Intractable Seizures. *Neurology.* 1995;45:224-230.

[11] Handforth A, Degiorgio Cm, Schachter Sc, Uthman Bm, Naritoku Dk, Tecoma Es Et `Al. Vagus Nerve Stimulation Therapy For Partial-Onset Seizures: A Randomized Active-Control Trial. *Neurology.* 1998;51(1):48-55.

[12] Van Der Loos Ml, Mulder Ph, Hartong Eg, Blom Mbj, Vergouwen Ac, De Keyzer H Et Al. Efficacy And Safety Of Lamotrigine As Add-On To Lithium In The Treatment Of Bipolar Depression: A Multi-Center, Double-Blind, Placebo-Controlled Trial. *Am J Psychiatry.* In Press.

[13] Foley Jo, Dubois F. Quantitative Studies Of The Vagus Nerve In The Cat. I. The Ratio Of Sensory Motor Studies. *J Comp Neurol.* 1937;67:49–67.

[14] Chae Jh, Nahas Z, Lomarev M, Denslow S, Lorberbaum Jp, Bohning De Et Al. A Review Of Functional Neuroimaging Studies Of Vagus Nerve Stimulation (Vns*). J Psychiatr Res.* 2003;37:443–455.

[15] Kraus T, Hosl K, Kiess O. Bold Fmri Deactivation Of Limbic And Temporal Brain Structures And Mood Enhancing Effect By Transcutaneous Vagus Nerve Stimulation. *J Neural Transm.* 2007;114(11):1485-1493.

[16] Drevets Wc. Neuroimaging And Neuropathological Studies Of Depression: Implications For The Cognitive-Emotional Features Of Mood Disorders. *Curr Opin Neurol.* 2001;11(2):240-9.

[17] Mayberg Hs. Positron Emission Tomography Imaging In Depression: A Neural Systems Perspective. *Neuroimaging Clin N Am.* 2003;13(4):805-815.

[18] Ramani R. Vagus Nerve Stimulation Therapy For Seizures. *J Neurosurg Anesthesiol.* 2008;20(1):29-35.

[19] Nemeroff Cb, Mayberg Hs, Krahl Se, Mcnamara J, Frazer A, Henry Tr Et Al. Vns Therapy In Treatment-Resistant Depression: Clinical Evidence And Putative Neurobiological Mechanisms. *Neuropsychopharmacology.* 2006;31(7):1345-55.

[20] Carpenter Ll, Moreno Fa, Kling Ma, Anderson Gm, Regenold Wt, Labiner Dm Et Al. Effect Of Vagus Nerve Stimulation On Cerebrospinal Fluid Monoamine Metabolites, Norepinephrine And A-Aminobutyric Acid Concentrations In Depressed Patients. *Biol Psychiatry.* 2004;56:418-426.

[21] Dorr Ae, Debonnel G. Effect Of Vagus Nerve Stimulation On Serotonergic And Noradrenergic Transmission. *J Pharmacol Exp Ther*. 2006;318(2):890-898.

[22] Devous Md, Husain M, Harris Ts, Rush Aj. *Effects Of Vns On Regional Cerebral Blood Flow In Depressed Subjects*. Poster Presented At The 42nd Annual New Clinical Drug Evaluation Unit Meeting. Boca Raton, Fl, 2002; 10–13.

[23] Zobel A, Joe A, Freymann N, Clusmann H, Schramm J, Reinhardt M Et Al. Changes In Regional Cerebral Blood Flow By Therapeutic Vagus Nerve Stimulation In Depression: An Exploratory Approach. *Psychiatry Res*. 2005;139(3):165-79.

[24] Hagen Mc, Sheikh Js, Adson D, Rittberg B, Abuzzahab Fs, Lee Jt Et Al. *Metabolic Changes In Treatment-Resistant Depression Responsive To Vns Therapy* Poster Presented At The 58th Annual Scientific Convention Of The Society Of Biological Psychiatry, San Francisco, Ca,2003: 5-17.

[25] Conway Cr, Chibnall, Jt, Fletcher Jw, Filla-Taylor J, Grossberg Gt, Li X. Et Al. Three Months Of Vagus Nerve Stimulation Is Associated With Increased Limbic And Paralimbic Activity (Fdg Pet) *In Treatment-Resistant Depressed Subjects*. Poster Presented At The 57th Annual Scientific Convention Of The Society Of Biological Psychiatry. Philadelphia, Pa, 2002:16–18.

[26] Rush Aj, George Ms, Sackeim Ha, Marangell Lb, Husain Mm, Giller C Et Al. Vagus Nerve Stimulation For Treatment Resistant Depression: A Multicenter Study. *Biol Psychiatry*. 2000;47:276-286.

[27] Sackeim Ha, Rush Aj, George Ms, Marangell Lb, Husain Mm, Nahas Z Et Al. Vagus Nerve Stimulation (Vns) For Treatment-Resistant Depression: Efficacy, Side Effects, And Predictors Of Outcome. *Neuropsychopharmacology*. 2001;25:713-728.

[28] Armitage R, Husain M, Hoffmann R, Rush Aj. The Effects Of Vagus Nerve Stimulation On Sleep EEG In Depression: A Preliminary Report. *J Psychosom Res*. 2003;54:475-482.

[29] Rush Aj, Marangell Lb, Sackeim Ha, George Ms, Brannan Sk, Davis Sm Et Al. Vagus Nerve Stimulation For Treatment-Resistant Depression: A Randomized, Controlled Acute Phase Trial. *Biol Psychiatr*. 2005;58:347-354.

[30] O'keane V, Dinan Tg, Scott L, Corcoran C. Changes In Hypothalamic-Pituitary-Adrenal Axis Measures After Vagus Nerve Stimulation Therapy In Chronic Depression. *Biol Psychiatr*. 2005;58:963-968.

[31] Neuhaus Ah, Luborzewski A, Rentzsch J, Brakemeier El, Opgen-Rhein C, Gallinat J Et Al. P300 Is Enhanced In Responders To Vagus Nerve Stimulation For Treatment Of Major Depressive Disorder. *J Affect Disord*. 2007;100:123–128.

[32] Marangell Lb, Rush Aj, George Ms, Sackeim Ha, Johnson Cr, Husain Mm Et Al. Vagus Nerve Stimulation (Vns) For Major Depressive Episodes: One Year Outcomes. *Biol Psychiatry*. 2002;51(4):280-7.

[33] Rush Aj, Sackeim Ha, Marangell Lb, George Ms, Brannan Sk, Davis Sm Et Al. Effects Of 12 Months Of Vagus Nerve Stimulation In Treatment-Resistant Depression: A Naturalistic Study. *Biol Psychiatry*. 2005;58(5),355-363.

[34] Nahas Z, Marangell Lb, Husain Mm, Rush Aj, Sackeim Ha, Lisanby Sh Et Al. Two-Year Outcome Of Vagus Nerve Stimulation (Vns) For Treatment Of Major Depressive Episodes. *J Clin Psychiatry.* 2005;66:1097-1104.

[35] George Ms, Rush Aj, Marangell Lb, Sackeim Ha, Brannan Sk, Davis Sm Et Al. A One-Year Comparison Of Vagus Nerve Stimulation With Treatment As Usual For Treatment-Resistant Depression. *Biol Psychiatr.* 2005;58:364-373.

[36] Schlaepfer Te, Frick C, Zobel A, Maier W, Heuser I, Bajbouj M Et Al. Vagus Nerve Stimulation For Depression: Efficacy And Safety In A European Study. *Psychol Med.* 2008;4:1-11.

[37] Janicak Md. Neuromodulation. *Cns Spectrums* 2008;13(5):370-372.

[38] Daban C, Martinez-Aran A, Cruz N, Vieta E. Safety And Efficacy Of Vagus Nerve Stimulation In Treatment-Resistant Depression. A Systematic Review. *J Affect Disord.* 2008;110(1-2):1-15.

[39] Sackeim H.A. (2004). Vagus Nerve Stimulation. *In: Brain Stimulation In Psychiatric Treatment.* Edited By Lisanby Sh. American Psychiatric Publishing, Inc. Washington, Dc; 99-142.

[40] Martinez Jm, Zboyan Ha. Vagus Nerve Stimulation Therapy In A Patient With Treatment-Resistant Depression: A Case Report Of Long-Term Follow-Up And Battery End-Of-Service. *Cns Spectr.* 2006;11:143-147.

[41] Critchley Hd, Lewis Pa, Orth M, Josephs O, Deichmann R, Trimble Mr Et Al. Vagus Nerve Stimulation For Treatment-Resistant Depression: Behavioral And Neural Effects On Encoding Negative Material. *Psychosom Med.* 2007;69:17-22.

[42] Conway, C.R. *Sustained Antidepressive Benefit After Interruption Of Vagus Nerve Stimulation Therapy.* Poster Presented At The Us Psychiatric And Mental Health Congress November 7–10 Las Vegas, Nevada Usa, 2005.

[43] Husain Mm, Stegman D, Trevino K. Pregnancy And Delivery While Receiving Vagus Nerve Stimulation For The Treatment Of Major Depression: A Case Report. *Ann Gen Psychiatry.* 2005;4:16.

[44] Marangell Lb, Suppes T, Zboyan Ha, Prashad Sj, Fischer G, Snow D Et Al. A 1-Year Pilot Study Of Vagus Nerve Stimulation In Treatment-Resistant Rapid-Cycling Bipolar Disorder. *J Clin Psychiatry.* 2008;69(2):183-9.

[45] Havel Pj. Peripheral Signals Conveying Metabolic Information To The Brain: Short-Term And Long-Term Regulation Of Food Intake And Energy Homeostasis. *Exp Biol Med.* 2001;226:963-977.

[46] Bodenlos Js, Kose S, Borckardt Jj, Nahas Z, Shaw D, O'neil Pm Et Al. Vagus Nerve Stimulation Acutely Alters Food Craving In Adults With Depression. *Appetite.* 2007;48:145-53.

[47] Pardo Jv, Sheikh Sa, Kuskowski Ma, Surerus-Johnson C, Hagen Mc, Lee Jt Et Al. Weight Loss During Chronic, Cervical Vagus Nerve Stimulation In Depressed Patients With Obesity: An Observation. *Int J Obes.* 2007;31(11):1756-1759.

[48] Rush Aj, Trivedi Mh, Wisniewski Sr, Nierenberg Aa, Stewart Jw, Warden D Et Al. Acute And Longer-Term Outcomes In Depressed Outpatients Requiring One Or Several Treatment Steps: A Star*D Report. *Am J Psychiatry.* 2006;163(11):1905-1917.

[49] Trivedi Mh, Fava M, Wisniewski Sr, Thase Me, Quitkin F, Warden D Et Al. Medication Augmentation After The Failure Of Ssris For Depression. *N Engl J Med.* 2006;354(12):1243-52.

[50] Sharma A, Chaturvedi R, Sharma A, Sorrell Jh. Electroconvulsive Therapy In Patients With Vagus Nerve Stimulation. *J Ect.* 2008; In Press

Index

A

D

E

H

I

J

K

L

M

N

O

P

Q

R

S

T

U

V

W

X

Y